Encyclopedia of Diabetes:
Clinical Aspects of Type 1 Diabetes

Volume 04

Encyclopedia of Diabetes:
Clinical Aspects of
Type 1 Diabetes
Volume 04

Edited by **Rex Slavin, Windy Wise and Roy Marcus Cohn**

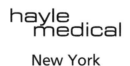

New York

Published by Hayle Medical,
30 West, 37th Street, Suite 612,
New York, NY 10018, USA
www.haylemedical.com

Encyclopedia of Diabetes: Clinical Aspects of Type 1 Diabetes
Volume 04
Edited by Rex Slavin, Windy Wise and Roy Marcus Cohn

International Standard Book Number: 978-1-63241-146-4 (Hardback)

Contents

Published by Hayle Medical,
30 West, 37th Street, Suite 612,
New York, NY 10018, USA
www.haylemedical.com

Encyclopedia of Diabetes: Clinical Aspects of Type 1 Diabetes
Volume 04
Edited by Rex Slavin, Windy Wise and Roy Marcus Cohn

© 2015 Hayle Medical

International Standard Book Number: 978-1-63241-146-4 (Hardback)

Encyclopedia of Diabetes: Clinical Aspects of Type 1 Diabetes Volume 04

Edited by **Rex Slavin, Windy Wise and Roy Marcus Cohn**

hayle
medical

New York

Encyclopedia of Diabetes:
Clinical Aspects of Type 1 Diabetes

Volume 04

Preface

Over the recent decade, advancements and applications have progressed exponentially. This has led to the increased interest in this field and projects are being conducted to enhance knowledge. The main objective of this book is to present some of the critical challenges and provide insights into possible solutions. This book will answer the varied questions that arise in the field and also provide an increased scope for furthering studies.

The book is compiled of up-to-the-minute information that elucidates recent knowledge of Type-1 Diabetes as an autoimmune disease. It also elaborates the obstacles that are still there with available treatments and probable solutions for the not too distant future. This book contains three sections namely, "Epidemiology and Etiology", "Genetics" and "Beta-Cell Function and Dysfunction".

I hope that this book, with its visionary approach, will be a valuable addition and will promote interest among readers. Each of the authors has provided their extraordinary competence in their specific fields by providing different perspectives as they come from diverse nations and regions. I thank them for their contributions.

Editor

Epidemiology and Etiology

The Epidemiology of Type 1 Diabetes Mellitus

Thomas Frese and Hagen Sandholzer

Additional information is available at the end of the chapter

1. Introduction

Type 1 diabetes mellitus (type 1 diabetes, insulin-dependent diabetes mellitus), one of the most common chronic diseases in childhood, is caused by insulin deficiency following auto-immune destruction of the pancreatic beta cells. Until the one and only therapeutic option – the life-long supplementation of insulin or its analogues – was established, affected children died within a short time. Although extensive investigations on the pathogenesis of type 1 diabetes have been performed, the underlying causes and mechanisms are still far from be-ing completely understood. The consequence is a lack of prevention strategies or causal therapies.

Great affords have been made to assess the incidence and prevalence of type 1 diabetes. The epidemiology of type 1 diabetes is estimated with different methods ranging from small cross-sectional studies to nationwide registries. Understanding the epidemiology of type 1 diabetes may identify risk factors, e.g. genetic predisposition or environmental factors, and may thereby elucidate the pathogenesis of type 1 diabetes. This could be one way to estab-lish possible preventive or causal therapeutic strategies. However, the findings on the possi-ble trigger factors of type 1 diabetes and its epidemiology are sometimes controversial or even contradictory.

In the present chapter, the incidence and prevalence of type 1 diabetes during the last decades will be described. Some fundamental facts about the estimation of type 1 diabe-tes epidemiology may facilitate understanding. The epidemiologic patterns of type 1 dia-betes regarding geographic differences, gender and age of the patients, as well as seasonal and ethnic factors in populations are summarized. The expected changes in type 1 diabetes epidemiology and its implications on future research directions and health care are mentioned.

2. Estimating the epidemiology of type 1 diabetes mellitus

The epidemiology of type 1 diabetes can be estimated in different ways. In principle, there is the possibility of estimating epidemiologic data by self-report of the patients, longitudinal- or cross-sectional studies or different-sized registries.

Data gained from self-reporting of diabetic patients have been shown to underestimate the true burden of diabetes (Forouhi, Merrick et al. 2006). Another possibility, but with similar limitations, is to assess data retrospectively (Mooney, Helms et al. 2004). Generally, longitudinal or cross-sectional studies are often locally or regionally performed. This limits the opportunity to get generalizable results because the epidemiology of type 1 diabetes is known to be heterogeneous regarding geography and ethnicity. Cross-sectional studies do not provide information on the time-dependent changes of the epidemiology. Additionally, many studies are limited to special settings, e.g. a general practice setting (Frese, Sandholzer et al. 2008), and although providing useful and necessary information, the reported data may not be representative for the epidemiology of type 1 diabetes.

Especially when estimating the incidence of type 1 diabetes, the latency of onset until diagnosis is important and influences the quality of estimated data. Also the validity of the chosen diagnosis should be critically reviewed. In a recent German investigation, 60 (10.3%) of 580 patients were reclassified at mean 2.4 years after the diagnosis of type 1 diabetes: 23 (38.3%) as type 1 diabetes; 9 (15%) as maturity onset diabetes of the young; 20 (33.3%) as "other specific diabetes forms", and 8 (13.3%) as "remission" of type 2 diabetes (Awa, Schober et al. 2011). The validity of the chosen diagnosis may differ depending on the data source that affords a correct differential diagnosis, e.g. between type 1 diabetes and malnutrition diabetes in developing countries or type 1 diabetes, type 2 diabetes and maturity onset diabetes of the young in industrial countries, as well as a correct encoding of diagnosis. This is because usual classification systems such as the International Classification of Primary Care or International Classification of Diseases cannot be assumed to be sufficiently complete and valid (Gray, Orr et al. 2003; Wockenfuss, Frese et al. 2009; Frese, Herrmann et al. 2012).

It is conclusive that reliable and valid – and thereby comparable – data on type 1 diabetes epidemiology have to be based on a complete and detailed assessment. Disease registries can be assumed to be probably the best method to estimate and manage standardized data. However, the availability, completeness, quality and accuracy of diabetes registers are again very variable (Forouhi, Merrick et al. 2006). Type 1 diabetes registries were established on different levels: local (Howitt and Cheales 1993), regional (Galler, Stange et al. 2010), national or multinational.

Much of our knowledge of the epidemiology of type 1 diabetes in young people has been generated by large collaborative efforts based on standardized registry data: the EURODIAB study in Europe and the DIAMOND project worldwide (Dabelea, Mayer-Davis et al. 2010). In order to provide reliable information about the incidence and geographical variation of type 1 diabetes throughout Europe, EURODIAB was established as a collaborative research project (Fuller 1989; Green, Gale et al. 1992). During a 15-year period, 1989 to 2003, 20 population-based EURODIAB registers in 17 countries registered 29,311 new cases of type 1 diabetes in children before their 15th birthday (Patterson, Dahlquist et al. 2009). The World Health Organization program, Multinational Project for Childhood Diabetes (Diabetes Mondiale or DIAMOND), has been developed to investigate and characterize global incidence and mortality of type 1 diabetes and the health care provided for type 1 diabetic patients. Both projects used similar ascertainment methodologies. However, DIAMOND ascertained some data retrospectively. This may have led to some underestimation of incidence rates. The completeness of case ascertainment varied from 35 to 100% in DIAMOND. Most European nations in DIAMOND had comparable (> 90%) rates of ascertainment to EURODIAB (Vehik and Dabelea 2010). DIAMOND reached the lowest completeness rates in Africa, Central and South America. This reflects a general problem when assessing type 1 diabetes epidemiology: data from developing countries are scarce and may not be fully representative due to low rates of completeness.

3. The incidence of type 1 diabetes mellitus

This section provides a comprehensive description of type 1 diabetes incidence, its changes over the last years, and its variability in populations and patient subgroups.

3.1. Geographic differences

Mean incidence rates of type 1 diabetes vary considerably depending on the geographic region (Galler, Stange et al. 2010). The worldwide incidence of type 1 diabetes is described to vary by at least 100- to 350-fold among different countries (Karvonen, Viik-Kajander et al. 2000). The highest incidence rates are found in Finland and Sardinia (Italy) and the lowest in South American countries, e.g. Venezuela and Brazil, and Asian countries, e.g. China or Thailand (Karvonen, Viik-Kajander et al. 2000; Borchers, Uibo et al. 2010; Panamonta, Thamjaroen et al. 2011). Apart from regions with low to intermediate incidence rates ranging between 5 and 20 per 100,000 children or adolescents per year, there are areas with incidence rates as high as 27 to 43 per 100,000 children or adolescents per year. Canada and Northern European countries, such as Finland and Sweden, have the highest incidence rates ranging between 30 and 40 per 100,000 children/adolescents per year. Incidence rates of countries in Central Europe (with the exception of Sardinia) vary from 8 to 18 per 100,000 children/adolescents per year. The incidence for type 1 diabetes in German children aged 0 to 14 years was estimated at 13 per 100,000 per year for 1987–1998 and at 15.5 per 100,000 per year for 1999–2003. The registry of the former German Democratic Republic, which was kept from 1960 until 1989, reported incidence rates between 7 and 14 per 100,000 children/adolescents per year (Galler, Stange et al. 2010). In Mediterranean countries, the incidence rates of type 1 diabetes also show wide variations, although for some of them, there are still no relevant and reliable data (Muntoni 1999). Summarizing the data on type 1 diabetes incidence, the polar-equatorial gradient does not seem to be as strong as previously assumed. The incidence of type 1 diabetes among different countries is presented in Table 1 and Table 2. When comparing the incidence of type 1 diabetes between countries, it is important to keep the size of the sample and the area of sampling in mind. This is because the incidence of type 1 diabetes may show strong variations among different regions from many countries as United States or Italy. Also a Romanian study revealed a wide geographic variation (6.71-fold) between the highest and the lowest incidence rates in different districts of the country (Ionescu-Tirgoviste, Guja et al. 2004).

While genetic factors are thought to explain some of the geographic variability in type 1 diabetes occurrence, they cannot account for its rapidly increasing frequency. Instead, the declining proportion of newly diagnosed children with high-risk genotypes suggests that environmental pressures are now able to trigger type 1 diabetes in genotypes that previously would not have developed the disease during childhood (Borchers, Uibo et al. 2010). The importance of environmental factors towards manifestation of type 1 diabetes is also supported by migration studies: For example a recently published study revealed that being born in Sweden, a country with high type 1 diabetes incidence, increases the risk for type 1 diabetes in children with a genetic origin in low-incidence countries (Soderstrom, Aman et al. 2012).

Country	Sampling Region	Incidence	AI of Incidence
Algeria	Oran	4.7	7.9 (1.85 to 14.00)
Australia	West	14.9	6.3 (2.11 to 10.50)
Australia[a]	New South Wales	19.4	2.8 (1.9 to 3.8)
Canada	Prince Edward Island	23.5	3.2 (-0.33 to 6.38)
Canada	Montreal	9.3	1.6 (-0.67 to 3.82)
China	Shanghai	0.7	7.4 (2.3 to 12.5)
Iceland	n.s.	9.0	2.3 (-2.38 to 6.96)
Israel	Yemenite Jews	5.0	3.2 (2.51 to 3.88)
Japan	Hokkaido	1.7	5.9 (4.14 to 7.63)
Libya	n.s.	8.7	6.3 (0.69 to 11.8)
New Zealand	Auckland	10.1	6.4 (4.20 to 8.52)
New Zealand	Canterbury	12.7	2.7 (.0.05 to 10.50)
Peru	Lima	0.5	7.7 (-1.0 to 16.4)
Thailand[b]	Northeast Thailand	0.6	n.s.
United States[c]	Colorado	19.4	2.3 (1.6 to 3.1)
United States	Hawaii	7.8	7.8 (1.8 to 14.9)
United States	Allegheny County	14.7	1.5 (0.21 to 2.83)
United States	Colorado	12.3	-0.2 (-2.52 to 2.19)

[a]Taplin, Craig et al. 2005

[b]Panamonta, Thamjaroen et al. 2011

[c]Vehik, Hamman et al. 2007

n.s.: not sepcified

Table 1. The incidence (per 100,000 per year) of type 1 diabetes and its annual increase (AI; with 95% confidence interval) in different non-European countries. If not otherwise indicated, data were adopted from the review of Onkamo, Vaananen et al. (1999). The analyzed time period differed from country to country.

Country	Sample	1st period	2nd period	AI
Austria	whole nation	9.0	13.3	4.3 (3.3 to 5.3)
Belgium	Antwerp	10.9	15.4	3.1 (0.5 to 5.8)
Bosnia[a]	Tuzla canton	8.9	-	15 (6.0 to 25)
Croatia[b]	two sources	6.9	-	9.0 (5.8 to 12.2)
Czech Republic	whole nation	8.7	17.2	6.7 (5.9 to 7.5)
Denmark[c]	whole nation	22.0	-	3.4 (1.9 to 5.0)
Estonia[d]	whole nation	10.1	16.9	3.3 (n.s.)
Finland	two regions	39.9	52.6	2.7 (1.4 to 4.0)
Germany	BadenWürttemberg	13.0	15.5	3.7 (2.9 to 4.5)
Germany	Düsseldorf	12.5	18.3	4.7 (3.1 to 6.3)
Hungary	18 counties	8.8	11.5	2.9 (1.9 to 3.9)
Italy[e]	Sardinia	37.7	49.3	2.8 (1.0 to 4.7)
Lithuana	whole nation	7.3	10.3	3.8 (2.2 to 5.3)
Luxembourg	whole nation	11.4	15.5	2.4 (-1.4 to 6.3)
Malta[f]	n.s.	14.7	-	0.5 (-2.1 to 3.2)
Montenegro[g]	whole nation	10.8	16.3	4.6 (0.4 to 9.6)
Norway	eight counties	21.1	24.6	1.3 (0.1 to 2.6)
Poland	Katowice	5.2	13.3	9.3 (7.8 to 10.8)
Romania	Bucharest	4.7	11.3	8.4 (5.8 to 11.0)
Slovakia	whole nation	8.2	13.6	5.1 (4.0 to 6.3)
Slovenia	whole nation	7.9	11.1	3.6 (1.6 to 5.7)
Spain	Catalonia	12.4	13.0	0.6 (-0.4 to 0.6)
Sweden	Stockholm county	25.8	34.6	3.3 (2.0 to 4.6)
United Kingdom	Northern Ireland	20.0	29.8	4.2 (3.0 to 5.5)
United Kingdom	Yorkshire	17.1	22.4	2.2 (1.1 to 3.4)
United Kingdom	Oxford	16.0	23.3	3.6 (2.6 to 4.6)

[a]Stipancic, La Grasta Sabolic et al. 2008, 1995-2003

[b]Tahirovic and Toromanovic 2007, 1995-2004

[c]Svensson, Lyngaae-Jorgensen et al. 2009, 1996-2005

[d]Teeaar, Liivak et al. 2010, 1983-1990 vs. 1999-2006

[e]Casu, Pascutto et al. 2004, 1989-1994 vs. 1995-1999

[f]Schranz and Prikatsky 1989, 1980-1987

[g]Samardzic, Marinkovic et al. 2010, 1997-2001 vs. 2002-2006

n.s.: not sepcified

Table 2. The incidence (per 100,000 per year) of type 1 diabetes and its annual increase (AI; with 95% confidence interval) in different European regions. If not otherwise indicated, data were adopted from Patterson, Dahlquist et al. (2009) and were estimated during the periods 1989-1993 and 1999-2003, respectively.

3.2. Changes over the last years

A global rise in the incidence of type 1 diabetes in children and adolescents has been report-ed over the past decades (Onkamo, Vaananen et al. 1999; Karvonen, Viik-Kajander et al. 2000; Soltesz 2003; Aamodt, Stene et al. 2007; Soltesz, Patterson et al. 2007). The world-wide annual increment of type 1 diabetes has already been summarized in the work of Onkamo, Vaananen et al. (1999). They found a statistically significant increase of incidence in 65% (24/37) of the examined populations. A non-statistically significant upward tendency was seen in another 12 populations, while a statistically significant decrease of type 1 diabetes incidence was not found. The global trend of the increase in the incidence of type 1 diabetes was 3.0% per year (95% CI 2.59-3.33; $p < 0.001$; Onkamo, Vaananen et al. 1999).

The United States stood apart from other nations in reporting a stable incidence of child-hood type 1 diabetes in the 1970s through the 1990s (Vehik and Dabelea 2010). The multi-center Search for Diabetes in Youth Study (SEARCH) reported that the 2002 to 2005 incidence of type 1 diabetes in non-Hispanic White younger than 14 years of age was 27.5/100,000 per year (Bell, Mayer-Davis et al. 2009). This exceeded the incidence predicted for 2010 by earlier data from Allegheny County, Pennsylvania (Dokheel 1993). A similar de-velopment was noticed by estimated data from Colorado (Vehik and Dabelea 2010).

For Europe, data from the EURODIAB-register suggest an annual increment of incidence of about 0.6-15% (see Table 2 for details; Patterson, Dahlquist et al. 2009). Earlier data regard-ing type 1 diabetes incidence from all 36 EURODIAB-centers were published by Green and Patterson (2001).

Regarding the strong differences in the annual increase in the incidence of type 1 diabetes between the countries, it must be mentioned that, besides the geographic differences, the in-cidence trend was found not to be continuously linear. Furthermore, the incidence trend in-creases exponentially. Predictions made by Onkamo et al. for the incidence rates in 2010 pointed to large increases, but, in retrospect, were too conservative, especially regarding younger children (Knip 2012).

3.3. Sex-dependent differences of type 1 diabetes mellitus incidence

Despite matched-pair investigations suggested that for some early childhood risk factors the odds ratio in boys were different from those in girls (Svensson, Carstensen et al. 2005), most of the published studies reported no significant difference between the type 1 diabetes inci-dence in boys and girls (Shaltout, Qabazard et al. 1995; Abellana, Ascaso et al. 2009; Svens-son, Lyngaae-Jorgensen et al. 2009; Samardzic, Marinkovic et al. 2010; Teeaar, Liivak et al. 2010). Other groups found small and thereby not relevant sex-related differences only for subgroups (Shaltout, Qabazard et al. 1995). A sex-related difference in incidence was found only in the 10- to 14-year age group with a significantly higher incidence in boys (18.77 vs. 14.7/100,000/year, $p = 0.015$; Bizzarri, Patera et al. 2010). However, a statistically significantly higher incidence in girls was reported by a Libyan (Kadiki and Roaeid 2002), a Thai (Pana-monta, Thamjaroen et al. 2011), and an Australian group (Taplin, Craig et al. 2005). The latter also found the average annual increase of incidence to be significantly higher in boys (3.8% vs. 1.9%, p = 0.046).

Taken together the reported studies suggest no sex-dependent differences in the incidence of type 1 diabetes. Type 1 diabetes can be assumed to be the only major organ-specific auto-immune disease not to show a strong female bias. The overall sex ratio is roughly equal in children diagnosed under the age of 15 years (Gale and Gillespie 2001). After the age of puberty, males are more frequently affected than females (Nystrom, Dahlquist et al. 1992).

3.4. Age-dependent differences of type 1 diabetes mellitus incidence

The following sections are intended to answer two questions: 1) does the incidence of type 1 diabetes differ between distinct age groups, and 2) what changes of the incidence of type 1 diabetes within these age groups occurred over the last years.

3.4.1. The age-dependent pattern of type 1 diabetes mellitus incidence

The incidence of type 1 diabetes shows an age-dependent pattern. It was reported to be significantly lower in the 0– to 4-year-old group than in the other groups (Bizzarri, Patera et al. 2010). Many studies from different countries reported an increase of the incidence with increasing age. The highest incidences were found in the 10 to 14-year-old age group (Karvonen, Viik-Kajander et al. 2000; Michaelis et al., 1993; Neu, Ehehalt et al. 2001; Taplin, Craig et al. 2005; Samardzic, Marinkovic et al. 2010).

3.4.2. The increase of incidence in different age groups

The increasing incidence of type 1 diabetes is evident. Although some groups found no age-dependent differences in the annual increment of type 1 diabetes incidence (Taplin, Craig et al. 2005; Svensson, Lyngaae-Jorgensen et al. 2009; Abduljabbar, Aljubeh et al. 2010), the majority of the published studies reported different increments of incidence after stratifying children and youths into different age groups: Michaelis et. al (1993) found an increment of incidence of about 12.6% in 0- to 9-year-old children, in 10- to 19-year-old children the increment was 3.8%. Similar results were reported by other German groups (Neu, Ehehalt et al. 2001; Ehehalt, Blumenstock et al. 2008): the relative increment of type 1 diabetes incidence was 5.7% per year in 0- to 4-year-old children, the other age groups showed smaller increments. The incidence of childhood-onset type 1 diabetes in Estonian children under 15 years of age increased annually by an average of 3.3% with the most rapid annual increase (9.3%) occurring in the youngest age group (Teeaar, Liivak et al. 2010). The EURODIAB register repeatedly confirmed that in Europe the annual increase of incidence is higher in younger children (0 to 4 years of age; Green and Patterson 2001; Patterson, Dahlquist et al. 2009).

3.5. Seasonal differences of type 1 diabetes mellitus incidence

When discussing seasonal differences in the epidemiology of type 1 diabetes, two different aspects must be mentioned: 1) different frequency of type 1 diabetes regarding the season of birth, and 2) the changing onset or diagnosis of type 1 diabetes through the year.

3.5.1. Seasonal changes in the incidence of type 1 diabetes mellitus

The seasonality of onset or diagnosis of type 1 diabetes has been extensively studied and the results, so far, are conflicting (Moltchanova, Schreier et al. 2009). However, an increment of type 1 diabetes incidence during the winter has been reported by manifold studies (for details: Padaiga, Tuomilehto et al. 1999) from different countries, e.g. Australia (Elliott, Lucas et al. 2010), the United States (Gorham, Barrett-Connor et al. 2009), Chile (Durruty, Ruiz et al. 1979; Santos, Carrasco et al. 2001), Sweden (Samuelsson, Carstensen et al. 2007; Ostman, Lonnberg et al. 2008), Norway (Joner and Sovik 1981), Greece (Kalliora, Vazeou et al. 2011), and the Czech Republic (Cinek, Sumnik et al. 2003). Recently, Jarosz-Chobot et al. (2011) reported that a significant increase in type 1 diabetes incidence among children over 4 years of age was observed in the autumn–winter season (p = 0.137 for the age group 0–4 years and p < 0.001 for the age groups 5-9 and 10-14 years). These findings were confirmed by other studies in Poland (Pilecki, Robak-Kontna et al. 2003; Zubkiewicz-Kucharska and Noczynska 2010). Other, partially incomparable, studies revealed no seasonal pattern in the onset or diagnosis of type 1 diabetes mellitus (Levy-Marchal, Papoz et al. 1990; Muntoni and Songini 1992; Ye, Chen et al. 1998) or reported seasonal changes only for subgroups (Michalkova, Cernay et al. 1995; Douglas, McSporran et al. 1999; Padaiga, Tuomilehto et al. 1999). Moltchanova et al. (2009) analyzed data from 105 centers in 53 countries: however, only 42 centers exhibited significant seasonality (p < 0.05) in the incidence of type 1 diabetes when the data were pooled for age and sex (Moltchanova, Schreier et al. 2009). Centers further away from the equator were on average more likely to exhibit seasonality (p < 0.001). Although the majority of the published data suggests seasonal-dependent changes in the incidence of type 1 diabetes mellitus, further research is needed to complete the picture. Especially populations living below the 30th parallel north should be studied, the populations themselves should be investigated more deeply, and the sample sizes should be increased to gain adequate power to detect seasonal changes in low-incidence populations.

According to the published literature, the seasonal changes in the incidence of type 1 diabetes are likely to be caused by changes of the (auto-)immune activity. The first point is that a reduced ultraviolet radiation exposure during the winter months may lead to reduced vitamin D levels. Thereby, the inhibitory effect of vitamin D on Th1-lymphocytes decreases. The second point is the stimulation of the immune system especially by viral infections during the winter months. The result of both could be a higher (auto-)immune activity that causes ß-cell destruction.

3.5.2. Effects of the season of birth on the incidence of type 1 diabetes mellitus

Possible influences of the season of birth are discussed for many autoimmune diseases, e.g. multiple sclerosis, Hashimoto thyreoditis, or Grave's disease (Krassas, Tziomalos et al. 2007). Spring births were associated with increased likelihood of type 1 diabetes, but possibly not in all United States regions (Kahn, Morgan et al. 2009). An Egyptian group reported that 48.3% of diabetic children were delivered during summer months (Ismail, Kasem et al. 2008). A German investigation showed children and adolescents with diabetes being significantly less often born during the months April-June and July-September (Neu, Kehrer et al. 2000). This seasonality pattern was different from those registered in Israel, Sardinia and Slovenia, in which the population with diabetes type 1 had most births during these months (1972; Neu, Kehrer et al. 2000). A Ukrainian group found that type 1 diabetes was some 30% more common among persons born in April than among persons born in December (Vaiserman, Carstensen et al. 2007). McKinney et al. analyzed data from 19 European countries, but found no uniform seasonal pattern of birth in childhood diabetes patients across European populations, either overall or according to sex and age (McKinney 2001). Small Turkish studies did not reveal any significant differences of the season of birth in type 1 diabetic vs. metabolically healthy children (Evliyaoglu, Ocal et al. 2002; Karaguzel, Ozer et al. 2007). The controversial results might be explained by the composition of most study samples: Laron et al. found a pattern in the seasonality of month of birth only in ethnically homogenous populations (such as Ashkenazi Jews, Israeli Arabs, individuals in Sardinia and Canterbury, New Zealand, and Afro-Americans), but not in heterogeneous populations (such as in Sydney, Pittsburgh and Denver; Laron, Lewy et al. 2005). Thereby, it becomes likely that ethnically heterogeneous populations comprising a mixture of patients with various genetic backgrounds and environmental exposures mask the different seasonality pattern of month of birth that many children with diabetes present when compared to the general population (Laron, Lewy et al. 2005).

Authors describing a relationship between season of birth and susceptibility for type 1 diabetes have attributed this to intrauterine infections, dietary intake of certain nutrients and possible toxic food components, short duration of breastfeeding, early exposure to cows' milk proteins, and vitamin D deficiency (Vaiserman, Carstensen et al. 2007). Since most of these factors vary with season, one would expect a difference in the seasonal birth pattern between the general population and those children who develop diabetes. A possible link between environmental factors and type 1 diabetes mellitus manifestation was provided by Badenhoop et al. They found HLA susceptibility genes to be in different proportions of patients either born in different seasons of the year or having manifested their disease in different historical periods over time (Badenhoop, Kahles et al. 2009).

3.6. Ethnic differences

It has been proposed that much of the current variation in the incidence of type 1 diabetes is due in part to differing distributions of ethnicity throughout the world. Many large studies of type 1 diabetes have provided evidence that the ethnic background is one of the most important risk factors for type 1 diabetes (Vehik and Dabelea 2010). It can be assumed that there is a genetically founded – and thereby ethnically associated – varying susceptibility for type 1 diabetes. The onset of the disease is then triggered by ubiquitous environmental factors (Knip, Veijola et al. 2005; Knip and Simell 2012). In general, susceptibility to type 1 diabetes is attributable to genes that link disease progression to distinct steps in immune activation, expansion, and regulation (Nepom and Buckner 2012).

One half of the genetic susceptibility for type 1 diabetes is explained by the HLA (human leukocyte antigen) genes (Knip and Simell 2012). It becomes conclusive that the main research focus is on ethnic variances in HLA-haplotypes and its association with type 1 diabetes (Lipton, Drum et al. 2011; Noble, Johnson et al. 2011). Based on the presence of two high-risk HLA-DQA1/B1 haplotypes, an investigation in the United States revealed that

Caucasians are at the highest and Latinos are at the second-highest risk for developing type 1 diabetes compared to all other ethnic groups (Lipton, Drum et al. 2011). However, there is accumulating evidence that the proportion of subjects with newly diagnosed type 1 diabetes and high-risk HLA genotypes has decreased over the last decades, whereas the proportion of those with low-risk or even protective HLA genotypes has increased (Hermann, Knip et al. 2003; Gillespie, Bain et al. 2004).

The second half of the genetic susceptibility for type 1 diabetes is caused by more than 50 non-HLA genetic polymorphisms (Knip and Simell 2012). Nowadays, there are more than 60 gene loci contributing to the susceptibility of developing type 1 diabetes (Morahan 2012), but this overwhelming list of type 1 diabetes risk genes exerts little influence on the clinical management of children that are at high risk. Conclusively, it is necessary to place the genetics of type 1 diabetes in a more amenable clinical context (Morahan 2012).

Despite the fact that there is consensus about the different genetic type 1 diabetes susceptibility among different ethnic groups, these differences cannot explain the complete variance of type 1 diabetes incidence and prevalence. Furthermore, the annual increment of type 1 diabetes incidence cannot be explained by changing genetic susceptibility. Together with the fact that many individuals are genetically highly susceptible for type 1 diabetes, it becomes conclusive that environmental factors play a crucial role in the onset of the disease and its epidemiology (Knip and Simell 2012).

4. The prevalence of type 1 diabetes mellitus

This section provides a comprehensive description of the type 1 diabetes prevalence, current prevalence trends, and its variability depending among populations and individuals of different age.

4.1. The geographic differences of type 1 diabetes mellitus prevalence

Banting and Best introduced the treatment of type 1 diabetes with insulin injections in the year 1922. Although their first patient (Leonard Thompson) died at the age of 27 from suspected pneumonia, other patients, even from this first treatment series, lived a long time (Teddy Ryder died at the age of 76, Jim Havens at the age of 59 and Elisabeth Ewans Hughes at the age of 73 years; Pliska, Folkers et al. 2005). This observation led to the assumption that the life expectancy of type 1 diabetic patients may be near to normal if the disease is properly treated. It was proven that the life expectation of type 1 diabetic patients has increased over the last decades (Ioacara, Lichiardopol et al. 2009; Miller, Secrest et al. 2012). Therefore, it becomes conclusive that the changes in incidence imply similar trends in the prevalence rates of type 1 diabetes and lead to an accumulation of the disease burden caused by type 1 diabetes and its complications. Recent studies suggest a doubling of type 1 diabetes prevalence within a 20-year period (Akesen, Turan et al. 2011; Ehehalt, Dietz et al. 2012). The International Diabetes Federation assumed that in 2011 about 490,100 children (aged 0 to 14 years) suffer from type 1 diabetes. This would correspond to a worldwide prevalence of (25.8 per 100,000 children aged 0 to 4 years). Following the Diabetes Atlas (International Diabetes Federation 2011), there 116,100 cases of type 1 diabetes in the Europe, 64,900 in the Middle East and North Africa region, 36,100 in the Africa, 94,700 in the North America and Caribbean, 36,100 in the South and Central America, 111,500 in the South-East Asia and 30,700 in the Western Pacific region. In accordance with incidence rates differing regionally within countries and also among different countries, the prevalence of type 1 diabetes mellitus varies in a broad range. The prevalence of type 1 diabetes in different countries is summarized in Table 3.

Country	Sampling Period	Prevalence
Finland	2000–2005	427.5
Sweden	2001–2005	270.5
Norway	1999–2003	182.4
United Kingdom	1989–2003	158.3
Canada	1990–1999	146.7
Denmark	1996–2005	141.2
Australia	1999–2008	137.8
United States	2002–2003	135.6
Germany	1989–2003	126.7
Netherlands	1996–1999	124.8
Czech Republic	1989–2003	117.5
New Zealand	1999–2000	115.9
Belgium	1989–2003	107.7
Ireland	1997	107.3
Austria	1989–2003	97.6
Portugal	1994–1998	95.5
Luxembourg	1989–2003	94.9
Slovak Republic	1989–2003	94.2
Iceland	1994–1998	91.1
Poland	1989–2003	85.7
France	1998–2004	84.5
Greece	1995–1999	80.2
Hungary	1989–2003	76.5
Spain	1989–2003	74.6
Switzerland	1991–1999	61.1
Italy	1990–1999	59.9
Turkey	1992–1996	19.8
Japan	1998–2001	15.7
Mexico	1990–1993	8.1
Korea	1990–1991	6.7

Table 3. The prevalence of type 1 diabetes in children younger than 15 years in different OECD countries. Data are based on estimations of the International Diabetes Federation (2009) and related to 100,000 children (0 to 14 years of age) of each country.

4.2. The age-related differences of type 1 diabetes mellitus prevalence

Regarding age dependents phenomena of type 1 diabetes incidence (see section 3.4) it becomes conclusive that 1) the prevalence of type 1 diabetes shows no sex-related differences
and increases with age due to accumulation of individuals suffering from the disease and 2)
the age-dependent increment of prevalence is not just linear but more likely exponential due
to an age-dependent increment of type 1 diabetes incidence. These assumptions have been
confirmed for example by the findings of the Australian Institute of Health and Welfare (see
Table 4) that were based on the Australian National Diabetes Register.

Age (years)	Persons	Prevalence
0 to 4	405	28.8 (26.0 to 31.6)
5 to 9	1,731	128.0 (122.0 to 134.1)
10 to 14	3,597	256.3 (247.9 to 264.7)
total	5,733	137.8 (134.2 to 141.4)

Table 4. The estimated prevalence (per 100,000 inhabitants of the respective age group with 95% confidence
interval) of type 1 diabetes among Australian children aged 0-14 years (Australian Institute of Health and Welfare
2011).

5. What the changing epidemiology implies for future research

The number of investigations concerning the epidemiology of type 1 diabetes is extensive.
However, the published results are controversial or even contradictory. There is consensus
about fundamental aspects, such as the increasing incidence and prevalence of type 1 diabetes. Thereby, it becomes clear that type 1 diabetes will become more and more of a burden.
Although most investigations and publications have been of high methodological quality,
they lack exact explanations of the described phenomena, and understanding the mechanisms and triggers of type 1 diabetes remains a mystery.

Future research should lead to improved methods of estimating the epidemiology of type 1
diabetes. Like this, more valid and thereby comparable data on type 1 diabetes epidemiology and risk factors have to be gained, but also more data on the epidemiology of type 1 diabetes over the whole lifespan are definitely needed (Knip 2012). Furthermore, future
research may lead to a better understanding of the underlying pathogenesis of type 1 diabetes by complementing the results of descriptive epidemiology with those of 'aetiological' epidemiology (Knip 2012) including the assessment of suspected environmental triggers and
risk factors as well as genetic background of the assessed individuals. Conclusively, future
research on type 1 diabetes cannot exclusively be performed with population-based approaches. Individualized approaches, e.g. metabolic profiling in both the pre-autoimmune

period and the preclinical period (Oresic, Simell et al. 2008), may provide clues to environmental triggers, such as infections or dietary changes, which likely cause disturbances in the intestinal microbiota and the immune system and contribute to the onset of type 1 diabetes. Thereby, children/adolescents at a high risk may be identified and possibilities for prevention of type 1 diabetes may be detected.

In part promising therapeutic approaches to type 1 diabetes as immunotherapy, stem cell-, β-cell- or islet of Langerhans-transplantation have to be assessed in future studies to find causal therapeutic strategies (Chatenoud, Warncke et al. 2012; Li, Gu et al. 2012; McCall, James Shapiro et al. 2012). Additionally, further research is needed in the field of chronic type 1 diabetes and the detection and treatment of its complications. The role of genetics in susceptibility to nephropathy, retinopathy and other diabetic complications still largely remains to be explored (Borchers, Uibo et al. 2010).

6. What the changing epidemiology implies for future health care

Until now, the treatment of type 1 diabetic patients has been the duty of pediatricians, internal specialists, or diabetologists. The consultation prevalence of type 1 diabetic patients in the general practitioners' consultation hour was low (Frese, Sandholzer et al. 2008). However, if the present trends continue, a doubling of new cases of type 1 diabetes in European children younger than 5 years is predicted between 2005 and 2020, and prevalent cases younger than 15 years will rise by 70% (Patterson, Dahlquist et al. 2009). Adequate health-care resources to meet these children's needs should be made available (Patterson, Dahlquist et al. 2009). It is important to ensure appropriate planning of services and that resources are in place to provide high-quality care for the increased numbers of children who will be diagnosed with diabetes in future years (Patterson, Dahlquist et al. 2009).

In Germany, the costs of pediatric diabetes care exceeded €110 million in 2007. Compared with estimates from the year 2000, average costs per patient had increased by 20% and direct total costs for German pediatric diabetes care by 47% (Bachle, Holl et al. 2012). The treatment costs rose because of new therapeutic strategies and an increase in diabetes prevalence. This illustrates that type 1 diabetes will be an increasing challenge for future health care.

Regarding future health care, it should be kept in mind that elderly and old patients with type 1 diabetes represent a growing population that requires thorough diabetes care. Especially type 1 diabetic patients older than 60 years will suffer from a longer diabetes duration, a doubled risk for severe hypoglycemia, and a higher percentage of cardiovascular complications (Schutt, Fach et al. 2012). In order to provide an adequate health care service, treatment strategies for adults and elderly persons suffering from type 1 diabetes have to be implemented in practice and the knowledge of involved physicians, especially general practitioners, has to be enhanced.

7. Summary

Data on the epidemiology of type 1 diabetes are based on standardized registry data, such as the Diabetes Mondiale (DIAMOND) Project worldwide and The Epidemiology and Prevention of Diabetes (EURODIAB) study in Europe. Some countries provide national registers. Regional or loco-regional registers as well as (cross-sectional) studies have added further data to the current knowledge. Epidemiologic data from developing countries are scarce and may not be fully representative.

The incidence of type 1 diabetes varies up to 100-fold among different countries. The highest incidences are found in northern countries, especially Finland. The lowest incidence rates were recorded in South American and Asian countries. When discussing type 1 diabetes incidence, also strong variations within countries have to be regarded and care should be taken when generalizing results from a regional sample to a general population. The incidence of type 1 diabetes increases worldwide exponentially. The mean of increment is 3.0% per year. Some assume that the incidence of type 1 diabetes in 2020 will be twice that of the year 2000. Before the age of puberty type 1 diabetes there is no sex-related difference in the incidence of type 1-diabetes. However some early childhood risk factors show different odds for boys and girls and after puberty males are more frequently affected by new onset of type 1 diabetes than females. Type 1 diabetes incidence increases with the age of the children/adolescents, but the annually increase of incidence is higher in younger children and those with moderate genetic susceptibility. There is evidence for a circannular variation with a peak of type 1 diabetes incidence during the winter months. Possible effects of the season of birth have to be further investigated with attention to the genetic background of assessed individuals. Genetic susceptibility explains some of the variation of type 1 diabetes incidence and prevalence with the highest risk in individuals with Caucasian or Latino background. As supported by migration studies, the increasing incidence of type 1 diabetes illustrates the importance of environmental risk factors as triggers of the disease.

Future research should focus on indentifying environmental and genetic risk factors of type 1 diabetes and its complications, preventive strategies and causal treatment options. The prevalence, which doubled worldwide over the last decades, will increase further and type 1 diabetes will shift more and more into the focus of general practitioners. It becomes conclusive that type 1 diabetes will be a burden for more and more patients and for the majority of health care systems.

Acknowledgment

This book chapter is dedicated to my much-valued teacher, Prof. Dr. Elmar Peschke.

Author details

Thomas Frese and Hagen Sandholzer

Department of Primary Care, Medical School, Leipzig, Germany

References

[1] Aamodt, G., Stene, L. C., et al. (2007). Spatiotemporal trends and age-period-cohort modeling of the incidence of type 1 diabetes among children aged < 15 years in Norway 1973-1982 and 1989-2003. *Diabetes Care*, 30(4), 884-889.

[2] Abduljabbar, M. A., Aljubeh, J. M., et al. (2010). Incidence trends of childhood type 1 diabetes in eastern Saudi Arabia. *Saudi Med J*, 31(4), 413-418.

[3] Abellana, R., Ascaso, C., et al. (2009). Geographical variability of the incidence of Type 1 diabetes in subjects younger than 30 years in Catalonia, Spain. *Med Clin (Barc)*, 132(12), 454-458.

[4] Akesen, E., Turan, S., et al. (2011). Prevalence of type 1 diabetes mellitus in 6-18-yr-old school children living in Istanbul, Turkey. Pediatr Diabetes 12(6), 567-571.

[5] Australian Institute of Health and Welfare (2011). Prevalence of Type 1 diabetes in Australian children, 2008. Canberra: Australian Institute of Health and Welfare.

[6] Awa, W. L., Schober, E., et al. (2011). Reclassification of diabetes type in pediatric patients initially classified as type 2 diabetes mellitus: 15 years follow-up using routine data from the German/Austrian DPV database. *Diabetes Res Clin Pract*, 94(3), 463-467.

[7] Bachle, C. C., Holl, R. W., et al. (2012). Costs of paediatric diabetes care in Germany: current situation and comparison with the year 2000. *Diabet Med*, 29(10):1327-1334.

[8] Badenhoop, K., Kahles, H., et al. (2009). MHC-environment interactions leading to type 1 diabetes: feasibility of an analysis of HLA DR-DQ alleles in relation to manifestation periods and dates of birth. *Diabetes Obes Metab*, 11(Suppl 1), 88-91.

[9] Bell, R. A., Mayer-Davis, E. J., et al. (2009). Diabetes in non-Hispanic white youth: prevalence, incidence, and clinical characteristics: the SEARCH for Diabetes in Youth Study. *Diabetes Care*, 32(Suppl 2), S102-111.

[10] Bizzarri, C., Patera, P. I., et al. (2010). Incidence of type 1 diabetes has doubled in Rome and the Lazio region in the 0- to 14-year age-group: a 6-year prospective study (2004-2009). *Diabetes Care*, 33(11), e140.

[11] Borchers, A. T., Uibo, R., et al. (2010). The geoepidemiology of type 1 diabetes. *Autoimmun Rev*, 9(5), A355-365.

[12] Casu, A., Pascutto, C., et al. (2004). Type 1 diabetes among sardinian children is increasing: the Sardinian diabetes register for children aged 0-14 years (1989-1999). *Diabetes Care*, 27(7), 1623-1629.

[13] Chatenoud, L., Warncke, K., Ziegler, A.G. (2012). Clinical immunologic interventions for the treatment of type 1 diabetes. *Cold Spring Harb Perspect Med*, 2(8), pii:a007716. doi: 10.1101/cshperspect.a007716

[14] Cinek, O., Sumnik, Z., et al. (2003). Continuing increase in incidence of childhood-onset type 1 diabetes in the Czech Republic 1990-2001. *Eur J Pediatr*, 162(6), 428-429.

[15] Dabelea, D., Mayer-Davis, E. J., et al. (2010). The value of national diabetes registries: SEARCH for Diabetes in Youth Study. *Curr Diab Rep*, 10(5), 362-369.

[16] Dokheel, T. M. (1993). An epidemic of childhood diabetes in the United States? Evidence from Allegheny County, Pennsylvania. Pittsburgh Diabetes Epidemiology Research Group. *Diabetes Care*, 16(12), 1606-1611.

[17] Douglas, S., McSporran, B., et al. (1999). Seasonality of presentation of type I diabetes mellitus in children. Scottish Study Group for the Care of Young Diabetics. *Scott Med J*, 44(2), 41-46.

[18] Durruty, P., Ruiz, F., et al. (1979). Age at diagnosis and seasonal variation in the onset of insulin-dependent diabetes in Chile (Southern hemisphere). *Diabetologia*, 17(6), 357-360.

[19] Ehehalt, S., Blumenstock, G., et al. (2008). Continuous rise in incidence of childhood Type 1 diabetes in Germany. *Diabet Med*, 25(6), 755-757.

[20] Ehehalt, S., Dietz, K., et al. (2012). Prediction model for the incidence and prevalence of type 1 diabetes in childhood and adolescence: evidence for a cohort-dependent increase within the next two decades in Germany. *Pediatr Diabetes*, 13(1), 15-20.

[21] Elliott, J. C., Lucas, R. M., et al. (2010). Population density determines the direction of the association between ambient ultraviolet radiation and type 1 diabetes incidence. *Pediatr Diabetes*, 11(6), 394-402.

[22] Evliyaoglu, O., Ocal, G., et al. (2002). No seasonality of birth in children with type 1 diabetes mellitus in Ankara, Turkey. *J Pediatr Endocrinol Metab*, 15(7), 1033-1034.

[23] Forouhi, N. G., Merrick, D., et al. (2006). Diabetes prevalence in England, 2001--estimates from an epidemiological model. *Diabet Med*, 23(2), 189-197.

[24] Frese, T., Herrmann, K., et al. (2012). Inter-rater reliability of the ICPC-2 in a German general practice setting. *Swiss Med Wkly*, (142), w13621.

[25] Frese, T., Sandholzer, H., et al. (2008). Epidemiology of diabetes mellitus in German general practitioners' consultation--results of the SESAM 2-study. *Exp Clin Endocrinol Diabetes*, 116(6), 326-328.

[26] Fuller, J. H. (1989). European Community Concerted Action Programme in Diabetes (EURODIAB). *Diabet Med*, 6(3), 278.

[27] Gale, E. A. & Gillespie, K. M. (2001). Diabetes and gender. *Diabetologia*, 44(1), 3-15.

[28] Galler, A., Stange, T., et al. (2010). Incidence of childhood diabetes in children aged less than 15 years and its clinical and metabolic characteristics at the time of diagnosis: data from the Childhood Diabetes Registry of Saxony, Germany. *Horm Res Paediatr*, 74(4), 285-291.

[29] Gillespie, K. M., Bain, S. C., et al. (2004). The rising incidence of childhood type 1 dia-
      betes and reduced contribution of high-risk HLA haplotypes. *Lancet*, 364(9446),
      1699-1700.

[30] Gorham, E. D., Barrett-Connor, E., et al. (2009). Incidence of insulin-requiring diabe-
      tes in the US military. *Diabetologia*, 52(10), 2087-2091.

[31] Gray, J., Orr, D., et al. (2003). Use of Read codes in diabetes management in a south
      London primary care group: implications for establishing disease registers. *BMJ*,
      326(7399), 1130.

[32] Green, A., Gale, E. A., et al. (1992). Incidence of childhood-onset insulin-dependent
      diabetes mellitus: the EURODIAB ACE Study. *Lancet*, 339(8798), 905-909.

[33] Green, A. & Patterson, C. C. (2001). Trends in the incidence of childhood-onset diabe-
      tes in Europe 1989-1998. *Diabetologia*, 44 (Suppl 3), B3-8.

[34] Hermann, R., Knip, M., et al. (2003). Temporal changes in the frequencies of HLA
      genotypes in patients with Type 1 diabetes--indication of an increased environmental
      pressure? *Diabetologia*, 46(3), 420-425.

[35] Howitt, A. J. & Cheales, N. A. (1993). Diabetes registers: a grassroots approach. *BMJ*,
      307(6911), 1046-1048.

[36] International Diabetes Federation (2011). IDF diabetes atlas. 5th edition, Brussels: In-
      ternational Diabetes Federation.

[37] Ioacara, S., Lichiardopol, R., et al. (2009). Improvements in life expectancy in type 1
      diabetes patients in the last six decades. *Diabetes Res Clin Pract*, 86(2), 146-151.

[38] Ionescu-Tirgoviste, C., Guja, C., et al. (2004). An increasing trend in the incidence of
      type 1 diabetes mellitus in children aged 0-14 years in Romania--ten years
      (1988-1997) EURODIAB study experience. *J Pediatr Endocrinol Metab*, 17(7), 983-991.

[39] Ismail, N. A., Kasem, O. M., et al. (2008). Epidemiology and management of type 1
      diabetes mellitus at the ain shams university pediatric hospital. *J Egypt Public Health
      Assoc*, 83(1-2), 107-132.

[40] Jarosz-Chobot, P., Polanska, J., et al. (2011). Rapid increase in the incidence of type 1
      diabetes in Polish children from 1989 to 2004, and predictions for 2010 to 2025. *Diabe-
      tologia*, 54(3), 508-515.

[41] Joner, G. & Sovik, O. (1981). Incidence, age at onset and seasonal variation of diabe-
      tes mellitus in Norwegian children, 1973-1977. *Acta Paediatr Scand*, 70(3), 329-335.

[42] Kadiki, O. A. & Roaeid, R. B. (2002). Incidence of type 1 diabetes in children (0-14
      years) in Benghazi Libya (1991-2000). *Diabetes Metab*, 28(6 Pt 1), 463-467.

[43] Kahn, H. S., Morgan, T. M., et al. (2009). Association of type 1 diabetes with month of
      birth among U.S. youth: The SEARCH for Diabetes in Youth Study. *Diabetes Care*,
      32(11), 2010-2015.

[44] Kalliora, M. I., Vazeou, A., et al. (2011). Seasonal variation of type 1 diabetes mellitus diagnosis in Greek children. *Hormones (Athens)*, 10(1), 67-71.

[45] Karaguzel, G., Ozer, S., et al. (2007). Type 1 diabetes-related epidemiological, clinical and laboratory findings. An evaluation with special regard to autoimmunity in children. *Saudi Med J*, 28(4), 584-589.

[46] Karvonen, M., Viik-Kajander, M., et al. (2000). Incidence of childhood type 1 diabetes worldwide. Diabetes Mondiale (DiaMond) Project Group. *Diabetes Care*, 23(10), 1516-1526.

[47] Knip, M. (2012). Descriptive epidemiology of type 1 diabetes--is it still in? *Diabetologia*, 55(5), 1227-1230.

[48] Knip, M. & Simell, O. (2012). Environmental triggers of type 1 diabetes. *Cold Spring Harb Perspect Med*, 2(7), a007690.

[49] Knip, M., Veijola, R., et al. (2005). Environmental triggers and determinants of type 1 diabetes. *Diabetes*, 54(Suppl 2), S125-136.

[50] Krassas, G. E., Tziomalos, K., et al. (2007). Seasonality of month of birth of patients with Graves' and Hashimoto's diseases differ from that in the general population. *Eur J Endocrinol*, 156(6), 631-636.

[51] Laron, Z., Lewy, H., et al. (2005). Seasonality of month of birth of children and adolescents with type 1 diabetes mellitus in homogenous and heterogeneous populations. *Isr Med Assoc J*, 7(6), 381-384.

[52] Levy-Marchal, C., Papoz, L., et al. (1990). Incidence of juvenile type 1 (insulin-dependent) diabetes mellitus in France. *Diabetologia*, 33(8), 465-469.

[53] Li, L., Gu, W., et al. (2012). Novel therapy for Type 1 diabetes - autologous hematopoietic stem cell transplantation. *J Diabetes*, doi, 10.1111/jdb.12002.

[54] Lipton, R. B., Drum, M., et al. (2011). HLA-DQ haplotypes differ by ethnicity in patients with childhood-onset diabetes. *Pediatr Diabetes*, 12(4 Pt 2), 388-395.

[55] McCall, M. & James Shapiro, A. M. (2012). Update on islet transplantation. *Cold Spring Harb Perspect Med*, 2(7), a007823.

[56] McKinney, P. A. (2001). Seasonality of birth in patients with childhood Type I diabetes in 19 European regions. *Diabetologia*, 44(Suppl 3), B67-74.

[57] Michalkova, D. M., Cernay, J., et al. (1995). Incidence and prevalence of childhood diabetes in Slovakia (1985-1992). Slovak Childhood Diabetes Epidemiology Study Group. *Diabetes Care*, 18(3), 315-320.

[58] Miller, R. G., Secrest, A. M., et al. (2012). Improvements in the life expectancy of type 1 diabetes: The Pittsburgh Epidemiology of Diabetes Complications Study cohort. *Diabetes*, 2012 Jul 30, Epub ahead of print.

[59] Moltchanova, E. V., Schreier, N., et al. (2009). Seasonal variation of diagnosis of Type 1 diabetes mellitus in children worldwide. *Diabet Med*, 26(7), 673-678.

[60] Mooney, J. A., Helms, P. J., et al. (2004). Seasonality of type 1 diabetes mellitus in children and its modification by weekends and holidays: retrospective observational study. *Arch Dis Child*, 89(10), 970-973.

[61] Morahan, G. (2012). Insights into type 1 diabetes provided by genetic analyses. *Curr Opin Endocrinol Diabetes Obes*, 19(4), 263-270.

[62] Muntoni, S. (1999). New insights into the epidemiology of type 1 diabetes in Mediterranean countries. *Diabetes Metab Res Rev*, 15(2), 133-140.

[63] Muntoni, S. & Songini, M. (1992). High incidence rate of IDDM in Sardinia. Sardinian Collaborative Group for Epidemiology of IDDM. *Diabetes Care*, 15(10), 1317-1322.

[64] Nepom, G. T. & Buckner, J. H. (2012). A functional framework for interpretation of genetic associations in T1D. *Curr Opin Immunol*, 2012 Jul 25, Epub ahead of print.

[65] Neu, A., Ehehalt, S., et al. (2001). Rising incidence of type 1 diabetes in Germany: 12-year trend analysis in children 0-14 years of age. *Diabetes Care*, 24(4), 785-786.

[66] Neu, A., Kehrer, M., et al. (2000). Seasonality of birth in children (0-14 years) with diabetes mellitus type 1 in Baden-Wuerttemberg, Germany. *J Pediatr Endocrinol Metab*, 13(8), 1081-1085.

[67] Noble, J. A., Johnson, J., et al. (2011). Race-specific type 1 diabetes risk of HLA-DR7 haplotypes. *Tissue Antigens*, 78(5), 348-351.

[68] Nystrom, L., Dahlquist, G., et al. (1992). Risk of developing insulin-dependent diabetes mellitus (IDDM) before 35 years of age: indications of climatological determinants for age at onset. *Int J Epidemiol*, 21(2), 352-358.

[69] Onkamo, P., Vaananen, S., et al. (1999). Worldwide increase in incidence of Type I diabetes--the analysis of the data on published incidence trends. *Diabetologia*, 42(12), 1395-1403.

[70] Oresic, M., Simell, S., et al. (2008). Dysregulation of lipid and amino acid metabolism precedes islet autoimmunity in children who later progress to type 1 diabetes. *J Exp Med*, 205(13), 2975-2984.

[71] Ostman, J., Lonnberg, G., et al. (2008). Gender differences and temporal variation in the incidence of type 1 diabetes: results of 8012 cases in the nationwide Diabetes Incidence Study in Sweden 1983-2002. *J Intern Med*, 263(4), 386-394.

[72] Padaiga, Z., Tuomilehto, J., et al. (1999). Seasonal variation in the incidence of Type 1 diabetes mellitus during 1983 to 1992 in the countries around the Baltic Sea. *Diabet Med*, 16(9), 736-743.

[73] Panamonta, O., Thamjaroen, J., et al. (2011). The rising incidence of type 1 diabetes in the northeastern part of Thailand. *J Med Assoc Thai*, 94(12), 1447-1450.

[74] Patterson, C. C., Dahlquist, G. G., et al. (2009). Incidence trends for childhood type 1 diabetes in Europe during 1989-2003 and predicted new cases 2005-20: a multicentre prospective registration study. *Lancet*, 373(9680), 2027-2033.

[75] Pilecki, O., Robak-Kontna, K., et al. (2003). Epidemiology of type 1 diabetes mellitus in Bydgoszcz region in the years 1997-2002. *Endokrynol Diabetol Chor Przemiany Materii Wieku Rozw*, 9(2), 77-81.

[76] Pliska, V., Folkers, G., et al. (2005). Insulin – eine Erfolgsgeschichte der modernen Medizin. *BioFokus Forschung für Leben* (69).

[77] Samardzic, M., Marinkovic, J., et al. (2010). Increasing incidence of childhood type 1 diabetes in Montenegro from 1997 to 2006. *Pediatr Diabetes*, 11(6), 412-416.

[78] Samuelsson, U., Carstensen, J., et al. (2007). Seasonal variation in the diagnosis of type 1 diabetes in south-east Sweden. *Diabetes Res Clin Pract*, 76(1), 75-81.

[79] Santos, J., Carrasco, E., et al. (2001). Incidence rate and spatio-temporal clustering of type 1 diabetes in Santiago, Chile, from 1997 to 1998. *Rev Saude Publica*, 35(1), 96-100.

[80] Schranz, A. G. & Prikatsky, V. (1989). Type 1 diabetes in the Maltese Islands. *Diabet Med*, 6(3), 228-231.

[81] Schutt, M., Fach, E. M., et al. (2012). Multiple complications and frequent severe hypoglycaemia in 'elderly' and 'old' patients with Type 1 diabetes. *Diabet Med*, 29(8), e176-e179.

[82] Shaltout, A. A., Qabazard, M. A., et al. (1995). High incidence of childhood-onset IDDM in Kuwait. Kuwait Study Group of Diabetes in Childhood. *Diabetes Care*, 18(7), 923-927.

[83] Soderstrom, U., Aman, J., et al. (2012). Being born in Sweden increases the risk for type 1 diabetes - a study of migration of children to Sweden as a natural experiment. *Acta Paediatr*, 101(1), 73-77.

[84] Soltesz, G. (2003). Diabetes in the young: a paediatric and epidemiological perspective. *Diabetologia*, 46(4), 447-454.

[85] Soltesz, G., Patterson, C. C., et al. (2007). Worldwide childhood type 1 diabetes incidence--what can we learn from epidemiology? *Pediatr Diabetes*, 8(Suppl 6), 6-14.

[86] Stipancic, G., La Grasta Sabolic, L., et al. (2008). Incidence and trends of childhood Type 1 diabetes in Croatia from 1995 to 2003. Diabetes Res Clin Pract 80(1), 122-127.

[87] Svensson, J., Carstensen, B., et al. (2005). Early childhood risk factors associated with type 1 diabetes – is gender important? *Eur J Epidemiol*, 20(5), 429-434.

[88] Svensson, J., Lyngaae-Jorgensen, A., et al. (2009). Long-term trends in the incidence of type 1 diabetes in Denmark: the seasonal variation changes over time. Pediatr Diabetes 10(4), 248-254.

[89] Tahirovic, H. & Toromanovic, A., (2007). Incidence of type 1 diabetes mellitus in children in Tuzla Canton between 1995 and 2004. *Eur J Pediatr*, 166(5), 491-492.

[90] Taplin, C. E., Craig, M. E., et al. (2005). The rising incidence of childhood type 1 diabetes in New South Wales, 1990-2002. *Med J Aust*, 183(5), 243-246.

[91] Teeaar, T., Liivak, N., et al. (2010). Increasing incidence of childhood-onset type 1 diabetes mellitus among Estonian children in 1999-2006. Time trend analysis 1983-2006. Pediatr Diabetes 11(2), 107-110.

[92] Vaiserman, A. M., Carstensen, B., et al. (2007). Seasonality of birth in children and young adults (0-29 years) with type 1 diabetes in Ukraine. *Diabetologia*, 50(1), 32-35.

[93] Vehik, K. & Dabelea, D. (2010). The changing epidemiology of type 1 diabetes: why is it going through the roof? *Diabetes Metab Res Rev*, 27(1), 3-13.

[94] Vehik, K., Hamman, R. F., et al. (2007). Increasing incidence of type 1 diabetes in 0- to 17-year-old Colorado youth. *Diabetes Care*, 30(3), 503-509.

[95] Wockenfuss, R., Frese, T., et al. (2009). Three- and four-digit ICD-10 is not a reliable classification system in primary care. *Scand J Prim Health Care*, 27(3), 131-136.

[96] Ye, J., Chen, R. G., et al. (1998). Lack of seasonality in the month of onset of childhood IDDM (0.7-15 years) in Shanghai, China. *J Pediatr Endocrinol Metab*, 11(3), 461-464.

[97] Zubkiewicz-Kucharska, A. & Noczynska, A., (2010). Epidemiology of type 1 diabetes in Lower Silesia in the years 2000-2005. *Pediatr Endocrinol Diabetes Metab*, 16(1), 45-49.

Chapter 2

Viruses and Type 1 Diabetes: Focus on the Enteroviruses

Didier Hober, Famara Sané, Karena Riedweg,
Ilham Moumna, Anne Goffard, Laura Choteau,
Enagnon Kazali Alidjinou and Rachel Desailloud

Additional information is available at the end of the chapter

1. Introduction

Type 1 diabetes (T1D) is one of the most common chronic diseases in developed countries and represents about 10% of all cases of diabetes. It is caused by a selective destruction of insulin-producing β cells in the pancreas. The disease has two subtypes: 1A, which includes the common, immune-mediated forms of the disease; and 1B, which includes nonimmune forms. In this review, we focus on subtype 1A, which for simplicity will be referred to as type 1 diabetes. [81, 34]. An increasing incidence rate of T1D has been observed for the last few decades especially in young individuals (less than five years old) [163]. The cause of T1D is still unknown. Several factors interact and lead to the development of the disease. An inflammatory islet infiltrate (insulitis) can be observed at the symptomatic onset of T1D, and reflects the immune response to β-cells [45]. T1D is an autoimmune disease, which implies a role of immune response effectors in the pathogenic processes and a failure of tolerance towards β-cell antigens.The susceptibility to T1D is influenced by genetic factors. More than 20 loci in addition to those located in the human leukocyte antigen (HLA) class II locus (especially DQ and DR) on chromosome 6 are involved. Another contribution to the pathogenesis of the disease could rely on epigenetic modifications (such as DNA methylation) and parent-of-origin effects [11]. Genetic modifications in the population cannot explain the rapidly increased incidence of T1D in most populations. Altogether, the incidence variation from one season to another, the relationship between immigration and disease development, and the differences in incidence in different parts of the world in neighboring populations with similar genetic profiles, suggest that the disease is a result of interaction of genetic and environmental factors [94].

Interplay between immune response, genetic and environmental factors such as nutriments, drugs, toxin and viruses play a role in the pathogenesis of the disease. Several teams paid attention to the relationship between viruses and type 1 diabetes, and their role in the patho-genesis of the disease. A novel subtype of type 1 diabetes called fulminant type 1 diabetes, without evidence of autoimmunity has been observed [61]. In that disease the role of viruses is strongly suspected as well, but is out of the scope of this chapter.

The relationship between type 1 diabetes in human beings and animals and various viruses belonging to different families has been investigated. Enteroviruses are among the viruses most able to be involved in the pathogenesis of autoimmune type 1diabetes.

After a presentation of the role of various viruses in the disease we will focus on enteroviruses, and then the clinical studies that were conducted to assess the relationship between enterovi-ruses and autoimmune T1D will be detailed. Thereafter the results of experimental investiga-tions aimed to elucidate the link between these viruses and the disease will be analyzed.

2. Various viruses have been associated with the development of type 1 diabetes

The role of viral infections in the pathogenesis of T1D has long been suspected and several viruses have been associated with T1D in various studies [160, 162]. In humans, observa-tions of acute diabetes succeeding to destruction of β-cells by cytopathic effect of viral infec-tion remain exceptional. Some viruses, as mumps, influenza B virus or human herpes virus 6 have already been reported in cases of acute T1D. Nevertheless, the fact that T1D devel-oped after the infection by such commun viruses suggest that factors within the host play more important roles than virus itself in the etiology of T1D [27, 59, 126].

The relationship between viral infection and T1D is mainly based on epidemiological argu-ments. The incidence of many allergic and autoimmune diseases has increased in developed countries (North-South gradient) over the past three decades, particularly in young chil-dren. Concomitantly, there was a clear decrease in the incidence of many infectious diseases in these countries, probably explained by the introduction of antibiotics, vaccination, and an improved hygiene and better socioeconomic conditions [6, 163].

Interestingly, viruses have been reported to be associated with T1D occurrence in animals. Experimental animal models, as BioBreeding (BB)-rat, nonobese diabetic (NOD) mouse or specific transgenic mouse strains, were used to investigate the mechanism by which viruses can modulate diabetogenesis.

2.1. Viruses and human type 1 diabetes

2.1.1. Rubella

Several reports have shown that congenital rubella was associated with induction of islet au-toantibodies in 10% to 20% of cases of congenital rubella, within 5 to 25 years [18, 56, 71].

The serum levels of antibodies against measles, mumps, and rubella (MMR) and autoanti-bodies against pancreas islet cells (ICA), islet cell surface, glutamic acid decarboxylase auto-antibodies (GADA), and insulin were determined in 386 school children between 11 and 13 years of age, before and 3 months after vaccination with combined MMR vaccine. It has been shown that children with rubella antibodies before vaccination had higher levels of ICA than seronegative children [98]. However, a study conducted in 2003 showed inconsis-tent results: in fact, no signs of β-cells autoimmunity (ie detection of ICA, insulin autoanti-bodies (IAA), antibodies to the tyrosine phosphatase related IA-2 molecule (IA-2 A) and glutamic acid decarboxylase (GADA)) were detected in 37 subjects with congenital rubella syndrome or exposed to rubella virus during fetal life [165]. The role of rubella in the trig-gering of T1D has been determined in hamsters. This study revealed that an autoimmune process and diabetes developed after rubella virus infection in neonatal hamsters [121]. Some authors suggested the molecular mimicry as a mechanism for rubella virus causing T1D, on the basis of co-recognition of β-cell protein determinants, such as GAD, and various rubella peptides by T-cells [118]. Recently, a clinical study has confirmed a significant asso-ciation between type 1 diabetes incidence and rubella in children in Italia [120].

2.1.2. Rotavirus

Rotavirus (RV), the most common cause of childhood gastroenteritis, has been suspected to trigger or exacerbate T1D in a few studies. Honeyman et al. showed a specific and highly significant association between RV seroconversion and increases in autoantibodies. Serum of 360 children with a parent or sibling with type 1 diabetes had been assayed for IAA, GA-DA, and IA-2A every 6 months from birth. In all children, 24 children had been classified as high-risk children because they developed diabetes or had at least 2 islet antibodies or 1 islet antibody detected on at least 2 occasions within the study period. In high-risk children, 86% developed antibodies to IA-2, 62% developed insulin autoantibodies, and 50% developed antibodies to GAD in association with first appearance or increase in RV IgG or IgA [70]. In 2002, Coulson et al demonstrated that rotavirus could infect pancreas in vivo [35]. In this study, nonobese diabetic (NOD) mice were shown to be susceptible to rhesus rotavirus in-fection. Pancreatic islets from NOD mice, nonobese diabetes-resistant mice, fetal pigs, and macaque monkeys supported various degrees of rotavirus growth. Human rotaviruses that were propagated in African green monkey kidney epithelial (MA104) cells in the presence of trypsin as previously described [128] replicated in monkey islets only [35]. In another study, the effect of RV infection on diabetes development, once diabetes was established, was de-termined on NOD and NOD8.3 TCR (transgenic for a T-cell receptor (TCR)) mice. The de-gree of diabetes acceleration was related to the serum antibody titer to RV. Thus, rotavirus infection aggravated insulitis and exacerbated diabetes, after β-cell autoimmunity was es-tablished [60]. Furthermore, rotavirus was also suspected to contain peptide sequences, in VP7 (viral protein 7), highly similar to T-cell epitopes in the islet autoantigens GAD and ty-rosine phosphatase IA-2, suggesting that T-cells directed against RV could induce or ampli-fy islet autoimmunity by molecular mimicry, in children with genetic susceptibility. Honeyman et al. also demonstrated that peptides in RV-VP7, similar to T-cell epitopes in IA-2 and GAD65, bound strongly to HLA-DRB1*04. The proliferative responses of T-cells to rotavirus peptide and islet autoantigen-derived peptides were significantly correlated [72]. Altogether, these observations suggested that RV infection could trigger or exacerbate islet autoimmunity by molecular mimicry.

2.1.3. Mumps

In 1992, Parkkonen et al showed that mumps virus was able to infect β-cells, leading to a minor decrease in insulin secretion in human fetal islet cultures [119]. The infection was invariably associated with an increase in the expression of human leucocyte antigen (HLA) class I molecules, mediated by soluble factors secreted by infected T cells, which could exaggerate the autoimmune process in pre-diabetic individuals by increasing the activity of autoreactive cytotoxic T cells [119]. Moreover, ICA have been observed in 14 out of 30 sera of children with mumps. In most children, the ICA persisted for no more than 2-4 months, although 2 children have been positive for 15 months. Nevertheless, no ICA-positive child acquired diabetic glucose metabolism, apart from one child who had persistent ICA and acquired diabetes mellitus three weeks after mumps infection [62]. Since the introduction of vaccination against MMR in most of occidental countries, several studies have reported on the relation between vaccination at childhood and the development of T1D [41, 78, 79]. Hyoty *et al.* demonstrated that vaccination against MMR in Finland was followed by a plateau in the rising incidence of T1D 6–8 years later suggesting a causal relation between these viral infections and the development of T1D [79]. However, the incidence of T1D continued to rise after the plateau. Other studies hypothesized that childhood vaccination would rather promote the development of T1D. No evidence has been found for the triggering effect of childhood vaccination on the development of T1D later in life [41, 78]. Hyoty et al. described a shared epitope, a 7 amino acid-long sequence (YQQQGRL), in mumps virus nucleocapsid and in MHC class II-associated invariant chain, which might cause immunological cross-reactivity between these molecules [80].

2.1.4. Human Endogenous Retroviruses

Human Endogenous Retroviruses (HERVs) are sequences which occupy about 10% of the human genome and are thought to be derived from ancient viral infections of germ cells. In some medical conditions, HERVs genes could be transcribed, expressed in protein and could be responsible of the development of autoantibodies that might react against host proteins. As a result, these mechanisms could lead to autoimmune diseases, such as T1D. HERVs may also dysregulate the immune response by being moved and inserted next to certain genes involved in immune regulation whose expression would be consequentially altered. Finally, HERVs are known to induce proinflammatory cytokines production, as IL-1β, IL-6, or TNF-α, by cells, such as monocytes [10]. The HERV-K18 variant has been shown to encode for a superantigen (SAg) that is recognized by T-cells with TCR Vβ7 chains and causes dysregulation of the immune system. HERV-K18 mRNA has been found to be enriched in tissues of patients with acute T1D. HERV-K18 transcription and SAg function in cells capable of efficient presentation are induced by proinflammatory stimuli and may trigger progression of disease to insulitis or from insulitis to overt diabetes [101]. The HERV-

K18 variant, which is transcriptionally silent, could be directly transactivated by EBV (Epstein Barr Virus) or HHV-6 (human herpes virus 6), or alternatively through the EBV or HHV-6- induced production of the IFN-α [143, 144].

Rubella virus, rotavirus, mumps virus and endogenous retroviruses are RNA viruses whose role in type 1 diabetes has been suspected. In addition to RNA viruses, it has been reported that DNA viruses as well could be involved in the development of the disease as described in the following paragraphs.

2.1.5. Cytomegalovirus

In 1988, Numazaki et al showed that cytomegalovirus (CMV) was able to infect tissue mon-olayer cultures of human fetal islets [112]. CMV infection apparently did not cause direct destruction of β-cells but was leading to changes in production of insulin [112]. Hille-brands et al. demonstrated that R(at)-CMV accelerated onset of diabetes without infecting pancreatic islets in BB-rats and suggested that virus-induced recruitment of peritoneal mac-rophages to the pancreas triggered the accelerated development of insulitis by enhancing activation of T-cells in pancreas [65]. In 2003, van der Werf et al indicated that R-CMV in-duced a very strong T-cell proliferative response in BB-rats suggesting that R-CMV might directly activate autoreactive T-cells resulting in accelerated onset of diabetes [161]. In 2010, Smelt et al demonstrated that RCMV induced a low, persistent infection in rat β-cells, as-sociated with an increasing β-cell immunogenicity, which might be an essential step in β-cells destruction and in the development or the acceleration of the onset of T1D [137]. Concerning the role of Human CMV (HCMV) in diabetogenesis, [64] postulated that there is T-cell cross-reactivity between Human CMV (HCMV) and GAD65 in pancreatic islet β-cell. HCMV-derived epitope could be naturally processed by dendritic cells and recog-nized by GAD65 reactive T-cells. Thus, HCMV may be involved in the loss of T-cell tolerance to autoantigen GAD65 by a mechanism of molecular mimicry leading to autoimmunity [64]. In 2008, Aarnisalo et al analysed specific anti-CMV IgG antibodies in 169 serum sam-ples from children who had developed the first T1D-associated autoantibody by the age of 2 years, and, in parallel, in 791 serum control from healthy children [1]. No associa-tion between perinatal CMV infection and progression to T1D was observed. This study con-cluded that perinatal CMV infections were not particularly associated with early serological signs of beta cell autoimmunity or progression to T1D in children with diabetes risk-asso-ciated HLA genotype [1]. However, serological, immunological, histological signs of auto-immunity and allograft rejection appeared concomitantly with early CMV infections in one type 1 diabetic patient receiving pancreas allograft. This observation suggests that persis-tent CMV infections might be relevant to the pathogenesis of type 1 diabetes [177].

2.1.6. Parvovirus B19

Several cases of autoimmune disease occurrence after an acute infection with parvovirus B19 have been reported. Kasuga et al. reported a case of a young adult who developed new onset T1D after an infection with parvovirus B19. Serum levels of B19 IgM and antibodies to the diabetic autoantigen IA-2 were significantly elevated. The authors noted homology in amino acid sequences between B19 and the extracellular domain of IA-2 [88, 113]. Munakata et al described the case of a 40-year-old Japanese woman, in which three autoimmune diseases occurred after acute parvovirus B19 infection: rheumatoid arthritis, T1D and Graves'disease [106]. Some authors attempted to explain these observations. Parvovirus B19 is known to promote a T-cell-mediated lymphoproliferative response, through the presentation by HLA class II antigen to CD4 cells and thus could theoretically generate T-cell-mediated autoimmunity [166]. Vigeant et al suggested that parvovirus B19 infection may lead to chronic modulation of the autoimmune response in predisposed individuals [164].

Although correlations between T1D and the occurrence of a viral infection that precedes the development of the autoimmune disease have been recognized, mechanisms by which viruses activate diabetogenic processes are still elusive and difficult to prove in humans. Studies of animal virus-induced T1D provide a lot of information concerning the possible role of virus infections in the induction of TID.

2.2. Viruses and animal type 1 diabetes

2.2.1. Encephalomyocarditis virus

A number of studies provide clear evidence that encephalomyocarditis virus (EMCV), belonging to the Cardiovirus genus of the Picornaviridae family, is able to induce very rapid onset of diabetes in mice. Based upon this evidence, EMCV-induced diabetes model has been proposed as a model of fulminant T1D [135]. Several studies determined the existence of two main variants of EMCV: the nondiabetogenic variant EMC-B virus, and the diabetogenic variant EMC-D virus. EMCV-D has preferential tropism for pancreatic β-cells and can induce diabetes in selective mouse strains, such as DBA/2 [102]. Nucleotide sequence analysis showed that EMC-D virus (7829 bases) differs from EMC-B virus (7825 bases) by only 14 nucleotides: two deletions of 5 nucleotides, 1 base insertion, and 8 point mutations. Further studies revealed that only the 776th amino acid, alanine (Ala-776), of the EMC virus polyprotein, located at position 152 of the major capsid protein VP1, is common to all diabetogenic variants. In contrast, threonine in this position (Thr-776) is common to all nondiabetogenic variants [176]. A single point mutation at nucleotide position 3155 or 3156 of the recombinant EMC viral genome, resulting in an amino acid change (Ala-776 in Thr-776), leads to the gain or loss of viral diabetogenicity [84]. A three-dimensional molecular modeling of the binding site of the EMC viral capsid protein VP1 revealed that the surface areas surrounding alanine (or glycine) at position 152 of the VP1 was more accessible, thus increasing the availability of the binding sites for attachment to β-cell receptors, resulting in viral infection and the development of diabetes [85]. Baek et al. showed that macrophages, especially mac-2 positive macrophages, were rapidly recruited in pancreas at the early stage of EMC-D virus infection, playing a central role in the process of pancreatic islets destruction in SJL/J mice [8, 9]. Recently, Mc Cartney et al. found that melanoma differentiation associated gene-5 (MDA5), a sensor of viral RNA eliciting IFN-I responses, IFN-α, and Toll-Like Receptor 3 (TLR3) were both required to prevent diabetes in mice infected with EMCV-D. In Tlr3-/- mice, a diabetes occured due to impaired tpe 1 IFN responses and β cell damage induced directly by virus, rather than autoimmune T cells. Mice lacking just 1 copy of Mda5 developed transient hyperglycemia when infected with EMCV-D. Thus, in the case of EMCV-D which infects and damages directly the pancreatic β cells, optimal functioning of viral sensors and type 1 IFN responses are required to prevent diabetes [102].

2.2.2. Kilham rat virus

Ellerman et al. demonstrated the ability of Kilham rat virus (KRV), an environmentally ubiq-uitous rat parvovirus, to precipitate autoimmune diabetes in BioBreeding Diabetes-Resistant (BBDR) rats that were not susceptible to spontaneous diabetes [47]. Chung et al. showed the important role of macrophages and macrophage-derived cytokines (IL-12, TNF-α, and IL-1β) in the KRV-induced autoimmune diabetes in the BBDR rats [29]. As it had been previ-ously shown, KRV did not directly infect β-cells. Thus, Choung et al. investigated the proc-ess by which KRV induced autoimmune pancreatic cells destruction. They discovered that it was rather due to a disrupted immune balance: Th1-like CD45RC+CD4+ and cytotoxic CD8+ T-cells were up-regulated whereas Th2-like CD45RC-CD4+ T-cells were down-regulated. Thus, KRV might be responsible for the activation of autoreactive T cells that are cytotoxic to beta cells, resulting in T cell-mediated autoimmune diabetes. In the same study, this group demonstrated that KRV-induced autoimmune diabetes in BBDR rats was not due to molecular mimicry [30]. Zipris et al. reported that infection by KRV or H-1, a close homo-logue virus of KRV, induced similar humoral and cellular immune responses in BBDR rats and Wistar Furth (WF) rats. Nevertheless, only KRV induced a decrease in splenic CD4+CD25+ T cells (regulatory T cells or Treg) able to suppress autoreactivity, in both rat strains. KRV was able to induce diabetes in BBDR rats but not in WF rats. The disease was associated with accumulation of non proliferating Treg in pancreatic lymph nodes. Together these data suggest a virus- and rat strain- specific mechanism of KRV-induced diabetes in genetically susceptible rats as BBDR rats, through an alteration of T cell regulation. It ap-pears that Treg are no longer able to inhibit autoreactive T cells activation [178]. It has also been shown that proinflammatory cytokines IL-6 and IL-12p40 were produced by spleen cells cultured in vitro in the presence of KRV in BBDR and WF rats. Ligation of TLR9 with CpG DNA induced the same pattern of cytokine production. In response to both KRV and CpG DNA, spleen cell populations enriched for B cells (CD45R+) secreted significantly more IL-12p40 than populations enriched for non B-cells (CD45R-). KRV was also able to stimu-late Flt-3L bone marrow-derived dendritic cells (DCs) to produce IL-12p40 in vitro. More-over, genomic DNA isolated from KRV, which is a single-strand DNA, induced the production of IL-12p40 in spleen cells from BBDR rats. Thus, the ligand within KRV that in-duces IL-12p40 secretion in spleen cells is viral DNA. Using appropriate inhibitors of TLR-signaling pathways, Zipris et al. indicated that the cytokine production by splenic cells was Protein Kinase R (PKR) and NF-κB dependent, whose activation leads to type I IFN produc-tion. KRV-induced secretion of IL-12p40 by BBDR spleen cells was inhibited by specific TLR9 inhibitors, as iCpG, and by chloroquine, which is a known inhibitor of endosomal acidification, essential step for the recruitment of TLR9 in the lysosomal compartment. Moreover, genomic DNA isolated from KRV induced the production of IL-12p40 in Flt-3L-induced DCs derived from wild-type BBDR rats but not TLR9-deficient mice. Finally, ad-ministration of chloroquine to virus-infected BBDR rats decreased the incidence of diabetes and decreased blood levels of IL-12p40. These data indicates that the TLR9 -signaling pathway is implicated in the KRV-induced innate immune activation and participates to the development of autoimmune diabetes in the BBDR rat [179, 13].

EMC and KRV are natural viral pathogens of rodent that brought a lot of information as far as the virus–induced pathogenesis of T1D. The role of these viruses in the human T1D has not been reported, however, the Ljungan virus is another rodent virus that has been suspected to be involved in human type 1diabetes.

2.2.3. Ljungan virus and human parechoviruses

The Ljungan virus (LV) is a RNA virus discovered in Sweden in the mid-1990s in rodents (Myodes glareolus; formerly Clethrionomys glareolus called "bank vole"). This virus belongs to the Parechovirus genus within the Picornaviridae family. Niklasson et al. described the occurrence of T1D in 67 wild bank voles after 1 month of captivity in laboratory: diabetic animals showed clinic signs of diabetes (persistent hyperglycemia with weight loss, ketosis, and hyperlipidemia) and specific β-cell destruction associated with signs of autoimmunity: increased levels of autoantibodies to GAD65, IA-2, and insulin. The disease was correlated with LV antibodies. Moreover, LV antigen was detected by immunocytochemistry in the islets of diabetic bank voles. In parallel, two groups of new onset diabetic children were studied: the first group represented a total of 53 children which were diagnosed with T1D between 1992 and 1995, and the second group was composed of 289 children with newly diagnosed T1D between 1995 and 2000. The study showed increased levels of LV antibodies in newly diagnosed T1D children indicating a possible zoonotic relationship between LV infection and human T1D [109].

In addtion to type 1 diabetes, viruses could be involved in the development of type 2 diabetes. Indeed, Niklasson et al. demonstrated that a type 2 diabetes-like disease could be induced by LV in a CD-1 mouse model. Pregnant CD-1 mice were infected with LV and kept under not stressful conditions. After weaning, puberty male mice were kept under stress (all males in the same cage) or not (animals in individual cage). All male mice received glucose (100 g/l) in the drinking water. Only animals infected in utero and kept under stress developed diabetes. Thus, in these animals, viral infection in utero, in combination with stress in adult life could induce diabetes in males [110]. In 2007, Blixt et al. investigated the functional characteristics of pancreatic islets, isolated from female and male bank voles considered as infected by LV. About 20% of all specimens were classified as glucose intolerance/diabetes (GINT/D) following a glucose tolerance test. Of these animals the majority became diabetic by 20 weeks of age, and GINT/D animals had increased serum insulin levels. Functional differences, concerning insulin content, capacity to synthesize (pro) insulin, secrete insulin and metabolize glucose, were observed between normal and GINT/D animals as well as between genders. The increased serum insulin level and the increased basal islet insulin secretion in GINT/D animals suggests that the animals had developed a type 2 diabetes probably due to LV infection associated with stress in laboratory [12].

Human parechoviruses, like LV, belong to the Parechovirus genus; they have also been implicated in the development of T1D in humans. In a recent nested case-control study, the

"Environmental Triggers of Type 1 Diabetes: The MIDIA study", stool samples from 27 children who developed islet autoimmunity (repeatedly positive for two or three autoantibodies) and 53 children matched for age and community of residence (control group) were analyzed for human parechovirus using a semi-quantitative real-time polymerase chain reaction every month from the 3rd to the 35th month. Sera of children were tested for autoantibodies against GAD, IA-2, and insulin every 3 months until the age of 1 year and every 12 months thereafter. There was no significant difference in the number of infection episodes between the two groups. There was also no significant difference in the prevalence of human parechovirus in stool samples throughout the study period, except in samples collected 3 months prior to seroconversion, in which 16/77 samples (20.8%) from cases had an infection as opposed to 16/182 (8.8%) samples from controls (OR = 3.17, p = 0.022) [148].

Various viruses were reported to be associated with human T1D: rubella and mumps virus, rotavirus, retrovirus, human parechovirus, cytomegalovirus and parvovirus B19 (table 1). In addition, viruses were reported to be associated with animal T1D: EMCV, KRV and LV, the role of which in human type 1 diabetes has also been studied (figure 2). Using animal models, as BB-rats, NOD mice or specific transgenic mouse strains, studies suggested different mechanisms by which viruses may be involved in the initiation or modulation of autoimmune process. These models suggested that a direct infection of islets, responsible for the release of autoantigens, could explain the activation of T-cells and the development of autoimmunity. Another hypothesis supported by some studies was the concept of molecular mimicry between virus and β-cells: a normal immune response against a viral antigen would become pathogenic for β cells due to the existence of structural homologies with the pancreatic antigen. In addition to their possible role in the activation of β-cell-reactive T cells, viruses can reduce the capacity of Treg cells to maintain tolerance. Together, these studies suggest that viruses through diffent mechanisms may trigger T1D and/or may participate in the amplification of the autoimmune process. In addition to the viruses presented in this section, the major candidates are enteroviruses. Therefore the rest of this review will be focused on these viruses.

	RNA virus		DNA virus
Human type 1 diabetes	*Togaviridae*	*Reoviridae*	*Herpesviridae*
	Rubella virus	Rotavirus	Cytomegalovirus
	Paramyxoviridae	*Retroviridae*	*Parvoviridae*
	Mumps virus	HERVs	Parvovirus B19
	Picornaviridae		
	Parechovirus		
	Enterovirus		
Animal type 1 diabetes	Encephalomyocarditis virus		Kilham rat virus
	Ljungan virus		

Table 1. Viruses involved in human and animal type 1 diabetes grouped according to their genome and their family (in red).

3. Presentation of enteroviruses

3.1. Classification of human enteroviruses

The Picornaviridae family consists of 9 genera: Erbovirus, Kobuvirus, Teschovirus, Aphtovirus, Cardiovirus Hepatovirus, Parechovirus, Enterovirus. Human pathogens are in the four last-mentioned genera. Human enteroviruses were previously classified on the basis of serologic criteria into 64 serotypes distributed as: poliovirus (PV), coxsackievirus A (CV-A), coxsackievirus B (CV-B), echovirus and other enteroviruses. The International Committee on Taxonomy of Viruses (ICTV) proposed a classification based on their phylogenetic relations encompassing 4 species, HEV-A, B, C, D, which include various serotypes (table 2). Recently, the former human rhinovirus species have been moved to the Enterovirus genus.

Species (number of serotypes)	Representatives
Human enteroviruses A (12)	Human coxsackievirus A2-8, A10, A12, A14, A16
	Human enterovirus 71
Human enteroviruses B (36)	Human coxsackievirus A9
	Human coxsackievirus B1-6
	Human echovirus 1–7, 9, 11–21, 24–27, 29–33
	Human enterovirus 69
Human enteroviruses C (11)	Human polioviruses 1-3
	Human coxsackieviruses A1, A11, A13, A15, A17–22, A24
Human enteroviruses D (2)	Human enterovirus 68, 70
Human rhinoviruses A (75)	
Human rhinoviruses B (25)	
Human rhinoviruses C (48)	
	Unclassified enteroviruses (over 50)

Table 2. Classification of human enteroviruses, adapted from www.picornaviridae.com

3.2. Structure of enterovirus particles

Picornaviridae particles are small (30 nm), icosahedral, non-enveloped viruses with a single-strand positive RNA genome (approxymatly 7 000- 8 500 nucleotides) (figure 1). The crystal structure of diverses representatives of the family have been solved [69, 2]. The fundamental capsid architecture is the same in all members of the family. The capsid is composed of 60 copies of each four structural proteins VP1 to VP4 in icosahedral symetry and protects the single strand genomic RNA and associated viral proteins [138]. In each case, VP1, VP2 and VP3 made of 240 to 290 residues (32.4-39.1 kDaltons) constitute the outer surface of the capsid. They are taking the form of eight-stranded antiparallel ß sheet structures with a "jelly roll" topology. In the case of enteroviruses and rhinoviruses, VP1 contains a cavity, or pocket, accessible from a depression on the outer surface of the virus capsid. VP4 is a shorter protein around 70 residues (7 kDaltons) lies across the inner face of the capsid with its N-terminus close to the icosahedral fivefold axis and its C-terminal close to the threefold axis [105]. The N-terminal residue of VP4 in all picornaviruses is covalently linked to the inner surface of the capsid defining a channel through the inner and outer surfaces.

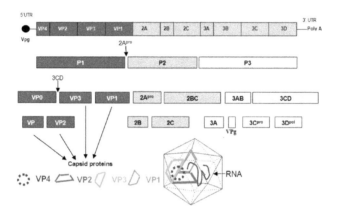

Figure 1. Organisation of the enterovirus genome, polyprotein processing cascade and architecture of enterovirus capsid The genome of enteroviruses contains one single open reading frame flanked by a 5'-and 3' untranslated regions (UTR). A small viral protein, VPg, is covalently linked to the 5' UTR. The 3'UTR encoded poly(A) tail. The translation of the genome results in a polyprotein which is cleaved into four structural proteins (dark gray) and seven non-structural proteins (light gray and yellow). The sites of cleavage by viral proteinases are indicated by arrows. The four structural proteins adopte an icosahedral symmetry with VP1, VP2 and VP3 located at the outer surface of the capsid and VP4 at the inner surface. The single strand genomic RNA is located inside the capsid.

3.3. Viral proteins of enterovirus: synthesis and functions

All picornaviruses have a similar genome organization consisting of a molecule of approximately 7,500 to 8,000 nucleotides (figure 1). The RNA genome is organized with one single large open reading frame preceded by a long 5'-untranslated region (5' UTR) [97]. It contains a 3' poly(A) tail with a variable length from 65 to 100 nt. The virion RNA has a virus-encoded peptide, VPg, covalently linked to the 5' end of the viral genome. Translation of the RNA genome yields a polyprotein of approximately 2,200 amino acids. An early cotranslational cleavage of the polyprotein by the viral 2A protease (2A^{pro}) releases a precursor protein P1 from the N terminus of the polyprotein. The P1 protein contains all the capsid protein sequences. Subsequent cleavage of P1 by the viral 3CD protease (3CD^{pro}) produces the capsid proteins VP1 and VP3 and the immature capsid protein VP0. Finally, the immature protein VP0 is cleaved to VP4 and VP2. There is no known protease requirement for this cleavage. From the P2 region, protein 2A may have an unidentified function in viral RNA synthesis. Protein 2B and its precursor 2BC have been suggested to be responsible for membranous alteration in infected cells. From the P3 region, two precursors are synthesized: 3AB and 3BC. The precursor 3AB is a multifunctional protein principally involved in the membrane association of replication complex. Protein 3A is a membrane binding protein that plays a role in inhibiting cellular protein secretion. Protein 3B (VPg) is a small peptide containing 21 to 23 amino acids, which is covalently linked with the 5'UTR. The precursor 3CD exhibits protease activity and is capable of processing the P1 precursor region. Protein 3C is the protease responsible for the majority of polyprotein cleavages. Protein 3D has the RNA-dependent-RNA polymerase activity and is one of the major components of the viral RNA replication complex.

3.4. Enterovirus lifecycle

The first stage of picornavirus infection of susceptible cells is mediated by the interactions of viral capsid with specific receptor on the cell membrane (figure 2). Receptors used by different picornaviruses include members of the immunoglobulin-like family, the low density lipoprotein receptor (LDLR) family (used by minor group of rhinovirus), the complement control family (used by certain rhinovirus), the integrin family of cell adhesion molecules (receptors for aphtovirus family) and the T cell immunoglobulin domain mucin-like domain receptors (TIM-1), receptor for hepatitis A virus, [159].

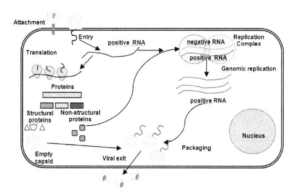

Figure 2. Enterovirus lifecycle.

The group of immunoglobulin-like molecules includes several well characterized receptors for viruses of the enterovirus genus. For example, intercellular adhesion molecule-1 (ICAM-1) is the receptor for major group human rhinoviruses (HRVs), the Coxsackie and adenovirus receptor (CAR), a component of the tight junction between cells in intact epithelium, is the common receptor for Adenoviruses and Coxsakieviruses. These molecules are all type 1 membrane glycoproteins encompasing, for CAR, two extracellular immunoglobulin-like (Ig-like) domains, a transmembrane domain, and a cytoplasmic domain. The first Ig-like domain is responsible for virus binding. The interactions of the receptor with virus capsid induce conformationnal modifications of capsid proteins and cellular receptor that initiate the process of viral entry and genome delivery to the cytoplasm. In brief, receptor binding triggers capsid rearrangements that result in the externalization of VP4 and the N-terminus of VP1. At the same time, released VP4 also interacts with the membrane. VP1 and/or VP4 form a membrane pore through which the genomic RNA is transported into the cytoplasm [159.].

The enterovirus genome is a positive stranded RNA that can be used as messenger RNA and immediately translated by the host cell to produce specific viral proteins. The viral genomic RNA is then transcribed into a complementary negative RNA, which is used as a template to synthezise new strands of genomic positive RNA. Enterovirus infection induces vesicles in infected cell that are localized in the perinuclear region of the cell and are thought to be the sites of RNA replication. These vesicles clusters where viral RNA can be detected have been refered to as replication complexs (RCs). Viral RNA replication occurs at the surface of vesicles. RCs derive from cellular membranes participating to endoplasmic reticulum-to-golgi traffick, hijacked by viral proteins [19]. The viral protein 3A plays a role in the formation of the RCs. Viral proteins synthesis and genomic RNA replication are catalyzed by RNA-dependent RNA polymerase 3D and several other viral proteins, 2B, 2C and 3AB, also participate in RNA replication [4]. It has been suggested that genome replication and encapsidation are coupled [111]. To date, the VPg protein has been implicated as a determinant of encapsidation.The encapsidation of the RNA is associated to the processing of the immature protein VP0 to yield VP4 and VP2. There is no known protease requirement for this cleavage, and it is thought to be autocatalytic, depending only on the capsid proteins themselves and perhaps the viral RNA. The cleavage of VP0 to form the virion is associated with a significant increase in the stability of the particle [68]. It is commonly accepted that enteroviruses exits the cell by lysis of the host cell. However, newly synthesized virus can be detected long before lysis. In addition, enteroviruses are able to establish persitent infection without killing the cell [32]. Both observations argue in favor of alternative exit pathways probably with activation of the apototic program in enterovirus-infected cells. Enteroviruses have a large distribution in the world. Fecal-oral route via the ingestion of contaminated water or food is the major way of enterovirus transmission. Enterovirus infections are generally asymptomatic, but some of them, especially the one due to coxsackievirus B (CV-B), have been associated with acute manifestations (around 20 diseases such as non-specific febrile disease, cutaneous symptoms, meningitis, encephalitis, pericarditis etc.). In addition, their role in chronic diseases, like chronic myocarditis, dilated cardiomyopathy, and T1D is strongly suspected [81].

4. Relationship between enteroviruses and autoimmune type 1 diabetes: clinical studies

Enterovirus infections are among the main environmental risk factors for autoimmune T1D and they have been diagnosed more frequently in T1D patients than in healthy subjects. In this section we report the different studies conducted to investigate the relationship between enteroviral infection and T1D. Theses studies have used different techniques to detect enteroviruses or their components (RT-PCR, cell culture, immunohistochemistry, in situ hybridization...) in blood (serum, plasma and leucocytes), stools, pancreas, intestine. Several studies throughout the world have displayed a relationship between enterovirus infection and the development of T1D (table 3).

We will present the detection of enteroviruses and/or their components in various biological samples in patients with clinical type 1 diabetes first, and thereafter in patients with signs of autoimmunity and/or risk of developing the disease.

4.1. Enterovirus in biological samples from patients with type 1 diabetes

4.1.1. Whole blood

The presence of enteroviral RNA in whole blood of adult patients with T1D has been reported by our group [5]. Viral RNA was detected by RT-PCR in 42% (5/12) of patients with newly diagnosed T1D (p <0.01 vs healthy subjects) and in 8% (1/12) of previously diagnosed T1D patients suffering from metabolic ketosis decompensation (P=0.07 vs patients with newly diagnosed T1D). RT-PCR was negative in the group of healthy subjects and patients with type 2 diabetes. Sequencing of amplified cDNA displayed that circulating enteroviral RNA in these patients had strong homologies with CVB (CVB3 in 4 patients with newly diagnosed T1D, CVB4 in another one, and in one previously diagnosed patient). This study demonstrated that enteroviral RNA could be detected in blood of adult patients at the onset or in the course of T1D.

An other study, performed also by our group, encompassed 56 patients with T1D (25 children whose average age was 13 years and 31 adults with an average age of 37 years), and 37 control subjects divided into 2 groups: the first comprising 24 subjects without any infectious, immunological or metabolic disease, the second group includes 13 patients with T2D [23]. The presence of IFN-α mRNA was detected by RT-PCR in whole blood of 42 out of 56 patients (75%) but in none of controls, and IFN-α was detected by a sensitive immunoassay in serum of 39 out of 56 patients. Enteroviruses-RNA sequences were detected in 50% (21/42) of patients with IFN-α in their blood, but not in patients without any IFN-α in their blood. The detection of enteroviral RNA was positive in 25% (3/12) of children with newly diagnosed T1D, 30% (4/13) of children with previously diagnosed T1D, 50% (10/20) of adult patients with newly diagnosed T1D and 36% (4/11) of adult patients with previously diagnosed T1D. Sequencing of amplified cDNA displayed that circulating enteroviral RNA in these 21 patients had strong homologies with CVB (CVB3 in 8 patients; CVB4 in 8 patients; CVB2 in 5 patients). The results of sequencing of circulating enteroviral RNA were concordant with the results of anti-CVB neutralizing antibodies assay. Otherwise, there was no significant relationship between enterovirus detection and age of patients or the pattern of disease (metabolic decompensation or not)

In Sweden, blood spots are routinely taken on days 2-4 of life for analysis of inherited metabolic diseases in all newborns and are stored in a biobank. From this biobank, a Swedish study investigated enteroviral RNA in blood spots from 600 children in the Swedish childhood diabetes register [39]. Six hundred healthy children were included as controls. Viral RNA was found in 27 out of 600 (4.5%) diabetic children compared to 14 out of 600 (2.3%) control children (p=0.04).

4.1.2. Serum and plasma

The polymerase chain reaction, targeting the 5' non coding region of enteroviral RNA was first used in an English study to detect viral genome in serum taken from 14 children at the onset of T1D and 45 control children matched for age, sex, date of specimen receipt and, as far as possible, geographic area [31]. In this study, a significant greater number of diabetic children had positive PCR results compared with controls (64% vs. 4%). Sequencing of enterovirus PCR products from six positive patients showed a significant homology with coxsackie B3 and B4 viruses, and some common patterns were observed among the sequences from infected diabetic children.

An English team investigated the relationship between enterovirus RNA and T1D in children [108]. One hundred ten children (aged 0-15 years with an average of 7.1 years) with newly diagnosed T1D were recruited. Detection of enterovirus RNA in serum collected in the week after diagnosis was based on a RT-PCR amplifying the 5' noncoding region of enterovirus genome. Hundred and eighty-two control children were matched to cases by age (average age: 6.6 years), sex and date of serum collection at the same hospital. The number of newly diagnosed children with a positive RT-PCR was significantly higher than in the control group (27% versus 4.9%, $p < 0.005$). Moreover, a significant proportion of diabetic children with a positive RT-PCR were of very young age. Indeed, enteroviruses were detected in 37% (20/54) of T1D children aged under 7 years, whereas only 4.6% (5/111) of corresponding control children were positive for enterovirus RNA ($p < 0.005$). For diabetic children older than 7 years, 17.8% (10/56) were found to be positive for enterovirus RNA sequences, while viral RNA was detected in only 5.6% (4/71) of corresponding controls ($p < 0.05$).

A French study evaluated the possible role of enteroviruses infections in the pathogenesis of T1D (Coutant et al., 2002). Sixteen newly diagnosed T1D children were included in this study. Forty nine control children matched for age, sex, date of venous collection and geographic area. A highly sensitive RT-PCR was used to investigate RNA in serum from patients and controls. Neutralzation antibodies to coxsackies viruses B1 to B6 were used to characterize the positive PCR samples. Enterovirus RNA was detected by PCR in only 2 of the 16 newly diagnosed T1D children and in only one of the 49 matched controls (p<0.1). Neutralization assay could not detect antibodies against coxsackiesviruses B1 to B6.

Two hundred and six newly diagnosed T1D children and 160 controls were included in an Australian study [37]. Enterovirus-RNA was found in either plasma or stool in 30% (62/206) of newly diagnosed T1D but only in 4 % (6/160) of controls (p<0.001). Case patients, positive for enterovirus RNA had lower C-peptide levels (p=0.04). Case children with enterovirus RNA levels were more likely to have a severe diabetic ketoacidosis (p = 0.03). Enteroviruses were detected in fewer children with HLA haplotype DRB1 * 03 DQB1 * 02 (p = 0.02) suggesting that the likely role of enteroviruses in the development of diabetes is important in some patients with specific genetic risk.

An Egyptian study included 70 diabetic children who were classified into 2 groups: the first group (I), 40 patients with newly diagnosed diabetic patients (less than one year), the second group (II), 30 children with diabetic patients with more than one year duration of disease [100]. In the control group there were 30 normal healthy children. Enterovirus infection was detected by viral culture of serum samples and confirmation of the results of tissue culture isolation was done by RT-PCR. In addition, anti-CVB IgM and IgG antibodies were searched by enzyme immuno assay. Enterovirus was isolated in group I (47.5%) and group II (23.3%). Neutralization test revealed that most of cases were coxsackievirus B4. In this study, coxsackievirus B IgM antibodies were significantly higher in diabetic patients of group I than those in group II (p<0.01) but there was no significant difference between group I and group II regarding IgG positivity.

A Japanese case-control study encompassed 61 patients with T1D aged 9 months to 40 years and 58 non diabetic subjects aged 1 month to 40 years whose serum was collected the same year [90]. A highly sensitive RT-PCR was used to investigate enterovirus RNA in serum samples. Moreover, neutralizing antibodies against Coxsackievirus and antibodies to GAD were measured and compared with the viral load and the enterovirus genotype. The detection of enterovirus was positive in 23 out of 61 patients (37.7%) and in 2 out of 58 controls (3.4%). The positivity of RT-PCR was decreasing by years gradually after the occurrence of T1D, there was neither gender nor age tendency. The sequence analysis of PCR amplicons displayed strong homologies with coxsackievirus B4 in 13 patients out of 23, and the level of neutralizing anti-CVB4 antibodies was significantly high in positive patients in RT-PCR. There was no relationship between the viral load in serum and antibodies against GAD.

A German group searched the enterovirus RNA by RT-PCR in the serum of diabetic children taken soon after the diagnosis of diabetes [104]. Seventeen out of 47 (36%) newly diagnosed diabetic cases were positive for enteroviral RNA whereas 2 out of 50 control subjects were positive (p<0.001).

Cuba is a country with a low incidence of T1D and with a high circulation of enteroviruses. In a Cuban study, the frequency of enteroviral RNA detection by RT-PCR was significantly higher in newly diagnosed T1D children whose diagnosis was made within 10 days before inclusion [26.5% (9/34)] compared to controls [2.9% (2/68)], matched for age, gender, geographic origin and date of serum collection (p = 0.0007) [127]. Enterovirus detection was more likely associated with severe diabetic ketoacidosis at onset (pH <7.1, p = 0.03) and high titres of autoantibodies against ICA (p <0.05).

4.1.3. Leucocytes and other biological samples

An English study included 17 newly diagnosed patients with T1D, 38 previously diagnosed patients with T1D (the median duration of T1D was 4 years) and 43 age and sex matched non-diabetic controls [53]. Enterovirus RNA was detected by PCR in peripheral blood mononuclear cells in 41 % of newly diagnosed patients with T1D, 39% of previously diagnosed patients and 31% of non diabetic controls. This study showed no difference between diabetic patients and controls regarding the frequency of infection by enterovirus. Whether enteroviruses acted as non-specific agents with an abnormal immune response of the host, is a question raised by the authors of this study.

In a Swedish group, Yin and colleagues used RT-PCR to detect enterovirus RNA in PBMC (peripheral blood mononuclear cells) from 24 newly diagnosed children patients [171]. The 24 control children were matched for age, sex and geographical location without evidence of ongoing infection. RT-PCR was performed with primers (groups A and B) corresponding to conserved areas in the 5'non-coding region. With group A primers, 50% (12/24) of newly diagnosed patients had a positive enterovirus RT-PCR, however, control children were negative (p<0.001). With group B primers, enterovirus sequences were detected in 46% (11/24) of newly diagnosed patients, and in 29 % (7/24) of control children, but the difference was not statistically significant. Taking into account the results obtained with the two sets of primers, the detection of enterovirus RNA was positive in 75% (18/24) of newly diagnosed patients and only in 29% (7/24) of control children.

One hundred and twelve diabetic children and 56 healty controls have been included in an Italian study [154]. Enterovirus common capsid antigens were detected by immunofuorescence in a panel of cell lines inoculated with total leucocytes from peripheral blood, and enteroviral RNA was detected in these cultures as well. Enteroviruses were detected by RT-PCR in 93/112 case children (83%) and 4/56 control children (7%), and directly in leukocytes at lower frequency. Thirteen cases of familial enterovirus infection were observed.

Enteroviral RNA has been searched in PBMC, plasma, throat and stools of 10 newly diagnosed children and 20 control children [132]. Viral RNA was found in PBMC of 4 patients (40%), in plasma of 2 patients (20%), and in stools in 1 patient, in contrast, no sample was positive in control children. All throat swabs from patients and controls were negative. According to the authors, a prolonged enteroviral infection could be suspected in these patients in front of a positive detection of viral RNA in PBMC and/or plasma together with a negative detection of viral RNA in stool and throat swabs.

4.1.4. Pancreas

A 10 years old child with a flu-like illness within 3 days prior to admission in hospital for diabetic ketoacidosis died on the 7th day of admission [175]. The autopsy showed infiltration of the pancreas islets by lymphocytes with necrosis of beta cells. The inoculation of mouse, monkey and human cell cultures with a homogenate of the patient's pancreas had led to the isolation of a CVB4. Serology showed an 8 fold increase in titer of neutralizing antibody to this virus between the second hospital day and day of death. Inoculation of mice with this viral isolate led to hyperglycemia, inflammation of the islets of Langerhans and necrosis of beta cells. Immunofluorescence detected viral antigen in beta cells of mouse pancreatic section. The virus isolate obtained from this patient is known as CVB4 E2.

A few years later, a British group [52], did not find VP1 by immunohistochemistry in pancreas beta cells of 88 patients who had died at clinical presentation of T1D. In contrast, by using the same method VP1 protein was found in cardiac myocytes from 12 of the 20 patients whose cause of death was an acute coxsackievirus B myocarditis, and in seven of these positive cases, insulitis was observed and VP1 was detected in islet endocrine cells, but rarely in exocrine pancreas. Together, these data suggested that the beta cell destruction in patients with fatal diabetes was unlikely related to a direct cytopathic effect of coxsackievirus B, however the role of viruses in the destruction of beta cells through an autoimmune mechanism can not be excluded.

A few years later, another group investigated the presence of enteroviral RNA in the pancreas of 2 children patients with fatal acute-onset T1D and 5 controls by using RT-PCR and Southern blot hybridization [17]. The detection of Enteroviral RNA, and other viral genome (cytomegalovirus, mumps and rubella) was negative in every case.

The relationship between enterovirus and T1D and the type of pancreatic cells infected with enteroviruses has been invesigated by a finish group [172]. The study included 12 newborn infants who died of fulminant infection with enteroviruses (myocarditis in most cases). Autopsy pancreases from 65 patients with T1D and 40 control subjects matched for age and sex were also studied for presence of enteroviral RNA by in situ hybridisation. Enteroviral RNA was detected in pancreas of 58% (7/12) of the 12 newborns; the enterovirus-positive cells were detected in numerous pancreatic islets and in some duct cells but not in exocrine pancreas. In situ hybridisation identified enteroviruses in 6% (4/65) of diabetic patients. Enteroviral RNA was located exclusively in islets. None of the control subjects was positive for enteroviral RNA.

More recently, an Italian team studied the relationship between enterovirus infection, inflammation of pancreatic beta cells, autoimmunity and beta cell function [43]. Six newly diagnosed T1D patients (1 week to 9 months) and 26 control organ donors were included in this study. Immunohistochemistry, electron microscopy, RT-PCR and sequencing, and virus isolation in cell culture were used to detect enteroviruses in pancreatic autopsic tissue. Enteroviral RNA was detected in 3 out of 6 diabetic patients but not in controls. Infection was specific of beta cells with non-destructive insulitis and with naturel killer cell infiltration. There was not apparent reduction of islet beta cells in these patients. The virus isolated from one of these 3 patients, identified as CVB4 was able to infect human pancreatic beta cells of nondiabetic multiorgan donors. Viral inclusions and signs of pyknosis were observed by electronic microscopy, and a loss of beta cell function was assessed by insulin secretion response to glucose, arginine and glibenclamide. These data show that enterovirus could infect beta cells in patients with T1D and that these viruses could be responsible for inflammation and functional abnormalities of these cells.

Recently, authors raised the issue of the relevance of pancreas tissue samples to display the relationship between enterovirus infection and type 1diabetes, since no enteroviral RNA was detected by RT-PCR in samples from pancreatic organ donors with diabetes [158]. Further investigation with pancreas from additionnal donors are needed to address the issue of the persistence of enteroviruses in this organ. Whether enteroviruses are present in pancreas tissue at the time of symptom onset should be investigated but tissue samples can not be easily obtained by biopsy in the case of this organ.

The prevalence of enteroviral capsid protein (VP1) in pancreatic autopsy tissue from 72 newly diagnosed T1D children and a large cohort of controls has been studied by immuno-histochemical staining by a british group [122]. The cell subtypes infected with enteroviruses were identified by immunofluorescence. The criterion of positivity was the presence of at least one intensely stained endocrine cell in an islet within any given section. According to this criterion, 61% (44/72) of diabetic children were positive in immunohistochemistry ver-sus 7.7% (3/39) of control children (p <0.001). There was no significant difference regarding age or gender between the VP1-positive and VP1-negative groups however the duration of diabetes seemed to be lower in the VP1-positive group (2.32 months vs 16.5 months; p=0.06).

4.1.5. Stools

Entroviruses are present in stools of infected individuals [125]. The hypothesis of the role of enteroviruses in T1D prompted researchers to look for these viruses in stools of patients.

An Italian group investigated enteroviruses in stools from 43 newly diagnosed diabetic chil-dren and 22 control children [42]. Stools and serum samples were collected within 2 months from the beginning of diabetes symptoms. In order to isolate enterovirus, stools were inoculat-ed to cell cultures and in suckling mice. Neutralizing antibodies to coxsackie virus B4 and anti-coxsackie viruses B1 to B6 complement fixing antibodies were measured. There was one case with high antibodies against coxsackie B4 virus but no enterovirus was isolated from stools.

A 16 month-old child with a predisposing HLA group (B18 DRw3) developed diabetes [21]. The disease outcame at hospital on the third day of steroid therapy for febrile purpura with-in the week of diphtheria/pertussis/tetanus and polio vaccination. Coxsackievirus B5 was isolated from stools and serologic studies showed a rise in titer of neutralizing antibodies directed to that isolate from less than 10 on the first day to 640 on the eleventh day. The sud-den onset of T1D in the course an acute coxsackievirus B5 infection suggests the potential involvement of this virus in the disease in that case.

4.1.6. Intestine

Different virological methods were used in a Finnish study to evaluate whether enterovirus-es can be found in small intestinal mucosa of 12 patients with T1D (age: 18 to 53, 2 out of them were male) and 10 non-diabetic subjects (age 23 to 71, 3 out of them were male) [114]. These individuals underwent gastroscopy for gastrointestinal symptoms and intestinal mu-cosa biopsies were taken for morphological analysis, which did not reveal any abnormality. To analyse the presence of enteroviruses in intestinal biopsy samples, immunohistochemis-try was used for detecting the viral protein VP1, and in situ hybridization. RT-PCR were used for detecting viral RNA. Six out of 12 (50%) diabetic patients were positive for entero-viral RNA by in situ hybridization, whereas all control subjects were negative (p = 0.015). Two of these positive patients had enteroviral RNA in the cells of lamina propria; four were positive in the epithelial cells of villi, in the crypts and in the cells of lamina propria. Immu-nohistochemistry was positive in 9 out of 12 (75%) of diabetic patients but only in 10% (1/10) of control subjects (p = 0.004): the protein VP1 was mainly localized in the epithelium. Viral RNA was found by RT-PCR in a frozen sample from one of the 4 diabetic patients who were positive in both in situ hybridization and immunohistochemistry. There was no relationship between the detection of enteroviral RNA in gut mucosa of diabetic patients and duration of diabetes, gender, HLA type or hyperglycemia.

The discrepancy in results obtained by RT-PCR and in situ hybridization could be explained by the fact that intestinal biopsy samples were obtained from two sites of the intestine, and by differences in samples preparation. These results display that subjects with T1D have enteroviral components in their gut mucosa.

4.2. Enterovirus in biological samples from individuals at high-risk of diabetes

A Finnish prospective study concerned children with prediabetic state, which were derived from a previous study "Childhood Diabetes in Finland" (DiMe) [99]. The study investigated enterovirus RNA in 93 serum samples from 11 prediabetic children who progressed to T1D during the follow-up. One hundred and eight serum samples from 34 control children who participated in the same cohort but did not develop autoimmunity against beta cells or T1D were examined. In this study, serum samples from 47 children with newly diagnosed T1D were also analysed. Antibodies against islet cells (ICA), glutamic acid decarboxylase (GADA), insulin (IAA) and the protein tyrosine phosphatase-related IA-2 protein (IA2-A) were analysed. Antibodies against coxsackie viruses B1 to B6 were measured by neutralization assay. Enterovirus RNA was found in 12 %(11/93) of follow-up samples from prediabetic children compared to only 2% (2/108) of follow-up samples from matched controls (p<0.01). Viral RNA was detected in none (0/47) of the serum samples obtained from diabetic children. The presence of enteroviral RNA was associated with a concomitant increase in ICA (p <0.01) and GADA (p <0.05), whereas no increase was observed in the rates of IAA and IA-2A. This study suggests that enterovirus genome can be found in serum of individuals and that it is associated with the induction of autoimmunity several years before the onset of symptoms. The presence of enterovirus RNA in serum of prediabetic children has been studied in Cuba [127]. This study encompassed 32 children positive for antibodies against ICA having a first-degree relative with T1D, 31 children, negative for antibodies against ICA having a diabetic first-degree relative, and 194 controls, who were matched for age, gender, geographic origin and date of serum collection. Enterovirus RNA was found in 15.6% (5/32) of islet autoantibody-positive first-degree relatives children, whereas all controls were negative for enteroviral genome (P = 0.003). Enterovirus RNA was found in 3.2% of 31 children, negative for antibodies against ICA having a diabetic first-degree relative, and in 1.6% of controls.

After seroconversion for islet antibodies (against GAD, insulin, IA-2), serum and rectal swabs were collected every 3-6 months until diagnosis of diabetes in the Diabetes and Autoimmunity Study in the Young (DAISY) encompassing 2,365 american genetically predisposed children for islet autoimmunity and T1D, according to HLA, and siblings or offspring of people with T1D (regardless of their genotype) [141]. Fifty of the 140 children who seroconverted to positivity for islet autoantibodies progressed to T1D. The prevalence of enteroviral RNA in serum and rectal swabs as displayed by RT-PCR declined with age and seemed to be higher at visits positive for multiple islet autoantibodies. The risk of progression to T1D following detection of enteroviral RNA in serum, in a 4-month interval, was significantly increased compared with negative detection. In contrast, the presence of enteroviral RNA in rectal swabs did not predict progression to T1D, which is in agreement with the results of the MIDIA study including 911 Norwegian children identified at birth with a HLA genotype conferring a risk of T1D [149].

Thirty height children with an increased genetic susceptibility to diabetes followed-up from birth who have progressed to T1D and 140 control children matched for sexe, date of birth, hospital district and HLA-DQ-conferred genetic susceptibility to T1D were included in the finnish type 1 Diabetes Prediction and Prevention study (DiPP) [115]. Serum samples were analysed for enterovirus RNA by RT-PCR: 5.1% of samples were enterovirus RNA positive in case children but only 1, 9% in control children (p<0. 01). In boys, the detection of enterovirus RNA during the 6 months preceding the discovery of autoantibodies was associated with a risk of diabetes (p<0.01).

Biological samples	Number of Cases/ Controls	Children/ adults patients	Positives cases/ Controls p value	Methods of detection	Reference	country
Whole blood	24/27	0/24	6/0 p <0.01	RT-PCR	Andréoletti et al., 1997	France
Whole blood	56/37	25/31	21/0 p *	RT-PCR	Chehadeh et al., 2000	France
Woole Blood	600/600	600/0	27/14 p=0.04	RT-PCR	Dahlquist et al., 2004	Sweden
Serum	14/45	14/0	9/2 p*	RT-PCR	Clements et al., 1995	England
Serum	110/182	110/0	30/9 p<0.005	RT-PCR	Nairn et al., 1999	England
Serum	16/49	16/0	2/1 p>0.05	RT-PCR	Coutant et al., 2002	France
Serum	70/30	70/0	26/0 p <0.05	Cell culture	Maha et al., 2003	Egypt
Serum	61/58	NI	23/2 p<0.05	RT-PCR	Kawashima et al., 2004	Japan
Serum	47/50	47/0	17/2 p<0.001	RT-PCR	Moya-Suri et al., 2005	Germany
Serum	34/68	34/0	9/2 p=0.0007	RT-PCR	Sarmiento et al., 2007	Cuba
Plasma stools	206/160	206/0	62/6 plasma or stools p<0.001	RT-PCR	Craig et al., 2003	Australia

Biological samples	Number of Cases/ Controls	Children/ adults patients	Positives cases/ Controls p value	Methods of detection	Reference	country
PBMC	24/24	24/0	18/7 p*	RT-PCR	Yin et al., 2002	Sweden
leucocytes	112/56	112/0	93/4 p*	RT-PCR	Toniolo et al., 2010	Italy
PBMC	10/20	10/0	4/0 p>0.05	RT-PCR	Schulte et al., 2010	Netherlands
plasma	10/20		2/0			
stools	10/20		1/0			
throat	10/20		0/0			
Pancreas	149/21	NI	0/7 p*	IHC	Foulis et al., 1990	England
Pancreas	65/40	0/65	4/0 p*	HIS	Ylipaasto et al., 2004	Finland
Pancreas	6/26	2/4	3/0	IHC Electronic microscope Cell culture RT-PCR	Dotta et al., 2007	Italy
Pancreas	72/39	NI	44/3 p<0.001	IHC	Richardson et al., 2009	England
Intestine	12/10	0/12	6/0 p=0.015 9/1 p=0.004	HIS IHC	Oikarinen et al., 2007	Finland

Table 3. Detection of enterovirus and/or their components (RNA, proteins) in biological samples of patients with type 1 diabetes. PBMC: Peripheral Blood Mononuclear Cells, RT-PCR: Retrotranscription Polymerase Chain Reaction, IHC: Immunohistochemistry, HIS: Hybridization in situ, NI: Not Indicated, p*: p value not mentioned.

5. Enterovirus and type 1 diabetes: Experimental approach

In previous sections of this review, clinical studies that were conducted to assess the relationship between enteroviruses and T1D have been presented. A significant association between enterovirus infection and T1D, particularly for studies that used molecular methods, has been displayed, and when identified the most often involved enteroviruses were coxsackieviruses B. Experimental studies have been performed to understand the possible link between enterovirus and T1D. In the present section, the results of in vivo studies on one hand and those of in vitro studies on the other hand are presented and analyzed.

5.1. In vivo studies in animal models

In order to analyse the hypothesis that enterovirus infections enhance or elicit autoimmune disorders such as T1D, a significant body of evidence is derived from investigations using animal models. Most of them used to explore research hypotheses regarding the relationship between enteroviruses and type 1 diabetes are mouse models (NOD, C57BL/k, C57BL/6, SJL/J, DBA/2, SWR/J, BALB/c, B10, CD-1...) [83]. Despite their limitation in diseases investigations, experimental models have greatly contributed to our knowledge of human diseases. The predominance of murine models for the investigation of the relationship between enteroviruses and T1D is due, among others, to a physiology relatively similar to that of human beings and the presence of specific receptors, the more prominent of them could be the coxsackievirus and adenovirus receptor (CAR) which is a receptor for coxsackievirus B [86]. Therefore experimental datas have been obtained from models based on infection with coxsackievirus B (CVB) (figure 3).

5.1.1. Enterovirus and immune system

Experimental in vivo studies have contributed improving our understanding of genetic and immunological implications, enteroviral tropism and mechanisms of pancreatic β-cells destruction in the context of enteroviral infection [83]. Enteroviruses generally infect the exocrine pancreas, but some strains preferentially infect islets. Some studies have addressed the role of CAR, the main receptor for CVB entry into host cell, in enteroviral tropism and target organ infection. CAR is expressed by intestine, pancreas and heart epithelial cells, as well as cardiomyocytes [54]. In transgenic mice CVB3 titers were markedly reduced in CAR-deficient tissues and pancreatic CAR deletion induced a strong attenuation of pancreatic CVB3 infection and pancreatitis [86].

The development of innate and adaptive immune responses is mediated by type I interferons (IFNs) produced early during viral infection to induce an antiviral state within target cells. Experimental studies have shown that mice deficient in type I IFNs receptor are more susceptible and die more rapidly than controls when infected with CVB3 [169, 40]. An efficient immune response depends on rapid recognition of viruses by the innate immune system and this recognition is primarily achieved by pattern-recognition receptors such as toll-like receptors (TLRs), retinoid-inducible gene 1-like receptors (RIG-1) and NOD-like receptors. It is noteworthy that interactions between NOD-like receptors and enteroviruses are still poorly understood.

Toll-like receptors are transmembrane glycoproteins expressed on the cytoplasmic membrane or in intracellular vesicals of several immune and non-immune cell populations; while RIG-I-like receptors, represented by RIG-I and the interferon-induced with helicase C domain 1 (IFIH-1), also called melanoma differentiation-associated gene 5 (MDA5) are expressed in the cytosol of most cell types [91]. Among TLRs, TLR3, known to be double-stranded RNA sensor on monocytes, is known to be crucial for the survival of mice infected with CVB4 [123]; and the production of cytokines by murine plasmocytoid dendritic cells have been shown to be closely linked with CVB detection and recognition by TLR7 [168]. The MDA5 is in turn essential for type I IFNs responses to CVB, since MDA5 knockout mice are deficient to type I IFN and are prone to early death when infected with CVB (Wang et al., 2010). Thus, pattern-recognition receptors activation by enteroviruses results on IFNs and chemokines production which could lead to an inflammatory state in infected tissues. Moreover, these inflammatory factors enhance the overexpression of MHC-I molecules, which could result in an increased exposure of infected cells to the immune system and could initiate an autoimmune process that could directly contribute to islet cells damage [173]. However an activation of MDA-5 with any other factor can not initiate autoimmunity, whereas IFN-I-induced MDA-5 accelerated a preexistent autoimmune process in an animal model [38].

Some studies in animals have highlighted the potent role of antibodies and immune cells during enteroviral infection. Results on mice have shown that gammaglobulins are essential in limiting the scope and severity of enteroviral infection by preventing viral persistence in infected tissues [103] and T lymphocytes can deeply limit virus replication in CVB3-induced myocarditis and pancreatitis [63].

5.1.2. Enteroviruses can induce diabetes in mice

Experiments have been conducted to evaluate the ability of CVB4 to elicit diabetes in mice. These studies have shown that the pancreas was a predominant site of virus replication and the target of a strong immune response.

A CVB4 strain isolated by Yoon et al. from the pancreas of a 10-year-old boy who died of diabetic ketoacidosis and called CVB4E2, have induced hyperglycaemia with inflammation of the Langerhans islets and β-cell necrosis when inoculated to susceptible mice SJL/J [175]. A similar result was obtain in the same SJL/J mice strain when inoculated with a CVB5 strain isolated from stools of a diabetic patient [121]. In another study, CVB4E2 has led to hyperglycaemia and the appearance of anti-GAD antibodies in the vast majority of mice, suggesting a potent role of enteroviruses in initiating or accelerating autoimmunity against β-cells [57]. Diabetes with viral replication in β-cells has been also obtained when CVB4 JVB strain was inoculated to susceptible mice [174]. In addition, diabetes has been obtained in mice infected by CVB3 and CVB5 when animals were first treated with sub-diabetogenic doses of streptozotocin, a highly specific β-cell toxin. Findings from that study have revealed that virus-induced diabetes can be facilitated by cumulative effects induced by genetic factors or environmental insults (chemicals, drugs, toxins), since CVB strains (B3 and B5) used in that study ordinarily produce little if any β-cell damage [153]. Furthermore, CVB4-induced abnormal thymic, splenic and peripheral lymphocytes repertoire maturation has been described in mice and these lymphocyte maturation disorders have preceded the onset of hyperglycemia in animals [22].

In a study, CD-1 mice have been infected with the diabetogenic strain CVB4E2 and followed during one year. Results from this study have revealed a prolonged presence of viral RNA in pancreas tissue, a significant decrease in insulin levels and islets cells destruction by two mechanisms: directly by cytotoxic effects of IFN-γ-stimulated peritoneal macrophages and by an antibody-dependent mechanism through islet cell autoantibody (ICA) [133]. In another study, infection of mice with CVB4 has led to a rapid development of the disease mediated by bystander activation of T cells [73], which would tend to confirm early findings that have shown that infection of normal mice with CVB4 causes an overt diabetes associated with low insulin levels consistent with islet cells destruction [33].

The mechanism behind this β-cell destruction has been explored in some studies. Analysis of the results from these studies reveals that the spontaneous development of diabetes in NOD mice can be accelerated by CVB4 infection though a "bystander" effect only if a sufficient number of pre-existing autoreactive T-cells was already present [134]. This observation was in agreement with another study which has shown that the overexpression of a TCR transgene specific to an islet autoantigen has induced diabetes onset 2-4 weeks after CVB4 inoculation in mice that do not develop diabetes spontaneously [73]. Islet cell destruction by autoreactive T-cells was the result of the release of sequestered islet antigens which followed β-cell inflammation and destruction caused by CVB infection [73, 2001]. Other studies have stated that β-cells are phagocyted by antigen-presenting cells like macrophages, rather than directly destroyed by a CVB-induced process [75, 133], because antigen-presenting cells isolated from CVB4-infected mice can induce diabetes if inoculated to non-infected mice [75].

Among T1D animal models, the NOD mouse remains far the most used and studied model. The NOD mice are susceptible to spontaneous T1D that develops over several weeks and share most aspects of human T1D [83]. In NOD mice, the disease occurs after T-cell-mediated destruction of β-cells [87, 170]. Some studies have revealed that CVB infection effects in NOD mice appear to be contingent upon the precise moment at which infection occurs [134, 156]. Thus, rapid T1D induction can be obtained when older NOD mice are inoculated with CVB and the disease occurs much more rapidly when mice islets are already developing autoimmune insulitis and high islet cells lytic viral replication are observed when à virulent strain is inoculated [156]. These findings suggest that CVB replicate more readily in aged NOD mice islet cells, especially if there is inflammation, than in those of younger animals.

Another factor seems to be the magnitude of effects of CVB4 infection onto β-cells, depending on the permissiveness of target cells, which is closely related to their sensitivity to IFNs. Indeed, coxsackievirus B4-infected-NOD mice which had defective IFNs responses have developed an acute form of type 1 diabetes, similar to the one in humans following severe enteroviral infection. Interferons act by inducing an antiviral state in target cells, including pancreatic β-cells, by reducing their permissiveness to viral entry and replication. The effect of IFNs is transmitted as an intracellular signal through the Jack-STAT signaling pathway [140]. In transgenic NOD mice that express the suppressor of cytokine signaling 1 (SOCS-1), a negative regulator of IFN action which inhibit the Jack-STAT signaling pathway, CVB4 infection has resulted in β-cell loss and diabetes onset. Similar results have been obtained during the same study in transgenic NOD mice of which β-cells were lacking IFN receptors. In addition to inducing on β-cells a lower permissiveness to CVB4 infection, IFNs contributed also to deeply decrease their sensitivity to NK cell-mediated destruction [50].

5.1.3. Molecular mimicry hypothesis

Glutamic acid decarboxylase 65kD (GAD65), a candidate autoantigen in the pathogenesis of T1D, is expressed in pancreatic β-cells. Some findings from mice have shown that CTL (cytotoxic T lymphocytes) are cytotoxic to islet cells [44] and that T cell responses to GAD65 were detectable in prediabetic NOD mice spleens prior to disease onset [89, 152]. One of the mechanisms proposed to explain enterovirus-induced autoimmunity in T1D model is based on the cross-reactivity between CVB antigens and β-cell endogenous proteins through molecular mimicry. Pancreatic β-cells infection by CVB will be followed by inflammatory response resulting in β-cell destruction and increased self-antigen presentation due to their phagocytosis by antigen-presenting cells (APCs). Since P2-C protein sequence of CVB partially resembles that of human GAD65, both autoreactive and antiviral T-cells activated upon CVB infection, might act as strong enhancers that may accelerate or aggravate the ongoing autoimmune process [28, 151].

Regardless T-cells cross reactivity effects, experiments on CVB4-infected NOD mice have provided the evidence that the release of β-cell antigens followed by their presentation by APCs (antigen presentation cells) such as macrophages can initiate or promote β-cell autoimmunity [75].

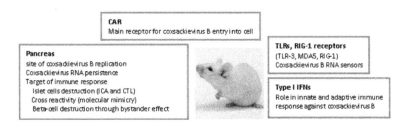

Figure 3. Information brought by animal models regarding coxsackievirus B infection and some aspects of type 1 diabetes pathogenesis

5.2. In vitro infection of β-cells and other cells with enteroviruses

Experiments have been conducted in vitro in order to analyse the hypotheses in favour of an association between enterovirus infections and T1D. Whether enteroviruses were able to infect the pancreatic tissue is a key issue concerning the relationship between enteroviruses and T1D. It has been shown that enteroviruses may be involved in the pathogenesis of T1D, either through direct β-cell infection or as triggers of the autoimmune processes. In particular, some results from in vitro experiments have suggested that enteroviruses, and especially CVB, may infect human β-cells and the infection may result in no apparent immediate effect or in functional impairment of β-cell [175, 174, 167, 124]. Most common enteroviruses in the environment can infect cultured human islets with β-cell destruction [93]. The figure 4 summarizes information brought by in vitro studies regarding coxsackievirus B infection which can be relevant for type 1 diabetes pathogenesis.

5.2.1. Enterovirus infection of β-cells

Persistent infection of human pancreatic islets by CVB associated with alpha interferon (IFN) synthesis was observed [23]. In this study conducted by our team, human pancreatic islets obtained from adult brain-dead donors and cultured in noncoated membrane inserts were infected with CVB3 and a diabetogenic (CVB4 E2) and a non-diabetogenic (CVB4 JVB) strain of CVB4. It was displayed that both α and β cells in human pancreatic islet can be persistently infected and long term CVB replication has been observed through the presence of infectious particles in culture supernatant fluids and intracellular viral negative-strand RNA up to 30 days post infection. This study showed that human islets challenged with CVB can synthesize IFN-α which is produced by infected β-cells only. These data support the hypothesis of a role of CVB in the high levels of type I IFNs that have been detected in pancreas or islets of patients with T1D [51, 76]. The viral persistence accompanied by synthesis of INF-α can enhance autoimmune processes leading to diabetes onset. The possibility that IFN-α could take part in T1D onset in genetically predisposed host have been tested in transgenic mice of which β-cells express this cytokine. It revealed that IFN-α was able to provoke the onset of the disease in transgenic animals, and that neutralizing IFN-α prevented inflammation and diabetes [142]. The expression of IFN-α in β-cells may lead to the development of diabetes in transgenic mice through the activation of autoimmune (islet-reactive) CD4+ TH1 cells [20].

Recent findings have shown that type I IFNs production can be induced in CVB infected human islet cells by intracellular viral RNA sensors such as TLR3, MDA-5 and RIG-1 genes [77]. These pattern-recognition receptors have also been told to upregulate the synthesis and production of chemokines. The sustaining of this process - IFNs and chemokines production – could be deleterious and involved in the development of autoimmunity, especially since persistent infection of islets cells in vitro by some CVB strains has been reported [23].

The infection of β-cells with CVB and the molecular pathways leading to CVB-induced β-cell death have been investigated. One study was aimed to evaluate the effects of different CVB4 strains on islets morphology and insulin release and another one compared inflammatory-related genes expression in CVB4-infected and uninfected isolated human islets. Results from these studies have revealed that even though the outcome of the infection differed, islet cells can be infected by all CVB4 strains. However, significant differences in viral titers and cell morphology were observed according to the phenotype of the strain: one with no cytopathic effect despite high virus titres (VD2921 stain), and the other with a pronounced cytopathic effect (V89-4557 strain), whereas a third one (JVB strain) have induced a significant increase of insulin release [55]. A microarray analysis of RNA from CVB4-infected human islets have shown specific induction of several inflammatory genes, some of them encoding proteins with potent biological activity such as IL-1β, IL-6, IL-8, MCP-1 and RANTES [117]. Recently, it has been reported that, except CVB1 and CVB3, all other CVB viruses induced a dose-dependent production of pro-inflammatory cytokines and chemokines in a rat insulinoma β-cell line (INS-1) [107].

The release of proinflammatory cytokines may strongly contribute to maintain a local pancreatic-islet inflammation that could result in an amplification of the immune attack against β-cells. In addition, the activation of MHC molecules in human fetal islet cells cultures infected by CVB4 could result in an increase exposure of infected cells to the immune system and support the autoimmune response against β-cells [119].

The inflammation of β-cells is supposed to be an early event in the pathogenesis of type 1diabetes [45]. An exaggerated inflammatory response to enterovirus may contribute to induce a prolonged inflammation state and β-cell loss, and could initiate or aggravate pathogenic processes of type 1 diabetes.

5.2.2. Enterovirus infection of thymus

It has been shown in mouse that CVB could infect the thymus with a disruption of organ functions that was associated with diabetes [22]. Further studies have been conducted to investigate the mechanisms and consequences of infection of thymus with CVB. The establishment of central T-cell tolerance is ensured by the thymus. Thymic epithelial cells (TEC) participate actively in the development of a biochemical environment needed for the maturation of immunocompetent T cells. Thymic epithelial cells are actively involved in the promotion of T-cell maturation by mediating negative and positive selection of thymocytes and by participating to the induction of tolerance [136].

In collaboration with Pr Vincent Geenen and his team (University of Lièges, Belgium) we investigated the hypothesis that T1D which is an autoimmune disease, can result from the disturbance of the central tolerance. Due to the role of thymus in induction and establishment of self-tolerance, enteroviral infection of TEC may result in interference and disturbance of T-cell ontogeny, which can induce or enhance the immune process leading to T1D. The infection of human TEC primary cultures with CVB4 and the resulting consequences on TEC function have been studied. Human TEC, isolated from thymus fragments obtained from children undergoing corrective surgery, were infected with CVB4 JVB and E2 strains. Findings from this study have revealed that a cytolytic virus such as CVB4 can infect persistently human TEC cultures without obvious cytopathic effect and this infection have led to a continuous increased production of cytokines IL-6, GM-CSF and LIF [14]. In order to evaluate the effect of enterovirus infection onto fetal thymus during pregnancy, intact explanted human foetal thymic organ cultures were infected with CVB4E2 strain. Results from this study have shown progressive thymocyte depletion and upregulation of MHC-I molecules expression on CD4+CD8+ double positive cells [15]. Another study was conducted on mouse to assess the effect of CVB infection on thymocytes maturation and differentiation. In this study, whole foetal thymus organ cultures obtained from 14 days foetal CD-1 mice were infected with CVB4E2 strain. Findings from that study have revealed in infected culture a disturbance of maturation and differentiation of T cells characterized by increased levels of mature CD4+ and CD8+ cells associated with decreased percentage of double positive cells [16].

Furthermore it was reported that CVB4 RNA can be found in thymus up to 70 days after per os infection of mice with CVB4E2. In vitro, CVB4 was able to infect and replicate in primary cultures of adult murine splenic and thymic cells [81].

The ability of enteroviruses such as CVB4 to infect the thymus during fetal life could have deleterious effects on thymus functions, since neonatal exposure to thymotropic virus could induce a virus-specific nonresponsiveness [95]. A global analysis of all these findings suggests that thymus organ can be infected by coxsackievirus B which can disturb the organ function with possible effects on the autoimmune processes leading to T1D.

5.2.3. Antibody-dependent enhancement of enterovirus infection

The antibody-dependent enhancement (ADE) of infection is a mechanism observed in vitro with various viruses and which can intervene in pathogenic processes induced by these viruses [145]. The ADE of CVB4 infection has been discovered by our group. It is caused by enhancing antibodies devoid of neutralizing activity and has been found in serum /plasma of T1D patients and controls. These antibodies, isolated from plasma by affinity chromatography, increase the CVB4-induced synthesis of IFN-α by human peripheral blood mononuclear cells (PBMC) in vitro [25]. It has been demonstrated that IFN-α synthesis by PBMC infected with CVB4 prealably incubated with specific antibodies is a result of the infection of monocytes that occurs by a mechanism involving the receptors CAR and those for the Fc portion of IgG molecule, FcγRII (Fcγ receptor II) and FcγRIII localised at the cell surface membrane [66]. CVB4 can strongly induce the production of IFN-α by PBMCs from patients with T1D compared with PBMC from healthy controls, which is due to anti-CVB4 enhancing antibodies bound to the cell surface membrane. In addition, a higher level of IFN-α was produced by PBMC of patients inoculated with CVB4 prealably incubated with plasma of patients [67]. The target of these antibodies has been identified as the enteroviral protein VP4 and it has been shown that the prevalence and the titres of anti-VP4 antibodies were higher in patients with T1D than in control subjects [26]. Specific anti-VP4 antibodies enhance the infection of PBMC with CVB4 [129]. The sequence of VP4 recognized by these antibodies was investigated and identified in competition experiments as amino acids 11 to 30 by using synthetic overlapping peptides spanning CVB4E2 VP4 protein [130]. The VP4 protein and a VP4 peptide have been used to detect anti-CVB4 enhancing antibodies by ELISA [26, 130]. The fact that enhancing anti-CVB4 antibodies bind the viral particles through VP4 is challenging, since, according the structural analysis of frozen enteroviruses by X-ray diffraction, the capsid protein VP4 is localized along the inner virion surface, like the amino-terminal sequences of the three external proteins VP1, VP2 and VP3. The explanation lies in the dynamic character of the virus structure at 37°C that would allow an exposure of these normally internal sequences and making a piece of the VP4 protein accessible to antibodies, as it has been shown in the case of the amino-terminal part of VP1 in the poliovirus system [96].

The increased infection of monocytes with CVB4 due to enhancing antibodies could lead, in vivo, in dissemination and worsening of histological lesions that may contribute to CVB4-induced disease, as described in a model of CVB3-induced myocarditis [131, 58, 92]. Furthermore, the enterovirus –induced production of IFN-α enhanced by antibodies, can play a pathogenic role. Indeed, chronic IFN-α synthesis or its abnormal activation in response to recurrent or repeated enteroviral infections can be associated with disorders leading to autoimmune diseases [23].

Further studies are needed to investigate the role of enhancing antibodies in the CVB-induced pathogenesis of T1D.

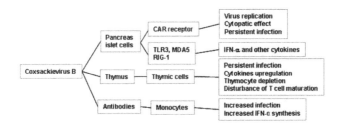

Figure 4. Information brought by in vitro studies regarding coxsackievirus B infection

5.3. Complex relationship between enteroviruses and type 1 diabetes

As mentioned above, the role of enteroviruses in T1D disease is strongly suspected. In contrast, a protective role of enteroviruses is suggested as well. Experimental data in favour of a protective role of these viruses have been reported. Indeed, some studies have shown that, rather than triggering an autoimmune process, CVB infections can provide significant protection against the development of T1D [155, 48]. Coxsackievirus B4, the human enterovirus most associated with an etiologic role in human T1D, has been reported to increase the rate of diabetes onset in older NOD mice but not in younger mice [134]. This result has been confirmed by other groups who provided evidence that disease induction required a pre-existing accumulation of β-cell specific autoreactive T cells within the pancreas, a phenomenon observed in older NOD mice, but not in younger mice [74, 156]. This protective effect may involve the virus strain, its virulence and replication rate, as well as the stage of autoimmune development, and the mechanism relies in long-term tolerance due to an increase in protective regulatory T cells with TGF-β production [49].

These findings support the concept that virus infections occurring early in childhood had a protective effect against T1D and are in agreement with the hygiene hypothesis [7, 157]. Indeed, it should be emphasized that there are significantly more enterovirus infections annually than new cases of T1D in population. The decreased enterovirus exposure rates following the increased hygiene levels might explain the high risk of developing the disease, since it has been revealed in epidemiological studies that T1D incidence is higher in developed countries than in developing ones, from less than 1 per 100,000 inhabitants in Asia to 14 in US and even more than 30 per 100,000 in Scandinavia [139].

6. Conclusion

Type 1 diabetes is a complex multifactorial disease. The involvement of enteroviruses as a major non-genetic etiological factor is a topic of reflexion for several research teams worldwide. Studies from these teams have shown that enteroviral infections, especially coxsackievirus B infections, are closely linked with T1D. Findings from experimental in vitro and in vivo studies have lightened the potent role that can play enteroviruses in inducing and/or worsening the disease. However, in certain particular conditions, enteroviruses can induce a protective effect in mouse model. Therefore, further studies are needed to understand the mechanisms behind this complex relationship between enteroviruses and T1D.

Declaration of interest

No conflict of interest

Acknowledgements

The authors thank Delphine Caloone for technical assistance and all their collaborators. The studies performed by the authors or in progress have been or are supported by EU FP5 VIR-DIAB Project (Contract QLK 2-CT-2001-01910), EU FP6 Integrated Project EURO-THY-MAIDE, (Contract LSHB-CT-2003-503410), EU FP7 PEVNET Project (FP7-HEALTH-2010-single-stage N° 261441), grants from Nord-Pas-de-Calais Région (ArCir convention 2004/018; BBS 2006), CHRU Lille, the ministère de l'Education nationale de la recherche et de la technologie, Université de Lille 2, France, and the comité mixte de coopération universitaire franco-tunisien (CMCU 2004 N○ 04/G0810 and CMCU 2008N808/G0808). Didier Hober was Fondation pour la Recherche Médicale 2008 prize winner. Didier Hober is a member of the VIrus in Diabetes International Study group (VIDIS group).

Author details

Didier Hober[1*], Famara Sané[1], Karena Riedweg[1], Ilham Moumna[1], Anne Goffard[1], Laura Choteau[1], Enagnon Kazali Alidjinou[1] and Rachel Desailloud[2]

*Address all correspondence to: didier.hober@chru-lille.fr

1 Université Lille 2, CHRU, Laboratoire de Virologie/ EA3610, 59037 Lille, France

2 UPJV CHU, Service d'Endocrinologie-Diabétologie-Nutrition, 80054 Amiens, France

References

[1] Aarnisalo, J., Veijola, R., Vainionpaa, R., Simell, O., Knip, M., & Ilonen, J. (2008). Cytomegalovirus infection in early infancy: risk of induction and progression of autoimmunity associated with type 1 diabetes. *Diabetologia* 51(5), 769-72.

[2] Acharya, R., Fry, E., Stuart, D., Fox, G., Rowlands, D., & Brown, F. (1989). The three-dimensional structure of foot-and-mouth disease virus at 2.9 A resolution. *Nature* 337(6209), 709-16.

[3] Ahmad, N., & Abraham, A. A. (1982). Pancreatic isleitis with coxsackie virus B5 infection. *Hum Pathol.* 13(7), 661-2.

[4] Andino, R., Boddeker, N., Silvera, D., & Gamarnik, A. V. (1999). Intracellular determinants of picornavirus replication. *Trends Microbiol.* 7(2), 76-82.

[5] Andreoletti, L., Hober, D., Hober-Vandenberghe, C., Belaich, S., Vantyghem, M. C., Lefebvre, J., & Wattre, P. (1997). Detection of coxsackie B virus RNA sequences in whole blood samples from adult patients at the onset of type I diabetes mellitus. *J Med Virol.* 52(2), 121-7.

[6] Bach, J.F. (2002). The effect of infections on susceptibility to autoimmune and allergic diseases. N *Engl J Med.* 347(12), , 911 EOF-20 EOF.

[7] Bach, J.F. (2005). Infections and autoimmune diseases. *J Autoimmun 25 Suppl.*, 74-80.

[8] Baek, H. S., & Yoon, J. W. (1990). Role of macrophages in the pathogenesis of encephalomyocarditis virus-induced diabetes in mice. *J Virol* 64(12), 5708-15.

[9] Baek, H. S., & Yoon, J. W. (1991). Direct involvement of macrophages in destruction of beta-cells leading to development of diabetes in virus-infected mice. *Diabetes* 40(12), 1586-97.

[10] Balada, E., Vilardell-Tarres, M., & Ordi-Ros, J. (2010). Implication of human endogenous retroviruses in the development of autoimmune diseases. *Int Rev Immunol* 29(4), 351-70.

[11] Beyan, H., Drexhage, R. C., van der Heul, Nieuwenhuijsen. L., de Wit, H., Padmos, R. C., Schloot, N. C., Drexhage, H. A., & Leslie, R. D. (2010). Monocyte gene-expression profiles associated with childhood-onset type 1 diabetes and disease risk: a study of identical twins. *Diabetes* 59(7), 1751-5.

[12] Blixt, M., Niklasson, B., & Sandler, S. (2007). Characterization of beta-cell function of pancreatic islets isolated from bank voles developing glucose intolerance/diabetes: an animal model showing features of both type 1 and type 2 diabetes mellitus, and a possible role of the Ljungan virus. *Gen Comp Endocrinol* 154(1-3), 41-7.

[13] Bortell, R., Pino, S. C., Greiner, D. L., Zipris, D., & Rossini, A. A. (2008). Closing the circle between the bedside and the bench: Toll-like receptors in models of virally induced diabetes. *Ann N Y Acad Sci*, 1150, 112-22.

[14] Brilot, F., Chehadeh, W., Charlet-Renard, C., Martens, H., Geenen, V., & Hober, D. (2002). Persistent infection of human thymic epithelial cells by coxsackievirus B4. *J Virol.* 76(10), 5260-5.

[15] Brilot, F., Geenen, V., Hober, D., & Stoddart, C. A. (2004). Coxsackievirus B4 infection of human fetal thymus cells. *J Virol.* 78(18), 9854-61.

[16] Brilot, F., Jaidane, H., Geenen, V., & Hober, D. (2008). Coxsackievirus B4 infection of murine foetal thymus organ cultures. *J Med Virol.* 80(4), 659-66.

[17] Buesa-Gomez, J., de la Torre, J. C., Dyrberg, T., Landin-Olsson, M., Mauseth, R. S., Lernmark, A., & Oldstone, M. B. (1994). Failure to detect genomic viral sequences in pancreatic tissues from two children with acute-onset diabetes mellitus. *J Med Virol.* 42(2), 193-7.

[18] Burgess, M. A., & Forrest, J. M. (2009). Congenital rubella and diabetes mellitus. *Diabetologia* 52(2), 369-70; author reply 373.

[19] Cameron, C. E., Suk, Oh. H., & Moustafa, I. M. (2010). Expanding knowledge of 3proteins in the poliovirus lifecycle. *Future Microbiol.* 5(6), 867-81.

[20] Chakrabarti, D., Hultgren, B., & Stewart, T. A. (1996). IFN-alpha induces autoimmune T cells through the induction of intracellular adhesion molecule-1 and B7.2. *J Immunol.* 157(2), 522-8.

[21] Champsaur, H., Dussaix, E., Samolyk, D., Fabre, M., Bach, C., & Assan, R. (1980). Diabetes and Coxsackie virus B5 infection. *Lancet* 1(8162), 251.

[22] Chatterjee, N. K., Hou, J., Dockstader, P., & Charbonneau, T. (1992). Coxsackievirus B4 infection alters thymic, splenic, and peripheral lymphocyte repertoire preceding onset of hyperglycemia in mice. *J Med Virol.* 38(2), 124-31.

[23] Chehadeh, W., Kerr-Conte, J., Pattou, F., Alm, G., Lefebvre, J., Wattre, P., & Hober, D. (2000a). Persistent infection of human pancreatic islets by coxsackievirus B is associated with alpha interferon synthesis in beta cells. *J Virol.* 74(21), 10153-64.

[24] Chehadeh, W., Weill, J., Vantyghem, M. C., Alm, G., Lefebvre, J., Wattre, P., & Hober, D. (2000b). Increased level of interferon-alpha in blood of patients with insulin-dependent diabetes mellitus: relationship with coxsackievirus B infection. *J Infect Dis.* 181(6), 1929-39.

[25] Chehadeh, W., Bouzidi, A., Alm, G., Wattre, P., & Hober, D. (2001). Human antibodies isolated from plasma by affinity chromatography increase the coxsackievirus B4induced synthesis of interferon-alpha by human peripheral blood mononuclear cells in vitro. *J Gen Virol.* 82(Pt 8), 1899-907.

[26] Chehadeh, W., Lobert, P. E., Sauter, P., Goffard, A., Lucas, B., Weill, J., Vantyghem, M. C., Alm, G., Pigny, P., & Hober, D. (2005). Viral protein VP4 is a target of human antibodies enhancing coxsackievirus B4and B3-induced synthesis of alpha interferon. *J Virol.* 79(22), 13882-91.

[27] Chiou, C. C., Chung, W. H., Hung, S. I., Yang, L. C., & Hong, H. S. (2006). Fulminant type 1 diabetes mellitus caused by drug hypersensitivity syndrome with human herpesvirus 6 infection. *J Am Acad Dermatol.* 54 (2 Suppl), S, 14-7.

[28] Christen, U., Edelmann, K. H., Mc Gavern, D. B., Wolfe, T., Coon, B., Teague, M. K., Miller, S. D., Oldstone, M. B., & von Herrath, M. G. (2004). A viral epitope that mimics a self antigen can accelerate but not initiate autoimmune diabetes. *J Clin Invest.* 114(9), 1290-8.

[29] Chung, Y. H., Jun, H. S., Kang, Y., Hirasawa, K., Lee, B. R., Van Rooijen, N., & Yoon, J. W. (1997). Role of macrophages and macrophage-derived cytokines in the pathogenesis of Kilham rat virus-induced autoimmune diabetes in diabetes-resistant Bio-Breeding rats. *J Immunol.* 159(1), 466-71.

[30] Chung, Y. H., Jun, H. S., Son, M., Bao, M., Bae, H. Y., Kang, Y., & Yoon, J. W. (2000). Cellular and molecular mechanism for Kilham rat virus-induced autoimmune diabetes in DR-BB rats. *J. Immunol* 165(5), 2866-76.

[31] Clements, G. B., Galbraith, D. N., & Taylor, K. W. (1995). Coxsackie B virus infection and onset of childhood diabetes. *Lancet* 346(8969), 221-3.

[32] Colbere-Garapin, F., Christodoulou, C., Crainic, R., & Pelletier, I. (1989). Persistent poliovirus infection of human neuroblastoma cells. *Proc Natl Acad Sci U S A* 86(19), 7590-4.

[33] Coleman, T. J., Gamble, D. R., & Taylor, K. W. (1973). Diabetes in mice after Coxsackie B 4 virus infection. *Br Med J.* 3(5870), 25-7.

[34] Concannon, P., Rich, S. S., & Nepom, G. T. (2009). Genetics of type 1A diabetes. *N Engl J Med.* 360(16), 1646-54.

[35] Coulson, B. S., Witterick, P. D., Tan, Y., Hewish, M. J., Mountford, J. N., Harrison, L. C., & Honeyman, M. C. (2002). Growth of rotaviruses in primary pancreatic cells. *J Virol* 76(18), 9537-44.

[36] Coutant, R., Carel, J. C., Lebon, P., Bougnères, P. F., Palmer, P., & Cantero-Aguilar, L. (2000). Detection of enterovirus RNA sequences in serum samples from autoantibody-positive subjects at risk for diabetes. *Diabet Med.* 19(11), 968-9.

[37] Craig, M. E., Howard, N. J., Silink, M., & Rawlinson, W. D. (2003). Reduced frequency of HLA DRB1*03DQB1*02 in children with type 1 diabetes associated with enterovirus RNA. *J Infect Dis.* 187(10), 1562-70.

[38] Crampton, S. P., Deane, J. A., Feigenbaum, L., & Bolland, S. (2011). IFIH1 gene dose effect reveals MDA-5 mediated chronic type I IFN gene signature, viral resistance and accelerated autoimmunity. *J Immunol, DOI:In Press.*

[39] Dahlquist, G. G., Forsberg, J., Hagenfeldt, L., Boman, J., & Juto, P. (2004). Increased prevalence of enteroviral RNA in blood spots from newborn children who later developed type 1 diabetes: a population-based case-control study. *Diabetes Care* 27(1), 285-6.

[40] Deonarain, R., Cerullo, D., Fuse, K., Liu, P. P., & Fish, E. N. (2004). Protective role for interferon-beta in coxsackievirus B3 infection. *Circulation* 110(23), 3540-3.

[41] De Stefano, F., Mullooly, J. P., Okoro, C. A., Chen, R. T., Marcy, S. M., Ward, J. I., Vadheim, C. M., Black, S. B., Shinefield, H. R., Davis, R. L., & Bohlke, K. (2001). Childhood vaccinations, vaccination timing, and risk of type 1 diabetes mellitus. *Pediatrics* 108(6), E112.

[42] Di Pietro, C., Del Guercio, M. J., Paolino, G. P., Barbi, M., Ferrante, P., & Chiumello, G. (1979). Type 1 diabetes and Coxsackie virus infection. *Helv Paediatr Acta* 34(6), 557-61.

[43] Dotta, F., Censini, S., van Halteren, A. G., Marselli, L., Masini, M., Dionisi, S., Mosca, F., Boggi, U., Muda, A. O., Prato, S. D., Elliott, J. F., Covacci, A., Rappuoli, R., Roep, B. O., & Marchetti, P. (2007). Coxsackie B4 virus infection of beta cells and natural killer cell insulitis in recent-onset type 1 diabetic patients. *Proc Natl Acad Sci U S A* 104(12), 5115-20.

[44] Dudek, N. L., Thomas, H. E., Mariana, L., Sutherland, R. M., Allison, J., Estella, E., Angstetra, E., Trapani, J. A., Santamaria, P., Lew, A. M., & Kay, T. W. (2006). Cytotoxic T-cells from T-cell receptor transgenic NOD8.3 mice destroy beta-cells via the perforin and Fas pathways. *Diabetes* 55(9), 2412-8.

[45] Eizirik, D. L., Colli, M. L., & Ortis, F. (2009). The role of inflammation in insulitis and beta-cell loss in type 1 diabetes. *Nat Rev Endocrinol.* 5(4), 219-26.

[46] Ejrnaes, M., von, Herrath. M. G., & Christen, U. (2006). Cure of chronic viral infection and virus-induced type 1 diabetes by neutralizing antibodies. *Clin Dev Immunol.* 13(2-4), 337-47.

[47] Ellerman, K. E., Richards, C. A., Guberski, D. L., Shek, W. R., & Like, A. A. (1996). Kilham rat triggers T-cell-dependent autoimmune diabetes in multiple strains of rat. *Diabetes* 45(5), 557-62.

[48] Filippi, C.M., & von Herrath, M.G. (2008). Viral trigger for type 1 diabetes: pros and cons. *Diabetes* 57(11), 2863-71.

[49] Filippi, C. M., Estes, E. A., Oldham, J. E., & von Herrath, M. G. (2009). Immunoregulatory mechanisms triggered by viral infections protect from type 1 diabetes in mice. *J Clin Invest* 119(6), 1515-23.

[50] Flodstrom, M., Maday, A., Balakrishna, D., Cleary, M. M., Yoshimura, A., & Sarvetnick, N. (2002). Target cell defense prevents the development of diabetes after viral infection. *Nat Immunol.* 3(4), 373-82.

[51] Foulis, A. K., Farquharson, M. A., & Meager, A. (1987). Immunoreactive alpha-interferon in insulin-secreting beta cells in type 1 diabetes mellitus. *Lancet* 2 (8573), 1423-7.

[52] Foulis, A. K., Farquharson, M. A., Cameron, S. O., Mc Gill, M., Schonke, H., & Kandolf, R. (1990). A search for the presence of the enteroviral capsid protein VP1 in pancreases of patients with type 1 (insulin-dependent) diabetes and pancreases and hearts of infants who died of coxsackieviral myocarditis. *Diabetologia* 33(5), 290-8.

[53] Foy, C. A., Quirke, P., Lewis, F. A., Futers, T. S., & Bodansky, H. J. (1995). Detection of common viruses using the polymerase chain reaction to assess levels of viral presence in type 1 (insulin-dependent) diabetic patients. *Diabet Med.* 12(11), 1002-8.

[54] Freimuth, P., Philipson, L., & Carson, S. D. (2008). The coxsackievirus and adenovirus receptor. *Curr Top Microbiol Immunol.* , 323, 67-87.

[55] Frisk, G., & Diderholm, H. (2000). Tissue culture of isolated human pancreatic islets infected with different strains of coxsackievirus B4: assessment of virus replication and effects on islet morphology and insulin release. *Int J Exp Diabetes Res.* 1(3), 165-75.

[56] Gale, E.A. (2008). Congenital rubella: citation virus or viral cause of type 1 diabetes? *Diabetologia* 51(9), 1559-66.

[57] Gerling, I., Chatterjee, N. K., & Nejman, C. (1991). Coxsackievirus B4-induced development of antibodies to 64000Mr islet autoantigen and hyperglycemia in mice. *Autoimmunity* 10(1), 49-56.

[58] Girn, J., Kavoosi, M., & Chantler, J. (2002). Enhancement of coxsackievirus B3 infection by antibody to a different coxsackievirus strain. *J Gen Virol.* 83(Pt 2), 351-8.

[59] Goto, A., Takahashi, Y., Kishimoto, M., Nakajima, Y., Nakanishi, K., Kajio, H., & Noda, M. (2008). A case of fulminant type 1 diabetes associated with significant elevation of mumps titers. *Endocr J.* 55(3), 561-4.

[60] Graham, K. L., Sanders, N., Tan, Y., Allison, J., Kay, T. W., & Coulson, B. S. (2008). Rotavirus infection accelerates type 1 diabetes in mice with established insulitis. *J Virol.* 82(13), 6139-49.

[61] Hanafusa, T., & Imagawa, A. (2007). Fulminant type 1 diabetes: a novel clinical entity requiring special attention by all medical practitioners. *Nat Clin Pract Endocrinol Metab* 3(1), 36-45; quiz 2p following 69.

[62] Helmke, K., Otten, A., & Willems, W. (1980). Islet cell antibodies in children with mumps infection. *Lancet* 2(8187), 211-2.

[63] Henke, A., Huber, S., Stelzner, A., & Whitton, J. L. (1995). The role of CD8+ T lymphocytes in coxsackievirus B3induced myocarditis. *J Virol.* 69(11), 6720-8.

[64] Hiemstra, H. S., Schloot, N. C., van Veelen, P. A., Willemen, S. J., Franken, K. L., van Rood, J. J., de Vries, R. R., Chaudhuri, A., Behan, P. O., Drijfhout, J. W., & Roep, B. O. (2001). Cytomegalovirus in autoimmunity: T cell crossreactivity to viral antigen and autoantigen glutamic acid decarboxylase. *Proc Natl Acad Sci U S A* 98(7), 3988-91.

[65] Hillebrands, J. L., van der Werf, N., Klatter, F. A., Bruggeman, C. A., & Rozing, J. (2003). Role of peritoneal macrophages in cytomegalovirus-induced acceleration of autoimmune diabetes in BB-rats. *Clin Dev Immunol.* 10(2-4), 133-9.

[66] Hober, D., Chehadeh, W., Bouzidi, A., & Wattre, P. (2001). Antibody-dependent enhancement of coxsackievirus B4 infectivity of human peripheral blood mononuclear cells results in increased interferon-alpha synthesis. *J Infect Dis.* 184(9), 1098-108.

[67] Hober, D., Chehadeh, W., Weill, J., Hober, C., Vantyghem, M. C., Gronnier, P., & Wattre, P. (2002). Circulating and cell-bound antibodies increase coxsackievirus B4in-

duced production of IFN-alpha by peripheral blood mononuclear cells from patients with type 1 diabetes. *J Gen Virol.* 83(Pt 9), 2169-76.

[68] Hogle, J.M. (2002). Poliovirus cell entry: common structural themes in viral cell entry pathways. *Annu Rev Microbiol.*, 56, 677-702.

[69] Hogle, J. M., Chow, M., & Filman, D. J. (1985). Three-dimensional structure of poliovirus at 2.9 A resolution. *Science* 229(4720), 1358-65.

[70] Honeyman, M. C., Coulson, B. S., Stone, N. L., Gellert, S. A., Goldwater, P. N., Steele, C. E., Couper, J. J., Tait, B. D., Colman, P. G., & Harrison, L. C. (2000). Association between rotavirus infection and pancreatic islet autoimmunity in children at risk of developing type 1 diabetes. *Diabetes* 49(8), 1319-24.

[71] Honeyman, M. C., & Harrison, L. C. (2009). Congenital rubella, diabetes and HLA. *Diabetologia* 52(2), 371-2; author reply 373.

[72] Honeyman, M. C., Stone, N. L., Falk, B. A., Nepom, G., & Harrison, L. C. (2010). Evidence for molecular mimicry between human T cell epitopes in rotavirus and pancreatic islet autoantigens. *J Immunol.* 184(4), 2204-10.

[73] Horwitz, M. S., Bradley, L. M., Harbertson, J., Krahl, T., Lee, J., & Sarvetnick, N. (1998). Diabetes induced by Coxsackie virus: initiation by bystander damage and not molecular mimicry. *Nat Med.* 4(7), 781-5.

[74] Horwitz, M. S., Fine, C., Ilic, A., & Sarvetnick, N. (2001). Requirements for viral-mediated autoimmune diabetes: beta-cell damage and immune infiltration. *J Autoimmun.* 16(3), 211-7.

[75] Horwitz, M. S., Ilic, A., Fine, C., Balasa, B., & Sarvetnick, N. (2004). Coxsackieviral-mediated diabetes: induction requires antigen-presenting cells and is accompanied by phagocytosis of beta cells. *Clin Immunol.* 110(2), 134-44.

[76] Huang, X., Yuang, J., Goddard, A., Foulis, A., James, R. F., Lernmark, A., Pujol-Borrell, R., Rabinovitch, A., Somoza, N., & Stewart, T. A. (1995). Interferon expression in the pancreases of patients with type I diabetes. *Diabetes* 44(6),658-64.

[77] Hultcrantz, M., Huhn, M. H., Wolf, M., Olsson, A., Jacobson, S., Williams, B. R., Korsgren, O., & Flodstrom-Tullberg, M. (2007). Interferons induce an antiviral state in human pancreatic islet cells. *Virology* 367(1), 92-101.

[78] Hviid, A., Stellfeld, M., Wohlfahrt, J., & Melbye, M. (2004). Childhood vaccination and type 1 diabetes. *N Engl J Med.* 350(14), 1398-404.

[79] Hyoty, H., Hiltunen, M., Reunanen, A., Leinikki, P., Vesikari, T., Lounamaa, R., Tuomilehto, J., & Akerblom, H. K. (1993a). Decline of mumps antibodies in type 1 (insulin-dependent) diabetic children and a plateau in the rising incidence of type 1 diabetes after introduction of the mumps-measles-rubella vaccine in Finland. Childhood Diabetes in Finland Study Group. *Diabetologia* 36(12), 1303-8.

[80] Hyoty, H., Parkkonen, P., Rode, M., Bakke, O., & Leinikki, P. (1993b). Common pep-
      tide epitope in mumps virus nucleocapsid protein and MHC class II-associated in-
      variant chain. *Scand J Immunol.* 37(5), 550-8.

[81] Jaidane, H., Gharbi, J., Lobert, P. E., Caloone, D., Lucas, B., Sane, F., Idziorek, T., Ro-
      mond, M. B., Aouni, M., & Hober, D. (2008). Infection of primary cultures of murine
      splenic and thymic cells with coxsackievirus B4. *Microbiol Immunol.* 52(1), 40-6.

[82] Jaidane, H., & Hober, D. (2008). Role of coxsackievirus B4 in the pathogenesis of type
      1 diabetes. *Diabetes Metab.* 34(6 Pt 1), 537-48.

[83] Jaidane, H., Sane, F., Gharbi, J., Aouni, M., Romond, M. B., & Hober, D. (2009). Cox-
      sackievirus B4 and type 1 diabetes pathogenesis: contribution of animal models. *Dia-
      betes Metab Res Rev.* 25(7), 591-603.

[84] Jun, H. S., Kang, Y., Notkins, A. L., & Yoon, J. W. (1997). Gain or loss of diabetogenic-
      ity resulting from a single point mutation in recombinant encephalomyocarditis vi-
      rus. *J Virol.* 71(12), 9782-5.

[85] Jun, H. S., Kang, Y., Yoon, H. S., Kim, K. H., Notkins, A. L., & Yoon, J. W. (1998). De-
      termination of encephalomyocarditis viral diabetogenicity by a putative binding site
      of the viral capsid protein. *Diabetes* 47(4), 576-82.

[86] Kallewaard, N. L., Zhang, L., Chen, J. W., Guttenberg, M., Sanchez, M. D., & Bergel-
      son, J. M. (2009). Tissue-specific deletion of the coxsackievirus and adenovirus recep-
      tor protects mice from virus-induced pancreatitis and myocarditis. *Cell Host Microbe*
      6(1), 91-8.

[87] Kanazawa, Y., Komeda, K., Sato, S., Mori, S., Akanuma, K., & Takaku, F. (1984). Non-
      obese-diabetic mice: immune mechanisms of pancreatic beta-cell destruction. *Diabeto-
      logia* 27 Suppl,, 113-5.

[88] Kasuga, A., Harada, R., & Saruta, T. (1996). Insulin-dependent diabetes mellitus asso-
      ciated with parvovirus B19 infection. *Ann Intern Med.* 125(8), 700-1.

[89] Kaufman, D. L., Clare-Salzler, M., Tian, J., Forsthuber, T., Ting, G. S., Robinson, P.,
      Atkinson, M. A., Sercarz, E. E., Tobin, A. J., & Lehmann, P. V. (1993). Spontaneous
      loss of T-cell tolerance to glutamic acid decarboxylase in murine insulin-dependent
      diabetes. *Nature*, 69-72.

[90] Kawashima, H., Ihara, T., Ioi, H., Oana, S., Sato, S., Kato, N., Takami, T., Kashiwagi,
      Y., Takekuma, K., Hoshika, A., & Mori, T. (2004). Enterovirus-related type 1 diabetes
      mellitus and antibodies to glutamic acid decarboxylase in Japan. *J Infect.* 49(2),
      147-51.

[91] Kemball, C. C., Alirezaei, M., & Whitton, J. L. (2010). Type B coxsackieviruses and
      their interactions with the innate and adaptive immune systems. *Future Microbiol.*
      5(9),, 1329-1347.

[92] Kishimoto, C., Kurokawa, M., & Ochiai, H. (2002). Antibody-mediated immune en-
      hancement in coxsackievirus B3 myocarditis. *J Mol Cell Cardiol* 34(9),, 1227 -1238 .

[93] Klemola, P., Kaijalainen, S., Ylipaasto, P., & Roivainen, M. (2008). Diabetogenic ef-
      fects of the most prevalent enteroviruses in Finnish sewage. *Ann N Y Acad Sci.*, 1150,
      210-2.

[94] Kondrashova, A., Reunanen, A., Romanov, A., Karvonen, A., Viskari, H., Vesikari,
      T., Ilonen, J., Knip, M., & Hyoty, H. (2005). A six-fold gradient in the incidence of
      type 1 diabetes at the eastern border of Finland. *Ann Med.* 37(1),, 67 -72 .

[95] Korostoff, J. M., Nakada, M. T., Faas, S. J., Blank, K. J., & Gaulton, G. N. (1990). Neo-
      natal exposure to thymotropic gross murine leukemia virus induces virus-specific
      immunologic nonresponsiveness. *J Exp Med.* 172(6), 1765-75.

[96] Li, Q., Yafal, A. G., Lee, Y. M., Hogle, J., & Chow, M. (1994). Poliovirus neutralization
      by antibodies to internal epitopes of VP4 and VP1 results from reversible exposure of
      these sequences at physiological temperature. *J Virol.* 68(6), 3965-70.

[97] Lin, J. Y., Chen, T. C., Weng, K. F., Chang, S. C., Chen, L. L., & Shih, S. R. (2009). Viral
      and host proteins involved in picornavirus life cycle. *J Biomed Sci.* 16, 103.

[98] Lindberg, B., Ahlfors, K., Carlsson, A., Ericsson, U. B., Landin-Olsson, M., Lernmark,
      A., Ludvigsson, J., Sundkvist, G., & Ivarsson, S. A. (1999). Previous exposure to mea-
      sles, mumps, and rubella--but not vaccination during adolescence--correlates to the
      prevalence of pancreatic and thyroid autoantibodies. *Pediatrics* 104(1), e12.

[99] Lonnrot, M., Salminen, K., Knip, M., Savola, K., Kulmala, P., Leinikki, P., Hyypia, T.,
      Akerblom, H. K., & Hyoty, H. (2000). Enterovirus RNA in serum is a risk factor for
      beta-cell autoimmunity and clinical type 1 diabetes: a prospective study. Childhood
      Diabetes in Finland (DiMe) Study Group. *J Med Virol.* 61(2), 214-20.

[100] Maha, M. M., Ali, M. A., Abdel-Rehim, S. E., Abu-Shady, E. A., El -Naggar, B. M., &
      Maha, Y. Z. (2003). The role of coxsackieviruses infection in the children of insulin
      dependent diabetes mellitus. *J Egypt Public Health Assoc.* 78(3-4), 305-18.

[101] Marguerat, S., Wang, W. Y., Todd, J. A., & Conrad, B. (2004). Association of human
      endogenous retrovirus K-18 polymorphisms with type 1 diabetes. *Diabetes* 53(3),
      852-4.

[102] Mc Cartney, S. A., Vermi, W., Lonardi, S., Rossini, C., Otero, K., Calderon, B., Gilfil-
      lan, S., Diamond, M. S., Unanue, E. R., & Colonna, M. (2011). RNA sensor-induced
      type I IFN prevents diabetes caused by a beta cell-tropic virus in mice. *J Clin Invest.*

[103] Mena, I., Perry, C. M., Harkins, S., Rodriguez, F., Gebhard, J., & Whitton, J. L. (1999).
      The role of B lymphocytes in coxsackievirus B3 infection. *Am J Pathol.* 155(4), 1205-15.

[104] Moya-Suri, V., Schlosser, M., Zimmermann, K., Rjasanowski, I., Gurtler, L., & Mentel,
      R. (2005). Enterovirus RNA sequences in sera of schoolchildren in the general popu-

lation and their association with type 1diabetes-associated autoantibodies. *J Med Microbiol.* 54(Pt 9), 879-83.

[105] Muckelbauer, J. K., Kremer, M., Minor, I., Diana, G., Dutko, F. J., Groarke, J., Pevear, D. C., & Rossmann, M. G. (1995). The structure of coxsackievirus B3 at 3.5 A resolution. *Structure* 3(7), 653-67.

[106] Munakata, Y., Kodera, T., Saito, T., & Sasaki, T. (2005). Rheumatoid arthritis, type 1 diabetes, and Graves' disease after acute parvovirus B19 infection. *Lancet* 366(9487), 780.

[107] Nair, S., Leung, K. C., Rawlinson, W. D., Naing, Z., & Craig, M. E. (2010). Enterovirus infection induces cytokine and chemokine expression in insulin-producing cells. *J Med Virol.* 82(11), 1950-7.

[108] Nairn, C., Galbraith, D. N., Taylor, K. W., & Clements, G. B. (1999). Enterovirus variants in the serum of children at the onset of Type 1 diabetes mellitus. *Diabet Med.* 16(6), 509-13.

[109] Niklasson, B., Heller, K. E., Schonecker, B., Bildsoe, M., Daniels, T., Hampe, C. S., Widlund, P., Simonson, W. T., Schaefer, J. B., Rutledge, E., Bekris, L., Lindberg, A. M., Johansson, S., Ortqvist, E., Persson, B., & Lernmark, A. (2003). Development of type 1 diabetes in wild bank voles associated with islet autoantibodies and the novel ljungan virus. *Int J Exp Diabesity Res.* 4(1), 35-44.

[110] Niklasson, B., Samsioe, A., Blixt, M., Sandler, S., Sjoholm, A., Lagerquist, E., Lernmark, A., & Klitz, W. (2006). Prenatal viral exposure followed by adult stress produces glucose intolerance in a mouse model. *Diabetologia* 49(9), 2192-9.

[111] Nugent, C. I., Johnson, K. L., Sarnow, P., & Kirkegaard, K. (1999). Functional coupling between replication and packaging of poliovirus replicon RNA. *J Virol,* 73(1), 427-35.

[112] Numazaki, K., Goldman, H., Wong, I., & Wainberg, M. A. (1988). Viral infection of human fetal islets of Langerhans. Replication of human cytomegalovirus in cultured human fetal pancreatic islets. *Am J Clin Pathol.* 90(1), 52-7.

[113] O'Brayan, T. A., Beck, M. J., Demers, L. M., & Naides, S. J. (2005). Human parvovirus B19 infection in children with new onset Type 1 diabetes mellitus. *Diabet Med.* 22(12), 1778-9.

[114] Oikarinen, M., Tauriainen, S., Honkanen, T., Oikarinen, S., Vuori, K., Kaukinen, K., Rantala, I., Maki, M., & Hyoty, H. (2008). Detection of enteroviruses in the intestine of type 1 diabetic patients.*Clin Exp Immunol.* 151(1), 71-5.

[115] Oikarinen, S., Martiskainen, M., Tauriainen, S., Huhtala, H., Ilonen, J., Veijola, R., Simell, O., Knip, M., & Hyoty, H. (2011). Enterovirus RNA in blood is linked to the development of type 1 diabetes. *Diabetes* 60(1), 276-9.

[116] Oldstone, M. B., Nerenberg, M., Southern, P., Price, J., & Lewicki, H. (1991). Virus infection triggers insulin-dependent diabetes mellitus in a transgenic model: role of anti-self (virus) immune response. *Cell* 65(2), 319-31.

[117] Olsson, A., Johansson, U., Korsgren, O., & Frisk, G. (2005). Inflammatory gene expression in Coxsackievirus B-4infected human islets of Langerhans. *Biochem Biophys Res Commun* 330(2), 571-6.

[118] Ou, D., Mitchell, L. A., Metzger, D. L., Gillam, S., & Tingle, A. J. (2000). Cross-reactive rubella virus and glutamic acid decarboxylase (65 and 67) protein determinants recognised by T cells of patients with type I diabetes mellitus. *Diabetologia* 43(6), 750-62.

[119] Parkkonen, P., Hyoty, H., Koskinen, L., & Leinikki, P. (1992). Mumps virus infects beta cells in human fetal islet cell cultures upregulating the expression of HLA class I molecules. *Diabetologia* 35(1), 63-9.

[120] Ramondetti, F., Sacco, S., Comelli, M., Bruno, G., Falorni, A., Iannilli, A., D'Annunzio, G., Iafusco, D., Songini, M., Toni, S., Cherubini, V., & Carle, F. (2011). RIDI study group. Type 1 diabetes and measles, mumps and rubella chilhood infections within the Italian Insulin-dependent diabetes Regitstry. *Diabet Med*, 1464-5491.

[121] Rayfield, E. J., Kelly, K. J., & Yoon, J. W. (1986). Rubella virus-induced diabetes in the hamster. *Diabetes* 35(11), 1278-81.

[122] Richardson, S. J., Willcox, A., Bone, A. J., Foulis, A. K., & Morgan, N. G. (2009). The prevalence of enteroviral capsid protein vp1 immunostaining in pancreatic islets in human type 1 diabetes. *Diabetologia* 52(6), 1143-51.

[123] Richer, M. J., Lavallee, D. J., Shanina, I., & Horwitz, M. S. (2009). Toll-like receptor 3 signaling on macrophages is required for survival following coxsackievirus B4 infection. *PLoS One* 4(1), e4127.

[124] Roivainen, M., Rasilainen, S., Ylipaasto, P., Nissinen, R., Ustinov, J., Bouwens, L., Eizirik, D. L., Hovi, T., & Otonkoski, T. (2000). Mechanisms of coxsackievirus-induced damage to human pancreatic beta-cells. *J Clin Endocrinol Metab* 85(1), 432-40.

[125] Salminen, K. K., Vuorinen, T., Oikarinen, S., Helminen, M., Simell, S., Knip, M., Ilonen, J., Simell, O., & Hyoty, H. (2004). Isolation of enterovirus strains from children with preclinical Type 1 diabetes. *Diabet Med.* 21(2), 156-64.

[126] Sano, H., Terasaki, J., Tsutsumi, C., Imagawa, A., & Hanafusa, T. (2008). A case of fulminant type 1 diabetes mellitus after influenza B infection. *Diabetes Res Clin Pract.* 79(3), e, 8-9.

[127] Sarmiento, L., Cabrera-Rode, E., Lekuleni, L., Cuba, I., Molina, G., Fonseca, M., Heng-Hung, L., Borroto, A. D., Gonzalez, P., Mas-Lago, P., & Diaz-Horta, O. (2007). Occurrence of enterovirus RNA in serum of children with newly diagnosed type 1 diabetes and islet cell autoantibody-positive subjects in a population with a low incidence of type 1 diabetes. *Autoimmunity* 40(7), 540-5.

[128] Sato, K., Inaba, Y., Shinozaki, T., Fujii, R., & Matumoto, M. (1981). Isolation of human rotavirus in cell cultures: brief report. *Arch Virol.* 69(2), 155-60.

[129] Sauter, P., Lobert, P. E., Lucas, B., Varela-Calvino, R., Alm, G., Wattre, P., & Hober, D. (2007). Role of the capsid protein VP4 in the plasma-dependent enhancement of the Coxsackievirus B4E2infection of human peripheral blood cells. *Virus Res.* 125(2), 183-90.

[130] Sauter, P., Chehadeh, W., Lobert, P. E., Lazrek, M., Goffard, A., Soumillon, M., Calo-one, D., Vantyghem, M. C., Weill, J., Fajardy, I., Alm, G., Lucas, B., & Hober, D. (2008). A part of the VP4 capsid protein exhibited by coxsackievirus B4 E2 is the target of antibodies contained in plasma from patients with type 1 diabetes. *J Med Virol.* 80(5), 866-78.

[131] Sauter, P., & Hober, D. (2009). Mechanisms and results of the antibody-dependent enhancement of viral infections and role in the pathogenesis of coxsackievirus B-induced diseases. *Microbes Infect.* 11(4), 443-51.

[132] Schulte, B. M., Bakkers, J., Lanke, K. H., Melchers, W. J., Westerlaken, C., Allebes, W., Aanstoot, H. J., Bruining, G. J., Adema, G. J., Van Kuppeveld, F. J., & Galama, J. M. (2010). Detection of enterovirus RNA in peripheral blood mononuclear cells of type 1 diabetic patients beyond the stage of acute infection. *Viral Immunol.* 23(1), 99-104.

[133] See, D. M., & Tilles, J. G. (1995). Pathogenesis of virus-induced diabetes in mice. *J Infect Dis.* 171(5), 1131-8.

[134] Serreze, D. V., Ottendorfer, E. W., Ellis, T. M., Gauntt, C. J., & Atkinson, M. A. (2000). Acceleration of type 1 diabetes by a coxsackievirus infection requires a preexisting critical mass of autoreactive T-cells in pancreatic islets. *Diabetes* 49(5), 708-11.

[135] Shimada, A., & Maruyama, T. (2004). Encephalomyocarditis-virus-induced diabetes model resembles "fulminant" type 1 diabetes in humans. *Diabetologia* 47(10), 1854-5.

[136] Singer, K. H., & Haynes, B. F. (1987). Epithelial-thymocyte interactions in human thymus. *Hum Immunol* 20(2), 127-44.

[137] Smelt, M. J., Faas, M. M., de Haan, B. J., Hofstede, J., Cheung, C. W., van der Iest, H., de Haan, A., & de Vos, P. (2010). Rat pancreatic beta cells and cytomegalovirus infection. *Pancreas* 39(1), 47-56.

[138] Smyth, M.S., & Martin, J.H. (2002). Picornavirus uncoating. *Mol Pathol.* 55(4), 214-9.

[139] Soltesz, G., Patterson, C. C., & Dahlquist, G. (2007). Worldwide childhood type 1 diabetes incidence--what can we learn from epidemiology? *Pediatr Diabetes 8 Suppl.*, 6, 6-14.

[140] Stark, G.R. (2007). How cells respond to interferons revisited: from early history to current complexity. *Cytokine Growth Factor Rev.* 18(5-6),, 419 -423 .

[141] Stene, L. C., Oikarinen, S., Hyoty, H., Barriga, K. J., Norris, J. M., Klingensmith, G., Hutton, J. C., Erlich, H. A., Eisenbarth, G. S., & Rewers, M. (2010). Enterovirus infec-

tion and progression from islet autoimmunity to type 1 diabetes: the Diabetes and Autoimmunity Study in the Young (DAISY). *Diabetes* 59(12), 3174-80.

[142]	Stewart, T. A., Hultgren, B., Huang, X., Pitts-Meek, S., Hully, J., & Mac, Lachlan. N. J. (1993). Induction of type I diabetes by interferon-alpha in transgenic mice. *Science* 260(5116), 1942-6.

[143]	Sutkowski, N., Conrad, B., Thorley-Lawson, D. A., & Huber, B. T. (2001). Epstein-Barr virus transactivates the human endogenous retrovirus HERV-K18 that encodes a superantigen. *Immunity* 15(4), 579-89.

[144]	Tai, A. K., Luka, J., Ablashi, D., & Huber, B. T. (2009). HHV-6A infection induces expression of HERV-K18encoded superantigen. *J Clin Virol.* 46(1), 47-8.

[145]	Takada, A., & Kawaoka, Y. (2003). Antibody-dependent enhancement of viral infection: molecular mechanisms and in vivo implications. *Rev Med Virol.* 13(6), 387-98.

[146]	Takeuchi, O., & Akira, S. (2008). MDA5/RIG-I and virus recognition. *Curr Opin Immunol.* 20(1), 17-22.

[147]	Taniguchi, T., Okazaki, K., Okamoto, M., Seko, S., Nagashima, K., Yamada, Y., Iwakura, T., & Seino, Y. (2005). Autoantibodies against the exocrine pancreas in fulminant type 1 diabetes. *Pancreas* 30(2), 191-2.

[148]	Tapia, G., Cinek, O., Rasmussen, T., Grinde, B., Stene, L. C., & Ronningen, K. S. (2011a). Longitudinal study of parechovirus infection in infancy and risk of repeated positivity for multiple islet autoantibodies: the MIDIA study. *Pediatr Diabetes* 12(1), 58-62.

[149]	Tapia, G., Cinek, O., Rasmussen, T., Witso, E., Grinde, B., Stene, L. C., & Ronningen, K. S. (2011b). Human enterovirus RNA in monthly fecal samples and islet autoimmunity in Norwegian children with high genetic risk for type 1 diabetes: the MIDIA study. *Diabetes Care* 34(1), 151-5.

[150]	The Juvenile Diabetes Research Foundation: The Network for Pancreatic Organ Donors with Diabetes. www.jdrfnpod.org.

[151]	Tian, J., Lehmann, P. V., & Kaufman, D. L. (1994). T cell cross-reactivity between coxsackievirus and glutamate decarboxylase is associated with a murine diabetes susceptibility allele. *J Exp Med.* 180(5), 1979-84.

[152]	Tisch, R., Yang, X. D., Singer, S. M., Liblau, R. S., Fugger, L., & Mc Devitt, H. O. (1993). Immune response to glutamic acid decarboxylase correlates with insulitis in non-obese diabetic mice. *Nature* 366(6450), 72-5.

[153]	Toniolo, A., Onodera, T., Yoon, J. W., & Notkins, A. L. (1980). Induction of diabetes by cumulative environmental insults from viruses and chemicals. *Nature* 288(5789), 383-5.

[154] Toniolo, A., Maccari, G., Federico, G., Salvatoni, A., Bianchi, G., & Baj, A. (2010). Are enterovirus infections linked to the early stages of type 1 diabetes? *American Society for Microbiology Meeting, San Diego, CA.*

[155] Tracy, S., Drescher, K. M., Chapman, N. M., Kim, K. S., Carson, S. D., Pirruccello, S., Lane, P. H., Romero, J. R., & Leser, J. S. (2002). Toward testing the hypothesis that group B coxsackieviruses (CVB) trigger insulin-dependent diabetes: inoculating non-obese diabetic mice with CVB markedly lowers diabetes incidence. *J Virol.* 76(23), 12097-111.

[156] Tracy, S., & Drescher, K. M. (2007). Coxsackievirus infections and NOD mice: relevant models of protection from, and induction of, type 1 diabetes. *Ann N Y Acad Sci.,* 1103, 143-51.

[157] Tracy, S., Drescher, K. M., Jackson, J. D., Kim, K., & Kono, K. (2010). Enteroviruses, type 1 diabetes and hygiene: a complex relationship. *Rev Med Virol.* 20(2), 106-16.

[158] Tracy, S., Drescher, K. M., & Chapman, N. M. (2011). Enteroviruses and type 1 diabetes. *Diabetes metab Res rev.* 27(8), 820-3.

[159] Tuthill, T. J., Groppelli, E., Hogle, J. M., & Rowlands, D. J. (2010). Picornaviruses. *Curr Top Microbiol Immunol,* 343, 43-89.

[160] van Belle, T.L., Coppieters, K.T., & von Herrath, M.G. (2011). Type 1 diabetes: etiology, immunology, and therapeutic strategies. *Physiol Rev.* 91(1), 79-118.

[161] van der Werf, N., Hillebrands, J. L., Klatter, F. A., Bos, I., Bruggeman, C. A., & Rozing, J. (2003). Cytomegalovirus infection modulates cellular immunity in an experimental model for autoimmune diabetes. *Clin Dev Immunol.* 10(2-4), 153-60.

[162] van der Werf, N., Kroese, F. G. M., Rozing, J., & Hillebrands, J. L. (2007). Viral infections as potential triggers of type 1 diabetes. *Diabetes Metab Res Rev.* (23), 169-83.

[163] Vehik, K., & Dabelea, D. (2011). The changing epidemiology of type 1 diabetes: why is it going through the roof? *Diabetes Metab Res Rev.* 27(1), 3-13.

[164] Vigeant, P., Menard, H. A., & Boire, G. (1994). Chronic modulation of the autoimmune response following parvovirus B19 infection. *J Rheumatol* 21(6), 1165-7.

[165] Viskari, H., Paronen, J., Keskinen, P., Simell, S., Zawilinska, B., Zgorniak-Nowosielska, I., Korhonen, S., Ilonen, J., Simell, O., Haapala, A. M., Knip, M., & Hyoty, H. (2003). Humoral beta-cell autoimmunity is rare in patients with the congenital rubella syndrome. *Clin Exp Immunol.* 133(3), 378-83.

[166] von, Poblotzki. A., Gerdes, C., Reischl, U., Wolf, H., & Modrow, S. (1996). Lymphoproliferative responses after infection with human parvovirus B19. *J Virol* 70(10), 7327-30.

[167] Vuorinen, T., Nikolakaros, G., Simell, O., Hyypia, T., & Vainionpaa, R. (1992). Mumps and Coxsackie B3 virus infection of human fetal pancreatic islet-like cell clusters. *Pancreas* 7(4), 460-4.

[168] Wang, J. P., Asher, D. R., Chan, M., Kurt-Jones, E. A., & Finberg, R. W. (2007). Cutting Edge: Antibody-mediated TLR7dependent recognition of viral RNA. *J Immunol.* 178(6), 3363-7.

[169] Wessely, R., Klingel, K., Knowlton, K. U., & Kandolf, R. (2001). Cardioselective infection with coxsackievirus B3 requires intact type I interferon signaling: implications for mortality and early viral replication. *Circulation* 103(5), 756-61.

[170] Wicker, L. S., Todd, J. A., & Peterson, L. B. (1995). Genetic control of autoimmune diabetes in the NOD mouse. *Annu Rev Immunol.*, 13, 179-200.

[171] Yin, H., Berg, A. K., Tuvemo, T., & Frisk, G. (2002). Enterovirus RNA is found in peripheral blood mononuclear cells in a majority of type 1 diabetic children at onset. *Diabetes* 51(6), 1964-71.

[172] Ylipaasto, P., Klingel, K., Lindberg, A. M., Otonkoski, T., Kandolf, R., Hovi, T., & Roivainen, M. (2004). Enterovirus infection in human pancreatic islet cells, islet tropism in vivo and receptor involvement in cultured islet beta cells. *Diabetologia* 47(2), 225-39.

[173] Ylipaasto, P., Kutlu, B., Rasilainen, S., Rasschaert, J., Salmela, K., Teerijoki, H., Korsgren, O., Lahesmaa, R., Hovi, T., Eizirik, D. L., Otonkoski, T., & Roivainen, M. (2005). Global profiling of coxsackievirus- and cytokine-induced gene expression in human pancreatic islets. *Diabetologia* 48(8), 1510-22.

[174] Yoon, J. W., Onodera, T., & Notkins, A. L. (1978). Virus-induced diabetes mellitus. XV. Beta cell damage and insulin-dependent hyperglycemia in mice infected with coxsackie virus B4. *J Exp Med.* 148(4), 1068-80.

[175] Yoon, J. W., Austin, M., Onodera, T., & Notkins, A. L. (1979). Isolation of a virus from the pancreas of a child with diabetic ketoacidosis. *N Engl J Med.* 300(21), 1173-9.

[176] Yoon, J. W., & Jun, H. S. (2006). Viruses cause type 1 diabetes in animals. *Ann N Y Acad Sci.*, 1079, 138-46.

[177] Zanone, M. M., Favaro, E., Quadri, R., Miceli, I., Giaretta, F., Romagnoli, R., David, E., Perin, P. C., Salizzoni, M., & Camussi, G. (2010). Association of cytomegalovirus infections with recurrence of humoral and cellular autoimmunity to islet autoantigens and of type 1 diabetes in a pancreas transplanted patient. *Transpl Int.* 23(3), 333-7.

[178] Zipris, D., Hillebrands, J. L., Welsh, R. M., Rozing, J., Xie, J. X., Mordes, J. P., Greiner, D. L., & Rossini, A. A. (2003). Infections that induce autoimmune diabetes in BBDR rats modulate CD4+CD25+ T cell populations. *J Immunol.* 170(7), 3592-602.

[179] Zipris, D., Lien, E., Nair, A., Xie, J. X., Greiner, D. L., Mordes, J. P., & Rossini, A. A. (2007). TLR9signaling pathways are involved in Kilham rat virus-induced autoimmune diabetes in the biobreeding diabetes-resistant rat. *J Immunol.* 178(2), 693-701.

Genetics

Chapter 3

Genes Involved in Type 1 Diabetes

Marina Bakay, Rahul Pandey and
Hakon Hakonarson

Additional information is available at the end of the chapter

1. Introduction

The prevalence of diabetes is increasing worldwide and to date it impacts the lives of approx-imately 200 million people (Steyn et al., 2009). It is estimated that by 2030, there will be 439 million adults affected by diabetes (International Diabetes Federation/diabetes prevalence: www.idf.org). Type 1 diabetes (T1D) represents approximately 10% of these patients and is most prevalent in populations of European ancestry, where there is ample evidence of increased annual incidence during the past five decades (Onkamo et al., 1999; EURODIAB ACE Study Group, 2000).

T1D is a complex trait that results from the interplay between environmental and genetic factors. Much evidence supports a strong genetic component associated with T1D. The epidemiological data showing differences in geographic prevalence is one clear indicator, with populations of European ancestry having the highest presentation rate. T1D has high con-cordance among monozygotic twins (33 to 42%) (Redondo et al., 2001) and runs strongly in families with sibling risk being approximately 10 times greater than in the general population (Clayton, 2009); this is in clear contrast to the "less genetic" type 2 diabetes, where the sibling risk ratio is relatively modest at 3.5 (Rich, 1990).

T1D develops at all ages and occurs through the autoimmune destruction of pancreatic β-cells with resulting lack of insulin production. The immune system participates in β-cell destruction through several of its components including natural killer (NK) cells, B lymphocytes, macro-phages, dendritic cells (DC), and antigen-presenting cells (APCs). Studies in human and animal models have shown that both innate and adaptive immune responses participate in disease pathogenesis, possibly reflecting the multifactorial nature of this autoimmune disorder.

In this review, we provide an update on genome-wide association studies (GWAS) discoveries to date and discuss the latest associated regions added to the growing repertoire of gene networks predisposing to T1D.

2. Genetic component in Type 1 diabetes

2.1. Before genome-wide association studies

Historically, prior to GWAS, only six loci had been fully established to be associated with T1D. The human leukocyte antigen (HLA) region on chromosome 6p21 was the first known candidate to be strongly associated with T1D in 1970s (Singal & Blajchman, 1973; Nerup et al., 1974; Cudworth & Woodrow, 1975). This cluster of homologous cell-surface proteins is divided into class I (A, B, C) and class II (DP, DQ, RD). The HLA genes encode highly polymorphic proteins, which are essential in self versus non-self immune recognition. The class I molecules are ubiquitously expressed and present intracellular antigen to CD8+ T cells. Class II molecules are expressed mainly on professional APCs: DCs, macrophages, B-lymphocytes and thymus epithelium. Class II molecules are composed of A and B chains, and present antigens to CD4+ T cells, which promote inflammation by secreting cytokines upon recognition of their specific targets. Approximately half of the genetic risk for T1D is conferred by the genomic region harboring the HLA class II genes primarily HLA-DRB1, -DQA1 and -DQB1 genes). In 1984, insulin (INS) gene encoded on chromosome 11p15 was identified as second loci linked with T1D (Bell et al., 1984). In 1996, the cytotoxic T-lymphocyte-associated protein 4 (CTLA4) gene encoded on chromosome 2q33 was recognized as third loci (Nistico et al., 1996). In 2004, a protein tyrosine phosphatase, non-receptor type 22 (PTPN22) gene encoded on chromosome 1p13, was found to be associated with susceptibility to T1D in another case-control study (Bottini et al., 2004). Vella et al., 2005 reported interleukin 2 receptor alpha (IL2RA) gene as fifth T1D loci on chromosome 10p15. In 2006, Smyth et al. identified the interferon-induced with helicase C domain 1 (IFIH1) gene on chromosome 2q24.3 as the sixth gene to be strongly associated with T1D.

2.2. GWAS of T1D

The advent of GWAS in the mid-2000s has changed the situation dramatically, increasing the pace and efficiency of discovery for the T1D associated loci, by a factor of ten. The critical platform for this work was laid by the HapMap project (International HapMap Consortium, 2003, 2005). The GWAS approach has been made possible by the development of high-density genotyping arrays. The genome is laid out in discrete linkage disequilibrium (LD) blocks with limited haplotype diversity within each of these blocks. Therefore, a minimal set of single nucleotide polymorphisms (SNPs) can detect almost all common haplotypes present, thus improving genotyping accuracy and reducing cost.

The first full-scale GWAS for T1D were published in 2007 by our group (Hakonarson et al., 2007) and The Wellcome Trust Case-Control Consortium (WTCCC, 2007). We examined a large pediatric cohort of European descent using the Illumina HumanHap 550 BeadChip platform.

The design involved 561 cases, 1,143 controls and 467 triads in the discovery stage, followed by a replication effort in 939 nuclear families. In addition to finding the "usual" suspects, including an impressive 392 SNPs capturing the very strong association across the major histocompatibility complex (MHC), we identified significant association with variation at the KIAA0350 gene, which we replicated in an additional cohort. The WTCCC study investigated seven common complex diseases including T1D by genotyping 2,000 cases and 3,000 controls with ~500,000 SNPs using the Affymetrix GeneChip, and reported a number of novel T1D loci, including the KIAA0350 genomic region (WTCCC, 2007). Todd et al., 2007 confirmed these findings, using 4,000 cases, 5,000 controls and 3,000 T1D families as well as association reported in the WTCCC study to the 12q13 region. In a separate effort we fast-tracked 24 SNPs at 23 distinct loci from our original study and established association to the 12q13 region with a combined P-value of 9.13×10^{-10} (Hakonarson et al., 2008); this was the same locus as reported by the WTCCC and Todd et al., 2007. The 12q13 region harbors several genes, including ERBB3, RAB5B, SUOX, RPS26 and CDK2. However, the causative variants at this locus remain unknown. Concannon et al., 2008 reported an association between SNP at the UBASH3A locus on 21q22.3 and T1D by using SNP genotyping data from a linkage study of affected sib pairs in nearly 2,500 multiplex families, a finding also corroborated by our efforts as well as association to the BACH2 gene (Grant et al., 2009).

2.3. Meta-analyses of T1D GWAS datasets

In order to get the most from GWAS and to increase the statistical power, several independent research groups carried out meta-analyses using datasets from different investigative groups. Cooper et al., 2008 performed the first meta-analysis by using T1D datasets from the WTCCC, 2007 and the Genetics of Kidneys in Diabetes (GoKind) study (Mueller et al, 2006; Manolio et al., 2007), and confirmed associations for PTPN22, CTLA4, MHC, IL2RA, 12q13, 12q24, CLEC16A and PTPN2. The SNPs with lowest nominal P-values were taken forward for further genotyping in an additional British cohort of 6,000 cases, 7,000 controls and 2,800 families. As a result, the IL2-IL21 association strengthened further and they found strong evidence for four additional loci: BACH2; a 10p15 region harboring the protein kinase C, theta gene (PRKCQ); a 15q24 region harboring nine genes including cathepsin H (CTSH) and a 22q13 region harboring tumor necrosis factor related protein 6 (C1QTNF6). Additional studies are required to elucidate the culprit genes and their mechanism at the 15q24 and 22q13 loci.

Barrett et al., 2009 meta-analysis uncovered in excess of 40 loci, including 18 novel regions, plus they confirmed a number of previously reported (Smyth et al., 2008; Fung et al., 2009; Cooper et al., 2009). The study included samples from WTCCC, 20070, the GoKind study (Mueller et al., 2006) and controls and family sets from Type 1 Diabetes Genetics Consortium (T1DGC). The meta-analysis observed association to 1q32.1 (which harbors the immunoregulatory interleukin genes IL10, IL19 and IL20), 9p24.2 contains only Glis family zinc finger protein 3 (GLIS3; first suggested by us in Grant et al., 2009), 12p13.31 which harbors a number of immunoregulatory genes including CD69 and 16p11.2 harboring IL27. These findings were further supported by our *in silico* replication efforts (Qu et al., 2010).

To identify additional genetic loci for T1D susceptibility, we examined associations in the largest meta-analysis to date between the disease and ~2.54 million genotyped and imputed SNPs in a combined cohort of 9,934 cases and 16,956 controls (Bradfield et al., 2011). Targeted follow-up of 53 SNPs in 1,120 affected trios uncovered three new loci associated with T1D that reached genome wide significance. The most significantly associated SNP (rs539514, $P = 5.66\times10^{-11}$) resided in an intronic region of the LMO7 (LIM domain only 7) gene on 13q22. The second most significantly associated SNP (rs478222, $P = 3.50\times10^{-9}$) resided in an intronic region of the EFR3B (protein EFR3 homolog B) gene on 2p23; however the region of linkage disequilibrium is approximately 800kb and harbors additional multiple genes, including NCOA1, C2orf79, CENPO, ADCY3, DNAJC27, POMC, and DNMT3A. The third most significantly associated SNP (rs924043, $P = 8.06\times10^{-9}$) was in an intergenic region on 6q27, where the region of association is approximately 900kb and harbors additional genes including WDR27, C6orf120, PHF10, TCTE3, C6orf208, LOC154449, DLL1, FAM120B, PSMB1, TBP and PCD2. These latest associations add to the growing repertoire of gene networks predisposing to T1D. Table 1 summarizes all T1D associated loci reported to date.

Reference	Sample Size	Replication Sample Size	Ethnic Group	Study Type	Main Findings
Hakonarson et al., 2007	467 trios, 561 cases, 1,143 controls	2,350 individuals in 549 families; 390 trios	European ancestry	GWAS	HLA-DRB1, HLA-DQA2, CLEC16A, INS, PTPN22
WTCCC 2007	1,963 cases, 2,938 controls	see Todd et al., 2007	European, British	GWAS	HLA-DRB1, INS, CTLA4, PTPN22, IL2RA, IFIH1, PPARG, KCNJ11, TCF7L2
Todd et al., 2007	see WTCCC 2007	2997 trios, 4,000 cases, 5,000 controls	European British	GWAS	PHTF1-PTPN22, ERBB3, CLEC16A, C12orf30
Hakonarson et al., 2008	467 trios, 561 cases, 1,143 controls	549 families, 364 trios	European ancestry	GWAS	SUOX - IKZF4
Concannon et al., 2008	2,496 families	2,214 trios, 7,721 cases, 9,679 controls	European ancestry	GWAS	INS, IFIH1, CLEC16A, UBASH3A
Cooper et al., 2008	3,561 cases, 4,646 controls	6,225 cases, 6,946 controls, 3,064 trios	European ancestry	GWAS meta-analysis	PTPN22, CTLA4, HLA, IL2RA, ERRB3, C12orf30, CLEC16A, PTPN2
Grant et al., 2009	563 cases, 1,146 controls, 483 case-parents trios	636 families, 3,303 cases, 4,673 controls	European ancestry	GWAS	EDG7, BACH2, GLIS3, UBASH3A, RASGRP1

Reference	Sample Size	Replication Sample Size	Ethnic Group	Study Type	Main Findings
Awata et al., 2009	735 cases, 621 controls	-	Japanese	TaqMan genotyping	ERBB3, CLEC16A
Zoledziewska et al., 2009	1037 cases, 1706 controls	-	European, Sardinian	TaqMan genotyping	CLEC16A
Fung et al., 2009	8010 cases, 9733 controls	-	European, British	TaqMan genotyping	STAT4, STAT3, ERAP1, TNFAIP3, KIF5A/PIP4K2C
Wu et al., 2009	205 cases, 422 controls	-	Han Chinese	TaqMan genotyping	CLEC16A
Barrett et al., 2009	7,514 cases, 9,045 controls	4,267 cases, 4,670 controls, 4,342 trios	European	GWAS meta-analysis	MHC, PTPN22, INS, C10orf59, SH2B3, ERBB3, CLEC16A, CTLA4, PTPN2, IL2RA, IL27, C6orf173, IL2, ORMDL3, GLIS3, CD69, IL10, IFIH1, UBASH3A, COBL, BACH2, CTSH, PRKCQ, C1QTNF6, PGM1
Wallace et al., 2010	7,514 cases, 9,045 controls	4,840 cases, 2,670 controls, 4,152 trios	European ancestry	GWAS meta-analysis	DLK1, TYK2
Wang et al., 2010	989 cases, 6197 controls	-	European ancestry	GWAS	PTPN22, IL10, IFIH1, KIAA0746, BACH2, C6orf173, TAGAP, GLIS3, L2R, INS, ERBB3, C14orf181, IL27, PRKD2, HERC2, CLEC16A, IFNG, IL26,
Reddy et al., 2011	1434 cases, 1864 controls	-	European ancestry, southeast USA	TaqMan genotyping	PTPN22, INS, IFIH1, SH2B3, ERBB3, CTLA4, C14orf181, CTSH, CLEC16A, CD69, ITPR3, C6orf173, SKAP2, PRKCQ, RNLS, IL27, SIRPG, CTRB2
Bradfield et al., 2011	9,934 cases, 16,956 controls	1,120 trios	European ancestry	GWAS meta-analysis	LMO7, EFR3B, 6q27, TNFRSF11B,

Reference	Sample Size	Replication Sample Size	Ethnic Group	Study Type	Main Findings
					LOC100128081, FOSL2
Asad et al., 2012	424 families, 3078 cases, 1363 controls	-	European, Scandinavians	Genotyping and sequencing	HTR1A, RFN180
Huang et al., 2012	16,179 individuals	-	European ancestry	Genomes-based imputation	CUX2, IL2RA

Table 1. T1D susceptibility loci identified to date.

2.4. Immune components in T1D

The immune system is well organized and well regulated with a basic function of protecting the host against pathogens. This places the immune system in a vital position between healthy and diseased states of the host. Its protective task is regulated by a complex regulatory mechanism involving a diverse army of cells and molecules of humoral and cellular factors working in concert to protect the body against invaders. The human immune system has two components: innate and adaptive. Innate immunity is comprised of physical, chemical, and microbiological barriers to the entry of antigen, and the elements of immune system (DC, macrophages, mast cells, NK cells, neutrophils, monocytes, complements, cytokines and acute phase proteins), which provide immediate host defense. Adaptive immunity is the hallmark of the immune system of higher animals with T and B cells as the key cellular players that provide more specific life-long immunity.

In T1D this system breaks down: insulin-producing β-cells are subjected to specific attack by the host immune system. To better understand the etiology of T1D, a plethora of research has been done to link the systematic destruction of β-cells and the role of the immune system. Linkage studies in 1970s revealed MHC as the first key contributor to T1D susceptibility. Further linkage analysis and candidate gene association studies revealed additional loci associated with T1D. Starting in 2007, GWAS have increased the number of loci be associated with T1D to almost 60. In Figure 1 we present 59 T1D susceptibility loci as where we have classified them into loci harboring non-immune (14) vs. immune (45) genes. Functional aspects of some genes are discussed below.

The complex crosstalk between innate and adaptive immune cells has major impact on the pathogenesis and development of T1D as illustrated in Figure 2. The initiation phase (Phase I) of T1D development takes place in the pancreas where conventional dendritic cells (cDCs) capture and process β-cell antigens. Apoptosis ('natural cell death') or viral infection can lead to β-cell death. Antiviral responses are mediated by invariant natural killer T (iNKT) cells; crossplay between iNKT and plasmacytoid DCs (pDCs) controls viral replication thus prevents subsequent inflammation, tissue damage, and downregulating T1D pathogenesis.

Migration of activated cDCs to the draining lymph node primes pathogenic islet antigen-specific T cells. This activation is promoted by macrophages through IL12 secretion. B cells present β-cell antigen to diabetogenic T cells and secrete autoantibodies in response. The activation of islet antigen-specific T cells can be inhibited by cDCs through engagement of programmed cell death ligand 1 (PDL1). The expansion phase (Phase II): iNKT cells can further promote the recruitment of tolerogenic cDCs and pDCs. These DCs promote expansion of regulatory T (TReg) cells through the production of indoleamine 2,3-dioxygenase (IDO), IL10, transforming growth factor-β (TGFβ) and inducible T cell co-stimulator ligand (ICOSL). Phase III: In the pancreas, β-cell can be killed by diabetogenic T cells and NK cells through the release of interferon-γ (IFNγ), granzymes and perforin, as well as by macrophages through the production of tumour necrosis factor (TNF), IL-1β and nitric oxide (NO). IL12 produced by cDCs sustains the effector functions of activated diabetogenic T cells and NK cells. TReg cells that inhibit diabetogenic T cells and innate immune cells through IL10 and TGFβ can prevent β-cell damage. Tolerogenic pDCs stimulated by iNKT cells could also control diabetogenic T cells through IDO production. Lastly, β-cells can inhibit diabetogenic T cells by expressing PDL1 and escape the cell death.

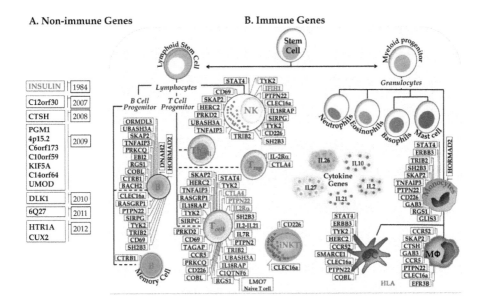

Figure 1. Immune and Non-immune T1D genes are depicted in a concept map representing the components of the immune system. The discovery of T1D susceptibility genes started as early as 1974 with just six genes identified by 2006 shown in red. The advent of GWAS led to flurry of novel genes associated with T1D reaching the excess of 40 by 2009 and almost 60 by 2012.

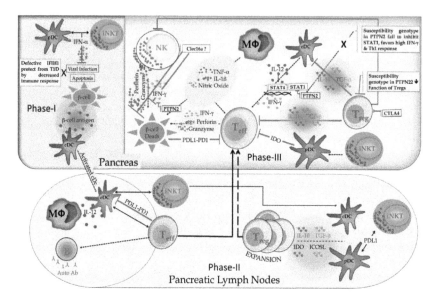

Figure 2. Pathogenesis model of T1D involves complex interactions between innate and adaptive immune cell types.

2.5. CLEC16A (16p13)

The C-type lectin domain family 16, member A (CLEC16A) gene encodes protein with C-type lectin domain structure, which makes it potentially related to the immune response (Robinson et al., 2006). It is established that C-type lectins function both as adhesion and pathogen recognition receptors (PPRs) (Cambi & Figdor, 2003). In addition, CLEC16A is almost exclusively expressed in immune cells including DCs, B-lymphocytes and NK cells. Our 2007 GWAS in a large pediatric cohort of European descent identified CLEC16A as a novel T1D susceptibility gene within a 233-kb linkage disequilibrium block on chromosome 16p13. Three common non-coding variants of the CLEC16A gene (rs2903692, rs725613 and rs17673553) reached genome-wide significance for association with T1D (Hakonarson et al., 2007). Subsequent replication studies in an independent cohort confirmed the association. Importantly, the allele of CLEC16A linked to protection from T1D was also associated with higher levels of CLEC16A expression in NK cells (Hakonarson et al., 2007).

The 2007 WTCCC study independently discovered CLEC16A (formally known as KIAA0350) as a T1D susceptibility locus associated with the non-coding variant rs12708716. This finding was confirmed immediately for T1D in populations of European descent (Todd et al., 2007, Cooper et al., 2008). To date, several SNPs (rs2903692, rs17673553, rs725613, rs12708716, rs12921922, rs12931878) within the CLEC16A gene have been reported to be associated with T1D in several populations: Sardinian (Zoledziewska et al., 2009), Spanish (Martinez et al., 2010), southeast USA (Reddy et al., 2011), Chinese (Wu et al., 2009; Sang et al., 2012), and

Japanese (Yamashita et al., 2011). Recently CLEC16A was also associated with adult-onset of autoimmune diabetes (Howson et al., 2011).

Several GWAS in different autoimmune diseases such as multiple sclerosis (MS) (Zuvich, 2011; Nischwitz et al., 2011), Addison's disease (Skinningsrud et al., 2008), systemic lupus erythematosus (SLE) (Gateva et al., 2009; Zhang et al., 2011), Celiac disease (Dubois et al., 2010), Crohn's disease (Márquez et al., 2009), selective immunoglobulin A deficiency (Jagielska et al., 2012), alopecia areata (Jagielska et al., 2012), rheumatoid arthritis (Martinez et al., 2010) and primary biliary cirrhosis (Mells et al., 2011; Hirschfield et al., 2012) also demonstrated association of the 16p13 loci with disease risk, implying that the 16p13 region contains a key regulator of the self-reactive immune response.

Recently, Davison et al., 2012 reported intron 19 of the CLEC16A gene behaves as a regulatory sequence, which affects the expression of a neighboring gene dexamethasone-induced (DEXI). While it is clear that intron 19 of CLEC16A is highly enriched for transcription-factor-binding events, more functional studies are needed to advance from GWAS to candidate causal genes and their biological functions.

To find causal variant of CLEC16A gene we sequenced the 16p13 region in 96 T1D patients and found 10 new non-synonymous SNPs resulting in one stop-codon, two splice site mutations, and 7 amino acid changes (unpublished data). The studies are under way to examine if these changes are correlated with CLEC16A expression and if these SPNs are present in control group.

Little is yet proven about CLEC16A functions. Kim et al., 2010 characterized ema as an endosomal membrane protein is required for endosomal trafficking and promotes endosomal maturation. Expression of human orthologue of ema 'CLEC16A' rescued the Drosophila mutant demonstrating conserved function of the protein. A recent study by the same group also reported its requirement for the growth of autophagosomes and proposed that the Golgi is a membrane source for autophagosomal growth, and that ema facilitates this process (Kim et al., 2012). Expression of CLEC16A rescued the autophagosome size defect in the ema mutant, suggesting that regulation of autophagosome morphogenesis may be one of the fundamental functions of CLEC16A. Another recent study elucidated the dynamic expression changes and localization of CLEC16A in lipopolysaccharide (LPS) induced neuroinflammatory processes in adult rats. CLEC16A expression was strongly induced in active astrocytes in inflamed cerebral cortex. *In vitro* studies indicated that the up-regulation of CLEC16A might be involved in astrocyte activation following LPS challenge (Wu et al., 2012).

2.6. Other novel T1D susceptibility loci (2011-2012)

In our latest effort to identify additional genetic loci for T1D, we examined associations in the largest meta-analysis to date between T1D and ~2.54 million SNPs in a combined cohort of 9,934 cases and 16,956 controls. Targeted follow-up of 53 SNPs in 1,120 affected trios uncovered three novel loci associated with T1D that reached genome-wide significance (Bradfield et al., 2011).

LMO7 (13q22): The most significantly associated SNP (rs539514, $P = 5.66 \times 10^{-11}$) resides in an intronic region of the LMO7 (LIM domain only 7) gene on 13q22 (Bradfield et al., 2011). LMO7 is a multi-domain mammalian protein with a calponin homology (CH) domain, a discs-large homologous regions (DHR) domain, and a LIM domain. Proteins of this family are involved in protein-protein interactions, regulation of cell adhesion and signaling (Ooshio et al., 2004; Yamada et al., 2004). The expression of LMO7 is cell type specific (Furuya et al., 2002; Kang et al., 2000; Lindvall et al., 2005; Bradfield et al., 2011; Rozenblum et al., 2002; Sasaki et al., 2003) and is essential for the development of muscle and heart tissues. Mice with homozygous deletions of LMO7 display retinal, muscular, and growth retardation (Semenova et al., 2003). LMO7 is upregulated in multiple cancers, especially at the metastatic stage; however under normal conditions its expression is low and limited to very few tissues (Furuya et al., 2002; Kang et al., 2000; Sasaki et al., 2003; Perou et al., 2000). In cultured rat ascites hepatoma cells, the upregulation of LMO7 correlates with the ability of transforming growth factor β (TGFβ) to enhance the invasiveness of these cells (Nakamura et al., 2005). Recent GWAS meta-analysis by Bradfield et al., 2011 identified LMO7 association with T1D. Although the function of LMO7 does not clearly relate to the etiology of T1D, LMO7 is expressed in pancreatic islets and thus is a possible biological candidate at this locus (Kutlu et al., 2009).

EFR3B (2q23): The second most significantly associated SNP among the new loci (rs478222, $P=3.50\text{x}10^{-9}$) resides in an intronic region of the EFR3B (protein EFR3 homolog B) gene on 2p23; however, the region of linkage disequilibrium is approximately 800 kb and harbors additional multiple genes, including NCOA1, C2orf79, CENPO, ADCY3, DNAJC27, POMC, and DNMT3A. EFR3B is an 817 amino acid protein that exists as three alternatively spliced isoforms and belongs to the EFR3 family. The gene encoding EFR3B maps to human chromosome 2p23.3. A number of genetic diseases have been linked to genes on chromosome 2 including Harlequin icthyosis, lipid metabolic disorder sitosterolemia, and Alstrom syndrome. Our recent study shows novel association of 2q23 locus with T1D risk. Location of SNP rs478222 in the intronic region of EFR3B gene makes it a good candidate, however the 2q23 region harbors additional multiple genes, including NCOA1, C2orf79, CENPO, ADCY3, DNAJC27, POMC, and DNMT3A.

Nuclear receptor coactivator 1 (NCOA1) protein is a member of the p160/steroid receptor coactivator (SRC) family. The product of this gene binds to a variety of nuclear hormone receptors in a ligand-dependent manner, suggesting that NCOA1 may play a role as a bridging molecule between nuclear hormone receptors and general transcription factors (Onate et al., 1995; Torchia et al., 1997).

C2orf79 is peptidyl-tRNA hydrolase domain containing 1 (PTRHD1) predicted protein with unknown function.

Centromere protein O (CENPO) gene encodes a component of the interphase centromere complex. The protein is localized to the centromere throughout cell division and is required for bipolar spindle assembly, chromosome segregation and checkpoint signaling during mitosis (Okada et al., 2006).

Adenylate cyclase 3 (ADCY3) gene encodes a membrane-associated enzyme. This protein catalyzes the formation of the secondary messenger cyclic adenosine monophosphate (cAMP) and is highly expressed in human placenta, testis, ovary, and colon (Ludwig & Seuwen,

2002). Wong et al., 2000 reported the presence of adenylyl cyclase 2, 3, and 4 in olfactory cilia. ADCY3 mutants failed olfaction-based behavioral tests indicating that ADCY3 and cAMP signaling are critical for olfactory-dependent behavior.

DnaJ/Hsp40 homolog, subfamily C, member 27 (DNAJC27) gene encodes 273 amino acid protein with RAB-like GTPase and DNAJ domains. EST database suggests high expression in nervous system and reproductive organs (Nepomuceno-Silva et al., 2004).

Pro-opiomelanocortin (POMC) gene encodes a polypeptide hormone precursor protein synthesized mainly in corticotroph cells of the anterior pituitary. POMC is essential for normal steroidogenesis and maintenance of adrenal weight. Mutations in this gene have been associated with early onset obesity, adrenal insufficiency, and red hair pigmentation (Krude et al., 1998; Hung et al., 2012).

DNA (cytosine-5)-methyltransferase 3 alpha (DNMT3A) gene encodes a protein that functions as a *de-novo* methyltransferase that can methylate unmethylated and hemimethylated DNA with equal efficiencies (Yanagisawa et al., 2002).

Additional fine gene mapping and functional studies are needed to determine causal variants for 2q23 region and their role in T1D.

Intergenic region 6q27: Intergenic region on 6q27 contained the third most significantly associated SNP (rs924043, $P=8.06\times10^{-9}$) in our recent study (Bradfield et al., 2011). The region of association is approximately 900kb and harbors multiple genes including PHF10, TCTE3, DLL1, FAM120B, PSMB1, TBP, and PDCD2. The 6q27 region also includes several genes of unknown function: C6orf208/LINC00574 (long intergenic non-protein coding RNA 574), T-complex-associated-testis-expressed 3 (TCTE3), LOC154449, WD repeat domain 27 (WDR27) and chromosome 6 open reading frame 120 (C6orf120).

Plant Homeo Domain (PHD) finger protein 10 (PHF10) encodes a subunit of an ATP-dependent chromatin-remodeling complex that functions in neural precursor cells (Yoo et al., 2009).

Delta-like 1-Drosophila (DLL1) is a human homolog of the Notch Delta ligand and a member of the delta/serrate/jagged family. It plays a role in mediating cell fate decisions during hematopoiesis and cell communication (Santos et al., 2007; Dontje et al., 2006). The protein is expressed in heart, pancreas and brain. Su et al., 2006 reported pancreatic regeneration in chronic pancreatitis requires activation of the notch-signaling pathway.

Family with sequence similarity 120B (FAM120B) gene encodes protein belonging to the constitutive coactivator of peroxisome proliferator-activated receptor gamma (PPARG) family. FAM120B functions in adipogenesis through PPARG activation in a ligand-independent manner (Li et al., 2007).

Proteasome (prosome, macropain) subunit, beta type, 1 (PSMB1) gene encodes a member of the proteasome B-type family, also known as the T1B family, that is a 20S core beta subunit (Trachtulec et al., 1997). This gene encodes TBP, the TATA-binding protein a transcription factor that functions at the core of the DNA-binding multiprotein transcription factor IID (TFIID). Binding of TFIID to TBP is the initial transcriptional step of the pre-initiation complex

(PIC) and plays a role in the activation of eukaryotic genes transcribed by RNA polymerase II (Keutgens et al., 2010).

Programmed cell death 2 (PDCD2) gene encodes a nuclear protein highly expressed in placenta, heart, pancreas, lung, and liver, and lowly expressed in spleen, lymph nodes, and thymus. Expression of this gene is known to be repressed by B-cell CLL/lymphoma 6 (BCL6); a transcriptional repressor (Agata et al., 1996).

In addition, despite not reaching the genome wide significance, our study observed evidence for association at three additional loci containing the candidate genes LOC100128081, TNFRSF11B and FOSL2 (Bradfield et al., 2011). Of these, it is notable that the tumor necrosis factor receptor superfamily, member 11B (TNFRSF11B) is a strongly associated locus with bone mineral density, also discovered in GWAS, and the locus harboring LOC100128081 has also been reported in the context of a GWAS of SLE. FOS-like antigen 2 (FOSL2) gene encodes a leucine zipper protein that dimerizes with the JUN family proteins and forms the transcription factor complex activator protein 1 (AP-1). The FOS proteins have been implicated as regulators of cell proliferation, differentiation, and transformation (Cohen et al., 1989).

CUX2 (12q24): Huang et al., 2012 re-analyzed the original 2007 WTCCC study by using the 1000 Genomes imputation and reported refined variant rs1265564 in Cut-like homeobox 2 (CUX2) region for association with T1D. CUX2 is expressed exclusively in neural tissues. The protein belongs to the CUT homeobox family and contains three CUT domains and a home-odomain; both domains are DNA-binding motifs (Gingras et al., 2005). CUX2 gene has been shown to directly regulate the expression of NeuroD (Iulianella et al., 2008). NeuroD/BETA2, a transcription factor of the insulin gene, is reported to be associated with T1D in Asian descent (Iwata et al., 1999; Kavvoura & Ioannidis, 2005). Thus CUX2 is a plausible candidate for exploration in T1D pathogenesis.

HTR1A (5p13-q13): Asad et al., 2012 confirmed the previously suggested association between the chromosome 5p13-q13 regions and T1D in Scandinavian families (Nerup et al., 2001). None of the previous GWAS have reported any association of 5p13-q13 with T1D. This recent study identified the 5-hydroxytryptamine receptor 1A (HTR1A) and the ring finger protein 180 (RFN180) genes to be associated with T1D in multiplex (Swedish and Danish) families. However, the conditional analysis indicated HTR1A has as a primary association with T1D. Both quantitative PCR and immunohistochemical analysis confirmed the presence of the HTR1A in human pancreas (Asad et al., 2012). The study suggests that HTR1A may affect T1D susceptibility by modulating the initial autoimmune attack or either islet regeneration, insulin release, or both. The HTR1A gene is known to encode for a G-protein coupled receptor specific for serotonin, which mediates cellular signaling via the amine serotonin (Barnes & Sharp, 1999). The HTR1A receptor is mainly known to mediate signal transduction in neurons in the central nervous system (Lesurtel et al., 2008). However, serotonin is also produced in pancreatic islets of several different species (Sundler et al., 1980). Studies in rodent islets show inhibition of insulin secretion by serotonin (Zawalich et al., 2004). Sumatriptan (serotonin agonist) has an inhibitory effect on insulin secretion in humans (Coulie et al., 1998). Mohanan et al., 2006 reported a decrease in expression of HTR1A with increased insulin release during pancreatic regeneration. HTR1A also plays a role in the immune system. High level of protein expression has been reported in activated T-cells and low in resting T-cells; down regulates adenylate cyclase, which in turn regulates T-cell cytokine production and cytotoxicity (Aune et al., 1993). Hence polymorphisms in the HTR1A gene may affect insulin release and T-cell activity, thereby increases the risk of developing T1D.

3. Conclusions

This chapter provides a summary of recent advances in the identification of multiple variants associated with T1D. Genome wide association studies have revolutionized the field of autoimmune mediated disorders. In T1D only six genetic factors were well established before GWAS. GWAS has contributed greatly by expanding the number of established genetic variants to 57 genes. Most of these genes are novel and were not in any investigator's favorite list. For the first time there is real consensus on the role of specific genetic factors underpinning T1D pathogenesis.

The discoveries of genetic factors involved in the pathogenesis of T1D through GWAS present the first step in a much longer process leading to cure. Genes uncovered using this approach are indeed fundamental to disease biology and will define the key molecular pathways leading to cure of T1D. However, such genome wide scans can lack coverage in certain regions where it is difficult to genotype so it is possible that other loci with reasonable effect sizes remain to be uncovered.

To date most of T1D-associated variants have been discovered utilizing cohorts of European ancestry because the SNP arrays were designed to optimally capture the haplotype diversity in this ethnicity. Novel SNP arrays are needed with the same degree of capture in diverse populations to elucidate the full role of each locus in a worldwide context.

The next challenge is to resolve the specific causal variants and determine how they affect the expression and function of these gene products. The Next-Generation Sequencing (NGS) technology has opened new avenues to elucidate the role of coding and noncoding RNAs in health and disease and would speed up the identification of causative gene variants in T1D.

No doubt, the *in vitro* and *in vivo* biology of these genes will be fascinating areas of exploration for many scientists. Only after fully uncovering the functional context of T1D associated genes; these findings will show promise of use for preventive strategies.

Acknowledgements

This research was financially supported by grant from National Institute of Health (DP3 DK085708-01) and an Institute Development Award to the Center for Applied Genomics from the Children's Hospital of Philadelphia.

Author details

Marina Bakay[1], Rahul Pandey[1] and Hakon Hakonarson[1,2]

1 Center for Applied Genomics, Children's Hospital of Philadelphia, Pennsylvania, USA

2 Department of Pediatrics, The University of Pennsylvania School of Medicine, Philadelphia, Pennsylvania, USA

References

[1] Agata, Y, Kawasaki, A, Nishimura, H, & Honjo, T. (1996). Expression of the PD-1 antigen on the surface of stimulated mouse T and B-lymphocytes. Int Immunol. 1996 May; , 8(5), 765-772.

[2] Asad, S, Nikamo, P, Gyllenberg, A, & Kockum, I. a novel type 1 diabetes susceptibility gene on chromosome 5PLoS One. 7(5)., 13-q13.

[3] Aune, T. M, Mcgrath, K. M, Sarr, T, & Kelley, K. A. (1993). Expression of 5HT1a receptors on activated human T cells. Regulation of cyclic AMP levels and T cell proliferation by 5-hydroxytryptamine. J Immunol 1993 Aug; , 151, 1175-1183.

[4] Awata, T, Kawasaki, E, & Tanaka, S. Japanese Study Group on Type 1 Diabetes Genetics ((2009). Association of type 1 diabetes with two loci on 12q13 and 16and the influence coexisting thyroid autoimmunity in Japanese. J Clin Endocrinol Metab. 2009 Jan; 94(1): 231-235., 13.

[5] Barnes NM & Sharp T ((1999). A review of central 5-HT receptors and their function. Neuropharmacology 1999 Aug; , 38(8), 1083-1152.

[6] Barrett, J. C, Clayton, D. G, & Concannon, P. Type 1 Diabetes Genetics Consortium ((2009). Genome-wide association study and meta-analysis find that over 40 loci affect risk of type 1 diabetes. Nat Genet. 2009 Jun; , 41(6), 703-707.

[7] Bell, G. I. Horita S & Karam JH ((1984). A polymorphic locus near the human insulin gene is associated with insulin-dependent diabetes mellitus. Diabetes, 1984 Feb; , 33(2), 176-183.

[8] Bottini, N, Musumeci, L, Alonso, A, & Mustelin, T. (2004). A functional variant of lymphoid tyrosine phosphatase is associated with type I diabetes. Nature genetics. 2004 Apr; , 36(4), 337-338.

[9] Bradfield, J. P, Qu, H. Q, Wang, K, & Hakonarson, H. meta-analysis of six type 1 diabetes cohorts identifies multiple associated loci. PLoS Genet. 2011 Sep; 7(9):e1002293.

[10] Cambi A & Figdor CG ((2003). Dual function of C-type lectin-like receptors in the immune system. Curr Opin Cell Biol. 2003 Oct; , 15(5), 539-46.

[11] Clayton, D. G. (2009). Prediction and interaction in complex disease genetics: experience in type 1 diabetes. PLoS genetics. 2009 Jul; 5(7):e1000540.

[12] Cohen, D. R, Ferreira, P. C, Gentz, R, & Curran, T. (1989). The product of a fos- related gene, Fra-1, binds cooperatively to the AP-1 site with Jun: transcription factor AP-1 is comprised of multiple protein complexes. Genes Dev. 1989 Feb; , 3(2), 173-184.

[13] Concannon, P, Onengut-gumuscu, S, & Todd, J. A. Type 1 Diabetes Genetics Consortium. ((2008). A human type 1 diabetes susceptibility locus maps to chromosome 21q22.3. Diabetes. 2008 Oct; , 57(10), 2858-2861.

[14] Cooper, J. D, Smyth, D. J, Smiles, A. M, & Todd, J. A. (2008). Meta-analysis of genome-wide association study data identifies additional type 1 diabetes risk loci. Nature genetics. 2008 Dec; , 40(12), 1399-401.

[15] Cooper, J. D, Walker, N. M, & Healy, B. C. Type I Diabetes Genetics Consortium. ((2009). Analysis of 55 autoimmune disease and type II diabetes loci: further confirmation of chromosomes 4q27, 12q13.2 and 12q24.13 as type I diabetes loci, and support for a new locus, 12q13.q14.1. Genes and immunity. 2009 Dec ;10 Suppl 1:S95-120., 3.

[16] Coulie, B, Tack, J, Bouillon, R, & Janssens, J. (1998). Hydroxytryptamine-1 receptor activation inhibits endocrine pancreatic secretion in humans. Am J Physiol 1998 Feb: 274(2 Pt 1): E, 317-320.

[17] Cudworth AG & Woodrow JC(1975). Evidence for HL-A-linked genes in "juvenile" diabetes mellitus. Br Med J. 1975 Jul 19; , 3(5976), 133-5.

[18] Davison, L. J, Wallace, C, Cooper, J. D, & Wallace, C. (2012). Long-range DNA looping and gene expression analyses identify DEXI as an autoimmune disease candidate gene. Hum Mol Genet. 2012 Jan 15; , 21(2), 322-33.

[19] Dontje, W, Schotte, R, Cupedo, T, & Blom, B. (2006). Delta-like1-induced Notch 1 signaling regulates the human plasmacytoid dendritic cell versus T cell lineage decision through control of GATA-3 and Spi-B. Blood 2006 Mar; , 107(6), 2446-2452.

[20] Dubois, P. C, Trynka, G, Franke, L, & Van Heel, D. A. (2010). Multiple common variants for celiac disease influencing immune gene expression. Nat Genet. 2010 Apr; , 42(4), 295-302.

[21] EURODIAB ACE Study Group(2000). Variation and trends in incidence of childhood diabetes in Europe. EURODIAB ACE Study Group. Lancet. 2000 Mar; , 355(9207), 873-876.

[22] Fung, E. Y, Smyth, D. J, Howson, J. M, & Todd, J. A. (2009). Analysis of 17 autoimmune disease-associated variants in type 1 diabetes identifies 6q23/TNFAIP3 as a susceptibility locus. Genes and immunity. 2009 Mar; , 10(2), 188-91.

[23] Furuya, M, Tsuji, N, Endoh, T, & Watanabe, N. (2002). A novel gene containing PDZ and LIM domains, PCD1, is overexpressed in human colorectal cancer. Anticancer Res. 2002 Nov-Dec; 22(6C): , 4183-4186.

[24] Gateva, V, Sandling, J. K, Hom, G, & Graham, R. R. replication study identifies TNIP1, PRDM1, JAZF1, UHRF1BP1 and IL10 as risk loci for systemic lupus erythematosus. Nat. Genet. 2009 Nov; , 41(11), 1228-1233.

[25] Gingras, H, Cases, O, Krasilnikova, M, & Nepveu, A. (2005). Biochemical characterization of the mammalian Cux2 protein. Gene 2005 Jan; , 344, 273-285.

[26] Grant, S. F, Qu, H. Q, Bradfield, J. P, & Hakonarson, H. (2009). Follow-up analysis of genome-wide association data identifies novel loci for type 1 diabetes. Diabetes. 2009 Jan; , 58(1), 290-295.

[27] Hakonarson, H, Grant, S. F, Bradfield, J. P, & Polychronakos, C. association study identifies KIAA0350 as a type 1 diabetes gene. Nature. 2007 Aug 2; , 448(7153), 591-594.

[28] Hakonarson, H, Qu, H. Q, Bradfield, J. P, & Polychronakos, C. (2008). A novel susceptibility locus for type 1 diabetes on Chr12q13 identified by a genome-wide association study. Diabetes. 2008 Apr; , 57(4), 1143-1146.

[29] Hirschfield, G. M, Xie, G, Lu, E, & Siminovitch, K. A. (2012). Association of primary biliary cirrhosis with variants in the CLEC16A, SOCS1, SPIB and SIAE immunomodulatory genes. Genes Immun. 2012 Jun; , 13(4), 328-335.

[30] Howson, J. M, Rosinger, S, Smyth, D. J, & Todd, J. A. (2011). Genetic analysis of adult-onset autoimmune diabetes. Diabetes. 2011 Oct; , 60(10), 2645-2653.

[31] Huang, J, Ellinghaus, D, Franke, A, & Li, Y. (2012). Genomes-based imputation identifies novel and refined associations for the Wellcome Trust Case Control Consortium phase 1 Data. Eur J Hum Genet. 2012 Jul; , 20(7), 801-805.

[32] Hung, C. N, Poon, W. T, Lee, C. Y, & Chan, A. Y. (2012). A case of early-onset obesity, hypocortisolism, and skin pigmentation problem due to a novel homozygous mutation in the proopiomelanocortin (POMC) gene in an Indian boy. J Pediatr Endocrinol Metab. 25(1-2): 175-179.

[33] International HapMap Consortium(2003). The International HapMap Project. Nature. 2003 Dec; , 426(6968), 789-796.

[34] International HapMap Consortium(2005). A haplotype map of the human genome. Nature. 2005 Oct 27; , 437(7063), 1299-1320.

[35] Iulianella, A, Sharma, M, Durnin, M, & Trainor, P. A. (2008). Cux2 (Cutl2) integrates neural progenitor development with cell-cycle progression during spinal cord neurogenesis. Development 2008 Feb; , 135(4), 729-741.

[36] Iwata, I, Nagafuchi, S, Nakashima, H, & Niho, Y. (1999). Association of polymorphism in the NeuroD/BETA2 gene with type 1 diabetes in the Japanese. Diabetes. 1999 Feb; , 48(2), 416-419.

[37] Jagielska, D, Redler, S, Brockschmidt, F. F, & Betz, R. C. (2012). Follow-Up Study of the First Genome-Wide Association Scan in Alopecia Areata: IL13 and KIAA0350 as

Susceptibility Loci Supported with Genome-Wide Significance. J Invest Dermatol. 2012 Apr.

[38] Kang, S, Xu, H, Duan, X, & Kennedy, G. C. (2000). PCD1, a novel gene containing PDZ and LIM domains, is overexpressed in several human cancers. Cancer Res. 2000 Sep; , 60(18), 5296-5302.

[39] Kavvoura FK & Ioannidis JP(2005). Ala45Thr polymorphism of the NEUROD1 gene and diabetes susceptibility: a meta-analysis. Hum Genet. 2005 Feb; , 116(3), 192-199.

[40] Keutgens, A, Zhang, X, Shostak, K, & Chariot, A. (2010). BCL-3 degradation involves its polyubiquitination through a FBW7-independent pathway and its binding to the proteasome subunit PSMB1. J Biol Chem. 2010 Aug 13; , 285(33), 25831-25840.

[41] Kim, S, Wairkar, Y. P, & Daniels, R. W. DiAntonio A. ((2010). The novel endosomal membrane protein Ema interacts with the class C Vps-HOPS complex to promote endosomal maturation. Cell Biol. 2010 Mar; , 188(5), 717-734.

[42] Kim, S, & Naylor, S. A. DiAntonio A. ((2012). Drosophila Golgi membrane protein Ema promotes autophagosomal growth and function. Proc Natl Acad Sci USA 2012 May; 109(18): E, 1072-1081.

[43] Krude, H, Biebermann, H, Luck, W, & Gruters, A. (1998). Severe early-onset obesity, adrenal insufficiency and red hair pigmentation caused by POMC mutations in humans. Nat Genet. 1998 Jun; , 19(2), 155-157.

[44] Kutlu, B, Burdick, D, Baxter, D, & Hood, L. (2009). Detailed transcriptome atlas of the pancreatic beta cell. BMC Med Genomics 2009 Jan; 2:3.

[45] Lesurtel, M, Soll, C, Graf, R, & Clavien, P. A. (2008). Role of serotonin in the hepato-gastro- Intestinal tract: an old molecule for new perspectives. Cell Mol Life Sci 2008 Mar; , 65(6), 940-952.

[46] Li, D. Kang Q & Wang DM. ((2007). Constitutive coactivator of peroxisome proliferator-activated receptor (PPAR-gamma), a novel coactivator of PPAR-gamma that promotes adipogenesis. Molec. Endocr. 2007 Oct; , 21(10), 2320-2333.

[47] Lindvall, J. M, Blomberg, K. E, Wennborg, A, & Smith, C. I. (2005). Differential expression and molecular characterisation of Lmo7, Myo1e, Sash1, and Mcoln2 genes in Btk-defective B-cells. Cell Immunol. 2005 May; , 235(1), 46-55.

[48] Ludwig, M, & Seuwen, K. (2002). Characterization of the human adenylyl cyclase gene family: cDNA, gene structure, and tissue distribution of the nine isoforms. J. Recept. Signal Transduct. Res. 2002 Feb-Nov; 22(1-4): 79-110.

[49] Manolio, T. A, Rodriguez, L. L, Brooks, L, & Collins, F. S. (2007). New models of collaboration in genome-wide association studies: the Genetic Association Information Network. Nature genetics. 2007 Sep; , 39(9), 1045-1051.

[50] Marquez, A, Varade, J, Robledo, G, & Urcelay, E. (2009). Specific association of a CLEC16A/KIAA0350 polymorphism with NOD2/CARD15(-) Crohn's disease patients. Eur J Hum Genet. 2009 Oct; , 17(10), 1304-1308.

[51] Martinez, A, Perdigones, N, Cénit, M. C, & Urcelay, E. (2010). Chromosomal region 16further evidence of increased predisposition to immune diseases. Ann Rheum Dis. 2010 Jan; 69(1): 309-311., 13.

[52] Mells, G. F, Floyd, J. A, Morley, K. I, & Anderson, C. A. (2011). Genome-wide association study identifies 12 new susceptibility loci for primary biliary cirrhosis. Nat. Genet. 2011 Mar; , 43(4), 329-332.

[53] Mohanan, V. V, Khan, R, & Paulose, C. S. (2006). Hypothalamic 5-HT functional regulation through 5-HT1A and 5-HT2C receptors during pancreatic regeneration. Life Sci 2006 Feb; , 78(14), 1603-1609.

[54] Mueller, P. W, Rogus, J. J, Cleary, P. A, & Warram, J. H. (2006). Genetics of Kidneys in Diabetes (GoKinD) study: a genetics collection available for identifying genetic susceptibility factors for diabetic nephropathy in type 1 diabetes. J Am Soc Nephrol. 2006 Jul; , 17(7), 1782-1790.

[55] Nakamura, H, Mukai, M, Komatsu, K, & Miyoshi, J. (2005). Transforming growth factor-beta1 induces LMO7 while enhancing the invasiveness of rat ascites hepatoma cells. Cancer Lett. 2005 Mar; , 220(1), 95-99.

[56] Nepomuceno-silva, J. L, De Melo, L. D, Mendonçã, S. M, & Lopes, U. G. (2004). RJLs: a new family of Ras-related GTP-binding proteins. Gene 2004 Mar; , 327(2), 221-232.

[57] Nerup, J, Platz, P, Andersen, O. O, & Svejgaard, A. (1974). HLA antigens and diabetes mellitus. Lancet. 1974 Oct; , 2(7885), 864-866.

[58] Nerup, J. Pociot F & European Consortium for IDDM Studies. ((2001). A genomewide scan for type 1-diabetes susceptibility in Scandinavian families: identification of new loci with evidence of interactions. Am J Hum Genet 2001 Dec; , 69(6), 1301-1313.

[59] Nischwitz, S, Cepok, S, Kroner, A, & Weber, F. (2011). More CLEC16A gene variants associated with multiple sclerosis. Acta Neurol Scand 2011 Jun; , 123(6), 400-406.

[60] Nistico, L, Buzzetti, R, Pritchard, L. E, & Todd, J. A. (1996). The CTLA-4 gene region of chromosome 2q33 is linked to, and associated with, type 1 diabetes. Belgian Diabetes Registry. Human molecular genetics. 1996 Jul; , 5(7), 1075-1080.

[61] Okada, M, Cheeseman, I. M, Hori, T, & Fukagawa, T. (2006). The CENP-H-I complex is required for the efficient incorporation of newly synthesized CENP-A into centromeres. Nature Cell Biol. 2006 May; , 8(5), 446-457.

[62] Onate, S. A, & Tsai, S. Y. Tsai MJ. & O'Malley BW. ((1995). Sequence and characterization of a coactivator for the steroid hormone receptor superfamily. Science 1995 Nov; , 270(5240), 1354-1357.

[63] Onkamo, P, Vaananen, S, Karvonen, M, & Tuomilehto, J. (1999). Worldwide increase in incidence of Type I diabetes--the analysis of the data on published incidence trends. Diabetologia. 1999 Dec; , 42(12), 1395-1403.

[64] Ooshio, T, Irie, K, Morimoto, K, & Takai, Y. (2004). Involvement of LMO7 in the association of two cell-cell adhesion molecules, nectin and E-cadherin, through afadin and alpha-actinin in epithelial cells. J. Biol. Chem. 2004 Jul; , 279(30), 31365-31373.

[65] Perou, C. M, Sørlie, T, Eisen, M. B, & Botstein, D. (2000). Molecular portraits of human breast tumours. Nature. 2000 Aug; , 406(6797), 747-752.

[66] Qu, H. Q, Bradfield, J. P, Li, Q, & Polychronakos, C. (2010). In silico replication of the genome-wide association results of the Type 1 Diabetes Genetics Consortium. Human molecular genetics. 2010 Jun 15; , 19(12), 2534-2538.

[67] Reddy, M. V, Wang, H, Liu, S, & She, J. X. (2011). Association between type 1 diabetes and GWAS SNPs in the southeast US Caucasian population. Genes Immun. 2011 Apr; , 12(3), 208-212.

[68] Redondo, M. J, Yu, L, Hawa, M, & Leslie, R. D. (2001). Heterogeneity of type I diabetes: analysis of monozygotic twins in Great Britain and the United States. Diabetologia. 2001 Mar; , 44(3), 354-362.

[69] Rozenblum, E, Vahteristo, P, Sandberg, T, & Kallioniemi, O. P. (2002). A genomic map of a 6-Mb region at 13q21-q22 implicated in cancer development: identification and characterization of candidate genes. Hum. Genet. 2002 Feb; , 110(2), 111-121.

[70] Rich, S. S. (1990). Mapping genes in diabetes. Genetic epidemiological perspective. Diabetes. 1990 Nov; , 39(11), 1315-1319.

[71] Robinson, M. J, Sancho, D, & Slack, E. C. Reis e Sousa C. ((2006). Myeloid C-type lectins in innate immunity. Nat Immunol. 2006 Dec; , 7(12), 1258-1265.

[72] Sang, Y, & Zong, W. Yan J & Liu M. ((2012). The Correlation between the CLEC16A Gene and Genetic Susceptibility to Type 1 Diabetes in Chinese Children. Int J Endocrinol. 2012:245384.

[73] Santos, M. A, Sarmento, L. M, Rebelo, M, & Demengeot, J. (2007). Notch1 engagement by Delta-like-1 promotes differentiation of B lymphocytes to antibody-secreting cells. Proc. Natl. Acad. Sci. USA 2007 Sep; , 104(39), 15454-15459.

[74] Sasaki, M, Tsuji, N, Furuya, M, & Watanabe, N. (2003). PCD1, a novel gene containing PDZ and LIM domains, is overexpressed in human breast cancer and linked to lymph node metastasis. Anticancer Res. 2003 May; 23(3B): , 2717-2721.

[75] Semenova, E, Wang, X, Jablonski, M. M, & Tilghman, S. M. (2003). An engineered 800 kilobase deletion of Uchl3 and Lmo7 on mouse chromosome 14 causes defects in viability, postnatal growth and degeneration of muscle and retina. Hum Mol Genet 2003 Jun; , 12(11), 1301-1312.

[76] Singal DP & Blajchman MA(1973). Histocompatibility (HL-A) antigens, lymphocyto-toxic antibodies and tissue antibodies in patients with diabetes mellitus. Diabetes. 1973 Jun; , 22(6), 429-432.

[77] Skinningsrud, B, Husebye, E. S, Pearce, S. H, & Undlien, D. E. (2008). Polymorphisms in CLEC16A and CIITA at 16are associated with primary adrenal insufficiency. J. Clin. Endocrinol. Metab., 2008 Sep; 93(9): 3310-3317., 13.

[78] Smyth, D. J, Cooper, J. D, Bailey, R, & Todd, J. A. association study of nonsynonymous SNPs identifies a type 1 diabetes locus in the interferon-induced helicase (IFIH1) region. Nature genetics. 2006 Jun; , 38(6), 617-619.

[79] Smyth, D. J, Plagnol, V, Walker, N. M, & Todd, J. A. (2008). Shared and distinct genetic variants in type 1 diabetes and celiac disease. The New England journal of medicine. 2008 Dec 25; , 359(26), 2767-2777.

[80] Steyn, N. P, Lambert, E. V, & Tabana, H. (2009). Conference on "Multidisciplinary approaches to nutritional problems". Symposium on "Diabetes and health". Nutrition interventions for the prevention of type 2 diabetes. Proc. Nutr. Soc. 2009 Feb; , 68(1), 55-70.

[81] Su, Y, Büchler, P, Gazdhar, A, & Friess, H. (2006). Pancreatic regeneration in chronic pancreatitis requires activation of the notch signaling pathway. J. Gastrointest. Surg. 2006 Nov; , 10(9), 1230-1241.

[82] Sundler, F, Hakanson, R, Loren, I, & Lundquist, I. (1980). Amine storage and function in peptide hormone-producing cells. Invest Cell Pathol. 1980 Jan-Mar; , 3(1), 87-103.

[83] Todd, J. A, Walker, N. M, Cooper, J. D, & Clayton, D. G. (2007). Robust associations of four new chromosome regions from genome-wide analyses of type 1 diabetes. Nature genetics. 2007 Jul; , 39(7), 857-864.

[84] Torchia, J, Rose, D. W, Inostroza, J, & Rosenfeld, M. G. (1997). The transcriptional co-activator p/CIP binds CBP and mediates nuclear-receptor function. Nature. 1997 Jun 12; , 387(6634), 677-684.

[85] Trachtulec, Z, Hamvas, R. M, Forejt, J, & Klein, J. (1997). Linkage of TATA-binding protein and proteasome subunit C5 genes in mice and humans reveals synteny conserved between mammals and invertebrates. Genomics. 1997 Aug; , 44(1), 1-7.

[86] Vella, A, Cooper, J. D, Lowe, C. E, & Todd, J. A. (2005). Localization of a type 1 diabetes locus in the IL2RA/CD25 region by use of tag single-nucleotide polymorphisms. Am J Hum Genet. 2005 May; , 76(5), 773-779.

[87] Wallace, C, Smyth, D. J, Maisuria-armer, M, & Clayton, D. G. (2010). The imprinted DLK1-MEG3 gene region on chromosome 14q32.2 alters susceptibility to type 1 diabetes. Nat Genet. 2010 Jan; , 42(1), 68-71.

[88] Wellcome Trust Case Control Consortium: WTCCC ((2007). Genome-wide association study of 14,000 cases of seven common diseases and 3,000 shared controls. Nature. 2007 Jun; , 447(7145), 661-678.

[89] Wang, K, Baldassano, R, Zhang, H, & Hakanarson, H. (2010). Comparative genetic analysis of inflammatory bowel disease and type 1 diabetes implicates multiple loci with opposite effects. Human molecular genetics. 2010 May; , 19(10), 2059-2067.

[90] Wong, S. T, Trinh, K, Hacker, B, & Storm, D. R. (2000). Disruption of the type III adenylyl cyclase gene leads to peripheral and behavioral anosmia in transgenic mice. Neuron. 2000 Sep; , 27(3), 487-497.

[91] Wu, X, Zhu, X, Wang, X, & Liu, Y. (2009). Intron polymorphism in the KIAA0350 gene is reproducibly associated with susceptibility to type 1 diabetes (T1D) in the Han Chinese population. Clin Endocrinol (Oxf). 2009 Jul; , 71(1), 46-49.

[92] Wu, X, Li, J, Chen, C, & Gao, Y. (2012). Involvement of CLEC16A in activation of astrocytes after LPS treated. Neurochem Res. 2012 Jan; , 37(1), 5-14.

[93] Yamada, A, Irie, K, Fukuhara, A, & Takai, Y. (2004). Requirement of the actin cytoskeleton for the association of nectins with other cell adhesion molecules at adherens and tight junctions in MDCK cells. Genes Cells 2004 Sep; , 9(9), 843-855.

[94] Yamashita, H, Awata, T, & Kawasaki, E. Japanese Study Group on Type 1 Diabetes Genetics. ((2011). Analysis of the HLA and non-HLA susceptibility loci in Japanese type 1 diabetes. Diabetes Metab Res Rev. 2011 Nov; , 27(8), 844-848.

[95] Yanagisawa, Y, & Ito, E. Yuasa Y & Maruyama K ((2002). The human DNA methyltransferases DNMT3A and DNMT3B have two types of promoters with different CpG contents. Biochim. Biophys. Acta 2002 Sep; , 1577(3), 457-465.

[96] Yoo, A. S, Staahl, B. T, Chen, L, & Crabtree, G. R. (2009). MicroRNA-mediated switching of chromatin-remodelling complexes in neural development. Nature. 2009 Jul; , 460(7255), 642-646.

[97] Zawalich, W. S, Tesz, G. J, & Zawalich, K. C. (2004). Effects of prior 5-hydroxytryptamine exposure on rat islet insulin secretory and phospholipase C responses. Endocrine. 2004 Feb; , 23(1), 11-16.

[98] Zhang, Z, Cheng, Y, Zhou, X, & Zhang, X. (2011). Polymorphisms at 16are associated with systemic lupus erythematosus in the Chinese population. J Med. Genet. 2011 Jan; 48(1): 69-72., 13.

[99] Zoledziewska, M, Costa, G, Pitzalis, M, & Marrosu, M. G. (2009). Variation within the CLEC16A gene shows consistent disease association with both multiple sclerosis and type 1 diabetes in Sardinia. Genes Immun. 2009 Jan; , 10(1), 15-17.

[100] Zuvich, R. L, Bush, W. S, Mccauley, J. L, & Haines, J. L. (2011). Interrogating the complex role of chromosome 16in multiple sclerosis susceptibility: independent genetic signals in the CIITA-CLEC16A-SOCS1 gene complex. Hum. Mol. Genet., 2011 Sep; 20(17): 3517-3524., 13.

Chapter 4

Update of Type 1 Diabetes

Mohamed M. Jahromi

Additional information is available at the end of the chapter

1. Introduction

Diabetes is one of the fastest growing diseases. World health organization estimates that approximately 340 million people have type 1 diabetes and this number increases by 3-5% each year so the type 1 diabetes population reached 25 million by 2010. Type 1 diabetes is an autoimmune disease that is caused as a result of destruction of pancreatic β-cells. Several factors may contribute to the pathogenesis of type 1 diabetes. Genetic susceptibility of type 1 diabetes is determined by polymorphisms/mutations in multiple genes in both human and animal models.

The Major Histocomapatibility Complex (MHC) accounts for approximately 40% of the familial aggregation of type 1 diabetes and the insulin gene for only 10 % suggesting the existence of additional loci. The gene for "Protein Tyrosine Phosphatase, Non-receptor type 22 (lymphoid)."PTPN22, the lymphocyte signaling molecule, on chromosome 1p13.3–p13.1 is a confirmed locus that contributes to multiple autoimmune disorders, including type 1 diabetes. Diabetes associated Cytotoxic T - Lymphocyte Antigen 4 (CTLA-4) locus polymorphisms in most populations have relative risks less than 1.5. A fundamental question is whether there are genetic polymorphisms that confer major risk for type 1 diabetes, other than the Human Leukocyte Antigen (HLA) DR and DQ alleles (class II HLA alleles). Recently, genes outside MHC region have considered playing an important role in the onset of diabetes.

As accumulative report suggest the role of olfactory receptor in the pathogenesis of diabetic microvascular and other diabetic complications, undoubtedly, this haplotype specific alteration of type 1 diabetes risk is an independent risk for the disease and can address the promising MHC-linked gene other than DR/DQ. Moreover, there is nothing to hinder for that this might be a signal that identify the role of olfactory receptor gene in the pathogenesis of type 1 diabetes in patients who are prone to diabetic complications.

Diabetes is one of the fastest growing diseases. Diabetes affects today an estimated 371 million people world-wide compared to 366 million by the end of 2011. Of course this includes 20 million to 40 million of patients with type 1 diabetes. While type 1 diabetes accounts for 5% to 20% of those with diabetes, it is associated with higher morbidity, mortality and health care cost than the more prevalent type 2 diabetes. Overall, 4.8 million people died and $ 471 billion were spent due to diabetes in 2012 [1-2].

New figures indicate that the number of people living with diabetes is expected to rise from 371 million in 2012 to 552 million by 2030, if no urgent action is taken. This equates to approximately three new cases every ten seconds or almost ten million per year. International diabetes federation also estimated that almost half of the people with diabetes are unaware that they have diabetes [2].

In some of the poorest regions in the world such as Africa, where infectious diseases have traditionally been the focus of health care systems, diabetes cases are expected to increase by 90% by 2030. At least 78% of people in Africa are undiagnosed and do not know they are living with diabetes (Figure 1):

• 80% of people with diabetes live in low and middle income countries.

• 78,000 children develop type 1 diabetes every year

• The greatest number of people with diabetes is between 40-59 years of age [2].

2. Why is there an increasing trend in the incidence of diabetes?

In the past, most diabetics were known to have a genetic tendency towards the disease. However, that trend has rapidly given way in the past few decades to other causes, at least from a statistical perspective. These genetically-independent trends that explain the growth in the incidence of diabetes can be summarized as follows: (a) overall growth in population, (b) increased life expectancy resulting in a higher ratio of aged population more prone to diabetes, (c) increasing obesity trends, (d) unhealthy diets and (e) sedentary lifestyles.

In other words, diabetes has increasingly become a lifestyle-related disease as it afflicts young and old, in developed and developing nations, around the world. As the number of patients grows across the globe, there has never been a stronger and more urgent need for therapeutic measures that arrest the growth of the disease and alleviate its secondary manifestations.

Middle East & North Africa: 1 in 9 adults in this region have diabetes; More than half of people with diabetes in this region don't know they have it. Europe: 1 out of every 3 dollars spent on diabetes healthcare was spent in this region; 21.2 million people in this region have diabetes and don't know it. Western Pacific: 1 in 3 adults with diabetes lives in this region; 6 of the top 10 countries for diabetes prevalence are Pacific Islands. South & Central America: Only 5% of all healthcare dollars for diabetes were spent in this region; 1 in 11 adults in this region has diabetes. Africa: Over the next 20 years, the number of people with diabetes in the region will almost double; This region has the highest mortality rate due to diabetes. South East Asia: 1

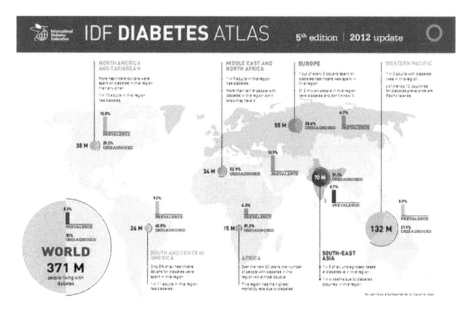

Figure 1. According to international diabetes federation5th edition; 2012the number of diabetes increases to 371 million. North America & Caribean: More healthcare dollars were spent on diabetes in this region than any other; 1 in 10 adults in this region has diabetes.

in 5 of all undiagnosed cases of diabetes is in this region; 1 in 4 deaths due to diabetes occurred in this region [2]

2.1. Pathogenesis

Type 1 diabetes develops slowly and progressive abnormalities in beta cell-function herald what appears to be a sudden development of hyperglycemia. Rising the hemoglobin A1c test (HbA1c) in the normal range[3], impaired fasting or glucose tolerance, as well as loss of first phase insulin secretion usually precede overt diabetes. The exact beta cell mass remaining at diagnosis is poorly defined and there are almost no studies of insulitis prior to diabetes onset [4]. For patients with long-term type 1 diabetes there is evidence of some beta cell function remaining (C-peptide secretion) though beta cell mass is usually decreased to less than 1% of normal [5]. At present methods to image/quantitate beta cell mass and insulitis are only beginning to be developed. In particular Positron Emission Tomography (PET) scanning utilizing a labeled amine (dihydrotetrabenazine) may provide the first method to image islet mass [6] and this is now being evaluated in man. A number of techniques are being evaluated to image insulitis [7].

A large body of evidence indicates that the development of type 1 diabetes is determined by a balance between pathogenic and regulatory T lymphocytes [8]. A fundamental question is whether there is a primary autoantigen for initial T cell autoreactivity with subsequent recognition of multiple islet antigens. A number of investigators have addressed in the Non-Obese Diabetic (NOD) mouse (spontaneously develops type 1 diabetes) the importance of immune reactivity to insulin with the dramatic finding that eliminating immune responses to insulin blocks development of diabetes and insulitis, and importantly immune responses to downstream autoantigens such as the Islet specific molecule Glucose-6-phosphatase catalytic subunit-Related Protein(IGRP) [9]. Knocking out both insulin genes (mice in contrast to humans have two insulin genes) with introduction of a mutated insulin with alanine rather than tyrosine at position 16 of the insulin B chain prevents development of diabetes [10]. Recognition of this B-chain peptide of insulin by T lymphocytes depends upon a "non-stringent" T cell receptor with conservation of only the alpha chain sequence (Valpha and Jalpha) and not the N-region of the alpha chain, or the Beta chain [11].

As in other immune diseases both genetic factors as well as environmental factors contribute in the pathogenesis of the disease (Figure 2). Environmental factors exert their effects ones genetic susceptibility factors already exist.

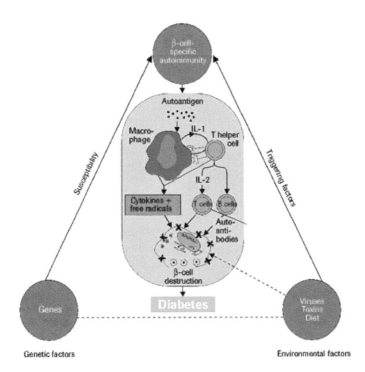

Figure 2. A schematic figure shows how environmental factors trigger TYPE 1 DIABETES onset in genetically suscepti-ble persons which ends to the process of β-cell-specific autoimmunity processes which lead to the destruction of pan-creatic β-cell. As antigen presenting cell is triggered by auto antigens it releases intiinfalmatory cytokines eg IL-1 that signals T-helper 1 class to activate B-cell and T cell in order to release autoantibodies to attach pancreatic β-cell.

3. Genetic factors

A mutation of the Forkhead bOX Protein 3 (FOXP3 gene, a transcription factor that controls the development of regulatory T cells is a cause of neonatal diabetes [12]. The syndrome is termed IPEX (Immune dysregulation, Polyendocrinopathy, Enteropathy, X-linked) syndrome. As reflected in the name, children with disorder suffer from overwhelming autoimmunity and usually die as infants. Of note bone marrow transplantation can reverse disease. IPEX syndrome is rare, as is neonatal diabetes. In the differential diagnosis of neonatal diabetes it must be recognized that half of children developing permanent neonatal diabetes have a mutation of the Kir6.2 molecule of the sulfonylurea receptor. These children with their non-autoimmune form of diabetes can be treated with oral sulfonylurea therapy.

Though more common than IPEX syndrome, the Autoimmune Polyendocrine Syndrome Type 1 (APS-1) syndrome is also rare. It results from a mutation of the "autoimmune regulator" AIRE gene, another transcription factor [13]. Approximately 15% of patients with this syndrome develop autoimmune diabetes. The leading hypothesis as to etiology (e.g. Addison's disease, mucocutaneous candidiasis, and hypoparathyroidism) is that AIRE controls expression of autoantigens and negative selection of autoreactive T lymphocytes within the thymus. A very recent dramatic discovery is the demonstration that essentially 100% of patients with Autoimmune Polyendocrine Syndrome type 1 (APS-1) have autoantibodies reacting with interferon alpha and other interferons. Such autoantibodies are extremely rare and essentially not found in patients with type 1 diabetes or Addison's disease outside of the syndrome.

Patients with type 1 diabetes and their relatives are at risk for development of thyroid autoimmunity, celiac disease, Addison's disease, pernicious anemia and a series of other autoimmune disorders [14]. Approximately 1/20 patients with type 1 diabetes have celiac disease by biopsy though the majority have no symptoms [15]. These asymptomatic individuals are usually detected with screening for transglutaminase autoantibodies. The level of transglutaminase autoantibodies relates to the probability of a positive biopsy and it is important for clinicians to know the threshold for likely positive biopsy for the assay they employ [16]. There remains controversy as to whether asymptomatic celiac disease when detected should be treated with a gluten free diet and large clinical trials are needed to address this question.

3.1. MHC genes

Type 1 diabetes has become one of the most intensively studied polygenic disorders. There are MHC as well as non-MHC genes or loci candidate to contribute in the genetic susceptibility to type 1 diabetes pathogenesis. According to the recent version of the National Center for Biotechnology Information (NCBI) map viewer these genes are located on all human chromosomes [17] (Figure 3). The strongest associations with both susceptibility and protection from type 1 diabetes are HLA DR and DQ molecules. For instance DQB1*0602 alleles are associated with dominant protection and DR3-DQ2 molecules (DQB1*0201) and DR4-DQ8 (DQB1*0302) with susceptibility [18].

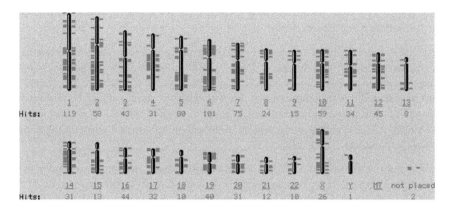

Figure 3. A schematic projection of type 1 diabetes susceptible genes location according to 2012 version of NCBI map viewer. Type 1 diabetes susceptible genes were reported on all chromosome of human[17].

Type 1 diabetes is a T cell organ specific autoimmune disease [19] with approximately 40% of the familial aggregation accounted for by the MHC region [20-21]. Nevertheless, it is generally assumed that the positive predictive value of MHC alleles is relatively low given the complex genetics and potential multiple environmental factors hypothesized to contribute to diabetes risk. However, approximately 1/2 to 1/3 of U.S. children who develop type 1 diabetes prior to age 15 have the highest risk DR/DQ genotype (HLA-DRB1*03-DQA1*0501-DQB1*0201/ DRB1*04-DQA1*0301-DQB1*0302, DR3-DQB1*02-01/DR4-DQB1*0302) [22-25]. Pursuing the hypothesis that additional major determinants of Type 1 diabetes risk (in addition to DR/ DQ genes) are within or close to the MHC region, highly conserved HLA-F [24-32].

Recently, OR gene have been associated with different diseases which support the hypothesis of the importance of OR in CNS in addition to smell [33]. Increasing studies suggest significant association among SNP in OR genes that link autoimmunity, psychiatric disorders, and smell impairment [33-36].

Interestingly, a large cluster of the human OR family 14, subfamily J and member 1gene (OR14J1) were found in proximity to the HLA-F, and so they were called "MHC-linked" OR-genes [1, 37-38]. Olfactory Receptor (OR) is our Central Nervous System (CNS) external messenger which translates the information from the odorant into neural pulses, a window for our mind. In addition, the important role of CNS in the pathogenesis of type 1 diabetes any variation in the genetic make-up of the OR might lead to the destruction of its function and notably malfunction of the CNS. The OR14J1C allele of OR gene in the conserved region of HLA-F showed a significant association with type 1 diabetes, except the known diabetogenic DQ/DR genes [39].

3.2. Non–MHC genes

Although important, the MHC susceptibility genes are not sufficient to induce type 1 diabetes, suggesting polygenic inheritance in most cases [40]. An important component of the susceptibility to type 1 diabetes resides in certain non-MHC genes that have an effect only in the presence of the appropriate MHC alleles.

In particular, polymorphisms of a promoter of the insulin gene and an amino acid change of PTPN22 are associated with the risk of TYPE 1 DIABETES in multiple populations [4-6]. A repeat sequence in the 5' region of the insulin gene is associated with greater insulin expression in the thymus and it is hypothesized that this contributes to decreasing the development of diabetes [7]. The polymorphism of the lymphocyte-specific tyrosine phosphatase gene influences T cell receptor signaling, and the same polymorphism is a major risk factor for multiple autoimmune disorders [8].

A polymorphism in the cytotoxic T-lymphocyte-associated antigen-4 gene was shown to be associated with the risk of type 1 diabetes in a meta-analysis of 33 studies involving over 5000 patients [9]. Other genes are implicated in risk for type 1 diabetes (eg, CTLA-4) [10] and other genetic loci, but their influence is very small, or so small that replication has been difficult.

Additional evidence for the role of non-MHC genes comes from studies in NOD (nonobese diabetic) mice. These mice develop spontaneous autoimmune diabetes with striking similarities to type 1 diabetes in humans [11]. Autoimmune infiltration of the islets of Langerhans (insulitis) begins at about 50 days of age and clinical diabetes appears at about 120 days.

Interferon (IFN-γ)+ T cells (Th1 cells) appear to be an important mediator of the insulitis in NOD mice, and destruction of the islet cells can be slowed by the administration of anti- IFN-γ antibodies. IFN-γ -inducing factor (IGIF; also called interleukin (IL)-18) and IL-12 are potent inducers of IFN-γ, and the progression of insulitis begins in parallel with increased release of these two cytokines(kent et al 2005). IGIF gene expression is upregulated in NOD mice, and the location of the IGIF gene suggests that it is a candidate gene for susceptibility to type 1 diabetes [41].Genetically altered (knockout) mice deficient in IL-18 had hyperphagia, obesity, hyperinsulinemia, and hyperglycemia; intracerebral administration of recombinant IL-18 decreased food intake and reversed hyperglycemia (Bach 2002). A new locus associated with type 1 diabetes, has been identified near the gene encoding the p40 subunit of IL12B in NOD mice [42].

It was initially thought that, in contrast to Th1 cells, Th2 cells (which produce IL-4, -5, -10, and -13) protected against the onset and progression of type 1 diabetes. However, Th2 cells also are capable of inducing islet-cell destruction, and therefore the onset and progression of type 1 diabetes are probably under the control of both Th1 and Th2 cells [1,43].

In our extensive cytokine gene polymorphisms effect on type 1 diabetes immunogenetics (44-46]we have shown clearly that a single nucleotide polymorphism (SNP) in the genetic of IL-4 gene, however, would contribute to the domination of T-h-1 cell to Th2 (IL-4) [46], lack of action of IL-4, the th2 cytokine initiator. Further, a Single Nucleotide Polymorphism (SNP) in the Transforming Growth Factor (TGF)-β gene ends up to lower production of TGF- β protein level. That may contribute to the lack of immunosuppressive effect of TGF- β in the pathogenesis of type 1 diabetes [47].

4. Environmental factors

During the last decades, the incidence of type 1 diabetes has increased significantly, reaching percentages of 3% annually worldwide. This increase suggests that besides genetic factors environmental perturbations (including viral infections) are also involved in the pathogenesis of type 1 diabetes.

There is a number of environmental factors contribute to the marked global variation in the incidence of type 1 diabetes. Evidence suggests that the incidence is lower in the tropics compared with further north or south of the equator.

Assuming that the observation that there is a direct relationship between incidence of type 1 diabetes and equatorial distance, a number of environmental factors appear to be protective against the development of an autoimmune pathological process. Ultra violet radiation results in increased levels of vitamin D, which is an important modulator of the immune system. Detailed studies have shown not only that lower levels of circulating vitamin D predispose to autoimmunity, but that vitamin D supplementation may also reduce the risk of developing type 1 diabetes (vitamin D). Further data are required to establish the clinical utility and cost-effectiveness of such interventions, including the demonstration of these positive effects over a longer period of time.

Other dietary considerations may also be important, with avoidance of cow's milk at an early age seemingly providing protection against autoimmunity. Again, it is unclear as to whether or not use of hydrolysed infant formulae instead of cow's milk for weaning will be of significant clinical benefit, as long-term prospective data of this type are lacking. However, the fact that cereal exposure at a young age may also provoke increased autoimmune activity reinforces the notion that antigen ingestion may affect immune system function.

The role for infectious agents in type 1 diabetes remains unclear, as there are variations on the hygiene hypothesis which suggest that certain infections may prove protective whereas others may be pathogenic. Certainly, evidence in animal models convincingly demonstrates an association between viral antigens and autoimmunity and human biopsies have shown viral particles in the pancreas of type 1 diabetes patients. However, there is a lack of data demonstrating a causal effect for viral infections. Furthermore, the intriguing prospect that parasitic infections may protect against type 1 diabetes requires further study, so that molecular mechanisms may be elucidated for therapeutic purposes.

Future research needs to be conducted on a large scale, with the inclusion of both randomised and prospective studies in order to establish the link between environmental factors and type 1 diabetes pathogenesis. In particular, long-term follow-up of infants is required to assess the true benefits of interventional trials. In addition, consideration of the interaction of genetics with environmental factors is necessary to complete the picture, as it is likely that both mechanisms are involved in determining geographical variation of disease [18, 48].

Environmental influences are another important factor in the development of type 1 diabetes. This has been illustrated in twin studies; less than 50 percent of monozygotic twins of probands with type 1 diabetes develop diabetes [49-50]. These observations are most likely explained by environmental factors such as viruses and dietary antigens.

5. Autoimmunity

Islet Cell Autoantibodies (ICAs) were first detected in serum from patients with autoimmune polyendocrine deficiency; they have subsequently been identified in 70 to 80 percent of patients with newly diagnosed type 1 diabetes and in prediabetic subjects (American Diabetic Association 1997). Measurement of serum ICA by staining of frozen sections of human pancreas was the major screening test used to identify subjects at risk for clinical diabetes but currently, large studies utilize a series of radioassays for autoantibodies reacting with specific islet autoantigens.

Children with type 1 diabetes who do not have islet-cell or other autoantibodies at presentation have a similar degree of metabolic decompensation as do children who have these antibodies, although those with more of the different types of antibodies appear to have the most accelerated islet destruction and a higher requirement for exogenous insulin during the second year of clinical disease [51]. A few patients without obvious evidence of islet autoimmunity have been described in whom the onset of hyperglycemia was abrupt, glycosylated hemoglobin values were normal, and serum pancreatic enzyme concentrations were high [52].

Autoantibodies to biochemically characterized beta-cell autoantigens: Insulin Autoantibodies (IAA), Auto-antibodies to the tyrosine phosphatases IA-2, Glutamic Acid Decarboxylase Autoantibodies (GADA), and zinc transporter 8 autoantibody (ZnT8A) [53] help to define type 1 diabetes a, if measured prior to or shortly after initiation of insulin therapy. IAA are masked by antibodies induced by exogenous insulin and become very hard to measure after just 10 to 14 days of insulin therapy. ZnT8A tend to disappear quickly after diagnosis of diabetes, while GADA and IA-2A tend to persist longer, but are rarely seen more than 5 years after diagnosis. Testing for at least two of these autoantibodies at diagnosis is now considered standard of care in type 1 diabetes. Good commercial assays exist for IA-2A, GADA, and ZnT8A, with the former two recently harmonized [54]. IAA are low-affinity antibodies and harder to measure; however, high-quality non-radioactive assays for IAA are close to being commercially available [55]. The search for additional islet autoantibodies and assay that would reliably detect autoreactive T-lymphocytes are active areas of research.

6. Complications

The management of type 1 diabetes and modalities for prevention of complications has evolved, such that the majority of patients with excellent care and education should avoid major microvascular complications. The finding from the Diabetes Control and Complications Trial (DCCT) follow-up study of "metabolic memory", namely long term benefit from early intensive glucose management is very encouraging [56]. Intensive management and strict guidelines for lipid lowering and early introduction of renoprotective medications are the norm. Laser therapy for advanced retinal disease is also the norm and "anti- Vascular endo-thelial growth factor (VEGF)" ocular therapy for macular edema is being extensively studied. Effective prevention of microvascular complications requires detection of early lesions, including determination of lipids, blood pressure, microalbuminuria, retinal exams. Preven-tative foot care and cardiovascular evaluation are also essential, with macrovascular disease a major problem for patients with long-term diabetes. Patients with type 1 diabetes have more severe progressive coronary artery atherosclerosis for any level of Low-density lipoprotein (LDL) cholesterol (57-586-57). Neuropathy remains difficult to treat [59] despite introduction of several newer medications.

Patients with diabetes and renal failure have a particularly poor prognosis when on dialysis. Every effort should be directed toward "early" renal transplantation in patients with type 1 diabetes and renal failure.

Genetic factors and key gene mutations have been implicated in the pathogenesis of diabetes. However, increasing evidence suggests that complex interactions between genes and the environment may play a major role in many common human diseases such as diabetes and its complications [39, 59-73]. Furthermore, the increased risk for both type 1 diabetes and type 2 diabetes can be controlled through medications, changes in dietary habits and increased exercise; subjects with diabetes continue to be plagued with numerous life-threatening complications. This continued development of diabetic complications even after achieving glucose control suggests a metabolic memory of prior glycemic exposure and indicates a missing link in diabetes etiology which recent studies have suggested may be attributed to epigenetic changes in target cells without alterations in gene coding sequences. Exploring a role for epigenetics in diabetic complications could allow for new insights clarifying the interplay between the environment and gene regulation and identify much needed new therapeutic targets.

Diabetic microvascular complications have been reported to be encountered with impairment in the olfactory system. Recently we have shown that polymorphism in the olfactory receptor, OR14J1C, may lead to an olfactory impairment that could be due to presence of microvascular diseases or other complication directly related to type 1 diabetes. The genetic alteration in the OR14J1 gene, A to C, could be linked to epigenetic processes [39].

6.1. What are common consequences of diabetes?

Over time, diabetes can damage the heart, blood vessels, eyes, kidneys, and nerves.

- Diabetes increases the risk of heart disease and stroke. 50% of people with diabetes die of cardiovascular disease (primarily heart disease and stroke).

- Combined with reduced blood flow, neuropathy in the feet increases the chance of foot ulcers and eventual limb amputation.

- Diabetic retinopathy is an important cause of blindness, and occurs as a result of long-term accumulated damage to the small blood vessels in the retina. After 15 years of diabetes, approximately 2% of people become blind, and about 10% develop severe visual impairment.

- Diabetes is among the leading causes of kidney failure. 10-20% of people with diabetes die of kidney failure.

- Diabetic neuropathy is damage to the nerves as a result of diabetes, and affects up to 50% of people with diabetes. Although many different problems can occur as a result of diabetic neuropathy, common symptoms are tingling, pain, numbness, or weakness in the feet and hands.

- The overall risk of dying among people with diabetes is at least double the risk of their peers without diabetes.

7. Conclusion

Type 1 diabetes has become perhaps the most intensively studied autoimmune illness results from autoimmune destruction of the insulin-producing ß-cells in the islets of Langerhans. This process occurs in genetically susceptible subjects, is probably triggered by one or more environmental agents, and usually progresses over many months or years during which the subject is asymptomatic and euglycemic. This long latent period is a reflection of the large number of functioning β-cells that must be lost before hyperglycemia occurs.

Polymorphisms in MHC genes and Non-MHC genes account for genetic susceptibility of the diseases. Genes in both the MHC and elsewhere in the genome have influence risk, but only HLA alleles have a large effect.

There are a number of autoantigens within the pancreatic ß-cells that may play important roles in the initiation or progression of autoimmune islet injury and its autoimmunity which might be a good prediction factor. Environmental factors that may affect risk include pregnancy-related and perinatal influences, viruses, and ingestion of cows' milk and cereals.

Author details

Mohamed M. Jahromi*

Address all correspondence to: mjahromi@yahoo.com

Pathology Department, Salmaniya Medical Complex, Ministry of Health, Manama, Kingdom of Bahrain

References

[1] Marian RowersChallenges in Diagnosing Type 1 diabetes in Different Populations. Diabetes Metab J. (2012). , 36, 90-97.

[2] http://wwwidf.org/diabetesatlas

[3] Stene, L. C, Barriga, K, Hoffman, M, et al. Normal but increasing hemoglobin A1c levels predict progression from islet autoimmunity to overt type 1 diabetes: Diabetes Autoimmunity Study in the Young (DAISY). Pediatr Diabetes (2006). , 7(5), 247-253.

[4] Gianani, R, Putnam, A, Still, T, et al. Initial results of screening of non- diabetic organ donors for expression of islet autoantibodies. J Clin Endocrinol Metab (2006). , 91, 1855-1861.

[5] Meier, J. J, Bhushan, A, Butler, A. E, Rizza, R. A, & Butler, P. C. Sustained beta cell apoptosis in patients with long-standing type 1 diabetes: indirect evidence for islet regeneration? Diabetologia (2005). , 48(11), 2221-2228.

[6] Souza, F, Simpson, N, Raffo, A, et al. Longitudinal noninvasive PET-based beta cell mass estimates in a spontaneous diabetes rat model. J Clin Invest (2006). , 116(6), 1506-1513.

[7] Turvey, S. E, Swart, E, Denis, M. C, et al. Noninvasive imaging of pancreatic inflammation and its reversal in type 1 diabetes. J Clin Invest (2005). , 115(9), 2454-2461.

[8] Chatenoud, L, & Bach, J. F. Regulatory T cells in the control of autoimmune diabetes: the case of the NOD mouse. Int Rev Immunol (2005).

[9] Krishnamurthy, B, Dudek, N. L, Mckenzie, M. D, et al. Responses against islet antigens in NOD mice are prevented by tolerance to proinsulin but not IGRP. J Clin Invest (2006). , 116(12), 3258-3265.

[10] Nakayama, M, Abiru, N, Moriyama, H, et al. Prime role for an insulin epitope in the development of type 1 diabetes in NOD mice. Nature (2005). , 435(7039), 220-223.

[11] Homann, D, & Eisenbarth, G. S. An immunologic homunculus for type 1 diabetes. Journal of Clinical Investigation (2006). , 116(5), 1212-1215.

[12] Wildin, R. S, & Freitas, A. IPEX and FOXP3: Clinical and research perspectives. J Autoimmun (2005). Suppl: , 56-62.

[13] Su, M. A, & Anderson, M. S. Aire: an update. Curr Opin Immunol (2004). , 16(6), 746-752.

[14] wwwncbi.nlm.nih.gov

[15] Barker, J. M, Yu, J, Yu, L, et al. Autoantibody "sub-specificity" in type 1 diabetes: Risk for organ specific autoimmunity clusters in distinct groups. Diab care (2005). , 28, 850-855.

[16] Hoffenberg, E. J, Emery, L. M, Barriga, K. J, et al. Clinical features of children with screening-identified evidence of celiac disease. peds (2004). , 113(5), 1254-1259.

[17] Liu, E, Li, M, Bao, F, et al. Need for quantitative assessment of transglutaminase au-
      toantibodies for celiac disease in screening-identified children. J Pediatr (2005). ,
      146(4), 494-499.

[18] Jahromi, M. M, & Eisenbarth, G. S. Genetic Determinants of type 1 diabetes Across
      Populations. Ann NY Acad Sci (2006). , 289-299.

[19] Kornete, J. M, & Piccirillo, C. A. Critical co-stimulatory pathways in the stability of
      Foxp3+ Treg cell homeostasis in Type I diabetes. Autoimmun Rev. (2011). , 11,
      104-111.

[20] Noble, J. A, Valdes, A. M, Cook, M, Klitz, W, Thomson, g, & Erlich, H. A. The role of
      HLA class II genes in insulin-dependent diabetes mellitus: molecular analysis of 180
      Caucasian, multiplex families.Am. J. Hum. Genet (1996). , 59, 1134-1148.

[21] Lambert, A. P, Gillespie, K. M, Thomson, G, Cordell, H. J, Todd, J. A, & Gale, E. A.
      and Bingley PJ. Absolute risk of childhood-onset type 1 diabetes defined by human
      leukocyte antigen class II genotype: a population-based study in the United King-
      dom. J. Clin. Endocrinol. Metab (2004). , 89, 4037-4043.

[22] Rewers, M, Bugawan, T. L, Norris, J. M, Blair, A, Beaty, B, Hoffman, M, et al. New-
      born screening for HLA markers associated with IDDM: diabetes autoimmunity
      study in the young (DAISY). Diabetologia (1996). , 39, 807-812.

[23] Johansson, S, Lie, B. A, Todd, J. A J. A, Pociot, F, Nerup, J, & Cambon-thomsen, A. et
      al. Evidence of at least two type 1 diabetes susceptibility genes in the HLA complex
      distinct from HLA-DQB1,-DQA1 and-DRB1. Genes Immun (2003). , 4, 46-53.

[24] Aly, T. A, Ide, A, Jahromi, M. M, Barker, J. M, Fernando, M. S, Babu, S. R, et al. Ex-
      treme Genetic Risk for Type 1A Diabetes. Proc Natl Acad Sci U S A (2006). , 103,
      14074-14079.

[25] Cheung, Y. H, Watkinson, J, & Anastassiou, D. Conditional meta-analysis stratifying
      on detailed HLA genotypes identifies a novel type 1 diabetes locus around TCF19 in
      the MHC. Hum Genet (2011). , 129, 161-176.

[26] Nejentsev, S, Howson, J. M, Walker, N. M, Szeszko, J, Field, S. F, Stevens, H. E, et al.
      The Wellcome Trust Case Control Consortium, Clayton DG, and Todd JA. Localiza-
      tion of type 1 diabetes susceptibility to the MHC class I genes HLA-B and HLA-A.
      Nature (2007). , 450, 887-892.

[27] Erlich, H, Valdes, A. M, Noble, J, Carlson, J. A, Varney, M, Concannon, P, et al. HLA
      DR-DQ haplotypes and genotypes and type 1 diabetes risk: analysis of the type 1 dia-
      betes genetics consortium families. Diabetes. (2008). , 57, 1084-1092.

[28] Aly, T. A, Baschal, E. E, Jahromi, M. M, Fernando, M. S, Babu, S. R, Fingerlin, T. E, et
      al. Analysis of Single Nucleotide Polymorphisms Identifies Major Type 1A Diabetes
      Locus Telomeric of the Major Histocompatibility Complex.Diabetes (2008). , 57,
      770-776.

[29] Baschal, E. E, Aly, T. A, Jasinski, J. M, Steck, A. K, Johnson, K. N, Noble, J. A, et al. The frequent and conserved DR3-B8-A1 extended haplotype confers less diabetes risk than other DR3 haplotypes. Diabetes Obes Metab (2009). , 11, 25-30.

[30] Concannon, P, Chen, W. M, Julier, C, Morahan, G, Akolkar, B, Erlich, H. A, et al. Genome-wide scan for linkage to TYPE 1 DIABETES in 2,496 multiplex families from the TYPE 1 DIABETES Genetics Consortium. Diabetes (2009). , 58, 1018-1022.

[31] Pociot, F, Akolkar, B, Concannon, P, Erlich, H. A, Julier, C, Morahan, G, et al. Genetics of TYPE 1 DIABETES: what's next? Diabetes (2010). , 59, 1561-1571.

[32] Zhang, B. Y, Zhang, J, & Liu, J. S. Block-Based Bayesian Epistasis Association Mapping With Application To Wtccc Type 1 Diabetes Data. Ann Appl Stat (2011). , 5, 2052-2077.

[33] Orozco, G, Barton, A, Eyre, S, Din, B, Worthington, J, Ke, X, Thomson, W, & Hla-dpb1-col, A. and three additional xMHC loci are independently associated with RA in a UK cohort. Genes and Immunity (2011). , 12, 169-175.

[34] NakaokaCui T, Tajima A, Oka A, Mitsunaga S, Kashiwase K, Homma Y, Sato S, Suzuki Y, Inoko H, Inoue I. A Systems Genetics Approach Provides a Bridge from Discovered Genetic Variants to Biological Pathways in Rheumatoid Arthritis. PLoS ONE ;(2011). e25389.

[35] Zhao, Y, Jiang, Z, & Guo, C. New hope for type 2 diabetics: targeting insulin resistance through the immune modulation of stem cells. Autoimmun Rev. (2011). , 11, 137-42.

[36] Takabatake, N, Toriyama, S, Takeishi, Y, Shibata, Y, Konta, T, Inoue, S, et al. A non-functioning single nucleotide polymorphism in olfactory receptor gene family is associated with the forced expiratory volume in the first second/the forced vital capacity values of pulmonary function test in a Japanese population. Biochem Biophys Res Commun. (2007). , 364, 662-667.

[37] Younger, R. M, Amadou, C, Bethel, G, Ehlers, A, Lindahl, K. F, Forbes, S, et al. Characterization of clustered MHC-linked olfactory receptor-genes in human and mouse. Genome Res (2001). , 11, 519-530.

[38] Santos, C. J, Uehara, S, Ziegler, A, & Uchanska-ziegler, B. Bicalho Mda G. Variation and linkage disequilibrium within odorant receptor gene clusters linked to the human major histocompatibility complex. Hum Immunol (2010). , 719, 843-850.

[39] Jahromi, M. M. HAPLOTYPE SPECIFIC ALTERATION OF DIABETES MHC RISK BY OLFACTORY RECEPTOR GENE POLYMORPHISM. Autoimmun Rev. (2012). May 8.

[40] Field, S. F, Howson, J. M, Smyth, D. J, Walker, N. M, Dunger, D. B, & Todd, J. A. Analysis of the type 2 diabetes gene, TCF7L2, in 13,795 TYPE 1 DIABETES cases and control subjects. Diabetologia (2007). , 2007, 212-213.

[41] Kent, S. C, Chen, Y, Bregoli, L, et al. Expanded T cells from pancreatic lymph nodes of type 1 diabetic subjects recognize an insulin epitope. Nature (2005). , 435(7039), 224-228.

[42] Ouyang, Q, Standifer, N. E, Qin, H, et al. Recognition of HLA Class I-Restricted {beta}-Cell Epitopes in TYPE 1 DIABETES. Diabetes (2006). , 55(11), 3068-3074.

[43] Achenbach, P, Warncke, K, Reiter, J, et al. TYPE 1 DIABETES risk assessment: improvement by follow-up measurements in young islet autoantibody-positive relatives. Diabetologia (2006). , 49(12), 2969-2976.

[44] Jahromi, M. M, Millward, B. A, & Demaine, A. G. The 5′ flanking G (-174) C region of the IL-6 gene polymorphism is highly associated with TYPE 1 DIABETES millitus. J Interferon and Cytokine Research; (2000). , 2000, 885-888.

[45] Cartwright, N, Demaine, A, Jahromi, M, Sanders, H, & Kaminski, E. A study of cytokine protein secretion, frequencies of cytokine expressing cells and IFN-G gene polymorphisms in normal individuals. J Transplantation (1999). , 10, 1546-1552.

[46] Jahromi, M. M, Millward, B. A, & Demaine, A. G. A CA repeat polymorphism of the interfron-γ gene is highly associated with TYPE 1 DIABETES: IFNG and IL-4 gene polymorphism and TYPE 1 DIABETES. J Interferon and Cytokine Research; (2000). , 20, 187-190.

[47] Jahromi, M. M, Millward, B. A, & Demaine, A. G. Significant Correlation between Association of Polymorphism in Codon 10 of the TGF-β1 T (29) C with TYPE 1 DIABETES and Patients with Nephropathy Disorder.J Interferon and Cytokine Research (2010).

[48] Alruhaili, M. Type 1 diabetes in the tropics: the protective effects of environmental factors. AJDM(2010). , 18, 1-8.

[49] American Diabetes AssociationReport of the Expert Committee on the Diagnosis and Classification of Diabetes Mellitus. Diab care (1997). , 20(7), 1183-1197.

[50] Wang, J, Miao, D, Babu, S, et al. Autoantibody negative diabetes is not rare at all ages and increases with older age and obesity. J Clin Endocrinol Metab (2007). , 92(11), 88-92.

[51] Gale, E. A. Latent autoimmune diabetes in adults: a guide for the perplexed. Diabetologia (2005). , 48(11), 2195-2199.

[52] Barker, J. M, Goehrig, S. H, Barriga, K, et al. Clinical characteristics of children diagnosed with TYPE 1 DIABETES through intensive screening and follow-up. Diab care (2004). , 27(6), 1399-1404.

[53] Fariba Vaziri-SaniAhmed J. Delli, Helena Elding-Larsson, Bengt Lindblad, Annelie Carlsson, Gun Forsander, Sten A. Ivarsson, Johnny Ludvigsson, Claude Marcus, and Åke Lernmark, on behalf of the Swedish Better Diabetes Diagnosis Study Group. A novel triple mix radiobinding assay for the three ZnT8 (ZnT8-RWQ) autoantibody

variants in children with newly diagnosed diabetes. J Immuno Methods (2011). , 371, 25-37.

[54] Bonifacio, E, Yu, L, Williams, A. K, Eisenbarth, G. S, Bingley, P. J, Marcovina, S. M, Adler, K, Ziegler, A. G, Mueller, P. W, Schatz, D. A, Krischer, J. P, Steffes, M. W, & Akolkar, B. Harmonization of glutamic acid decarboxylase and islet antigen-2 auto-antibody assays for national institute of diabetes and digestive and kidney diseases consortia. J Clin Endocrinol Metab. (2010). , 95, 3360-3367.

[55] Yu, L, Miao, D, Scrimgeour, L, Johnson, K, Rewers, M, & Eisenbarth, G. S. Distin-guishing persistent insulin autoantibodies with differential risk: nonradioactive biva-lent proinsulin/insulin autoantibody assay. Diabetes. (2012). , 61, 179-186.

[56] Patricia, A. Cleary, Trevor J. Orchard, Saul Genuth, Nathan D. Wong, Robert Detra-no, Jye-Yu C. Backlund, Bernard Zinman, Alan Jacobson, Wanjie Sun, John M. La-chin, and David M. Nathan, for the DCCT/EDIC Research Group. The Effect of Intensive Glycemic Treatment on Coronary Artery Calcification in Type 1 Diabetic Participants of the Diabetes Control and Complications Trial/Epidemiology of Diabe-tes Interventions and Complications (DCCT/EDIC) Study. Diabetes (2006). , 55, 3556-3565.

[57] Herold, K. C, Gitelman, S. E, Masharani, U, et al. A Single Course of Anti-CD3 Mono-clonal Antibody hOKT3{gamma}1(Ala-Ala) Results in Improvement in C-Peptide Re-sponses and Clinical Parameters for at Least 2 Years after Onset of TYPE 1 DIABETES. diab (2005). , 54(6), 1763-1769.

[58] Sustained effect of intensive treatment of TYPE 1 DIABETES mellitus on develop-ment and progression of diabetic nephropathy: the Epidemiology of Diabetes Inter-ventions and Complications (EDIC) studyJAMA (2003). , 290(16), 2159-2167.

[59] Genuth, S. Insights from the diabetes control and complications trial/epidemiology of diabetes interventions and complications study on the use of intensive glycemic treatment to reduce the risk of complications of TYPE 1 DIABETES. Endocr Pract (2006). Suppl , 1, 34-41.

[60] Cleary, P. A, Orchard, T. J, Genuth, S, et al. The Effect of Intensive Glycemic Treat-ment on Coronary Artery Calcification in Type 1 Diabetic Participants of the Diabe-tes Control and Complications Trial/Epidemiology of Diabetes Interventions and Complications (DCCT/EDIC) Study. Diabetes (2006). , 55(12), 3556-3565.

[61] Nathan, D. M, Cleary, P. A, Backlund, J. Y, et al. Intensive diabetes treatment and cardiovascular disease in patients with TYPE 1 DIABETES. N Engl J Med (2005). , 353(25), 2643-2653.

[62] Martin, C. L, Albers, J, Herman, W. H, et al. Neuropathy among the diabetes control and complications trial cohort 8 years after trial completion. Diabetes Care (2006). , 29(2), 340-344.

[63] King, G. L, & Loeken, M. R. Hyperglycemia-induced oxidative stress in diabetic complications. Histochem Cell Biol. (2004). , 122, 333-338.

[64] Hoeldtke, R. D, Bryner, K. D, & Vandyke, K. Oxidative stress and autonomic nerve
function in early type 1 diabetes. Clin Auton Res (2011). , 21, 19-28.

[65] Brands, A. M, Kessels, R. P, De Haan, E. H, Kappelle, L. J, & Biessels, G. J. Cerebral
dysfunction in type 1 diabetes: effects of insulin, vascular risk factors and blood-glu-
cose levels. Eur J Pharmacol. (2004). , 490, 159-168.

[66] Sima, A. A, Zhang, W, Muzik, O, Kreipke, C. W, Rafols, J. A, & Hoffman, W. H. Sequential abnormalities in type 1 diabetic encephalopathy and the effects of C-Peptide. Rev Diabet Stud (2009). , 6, 211-222.

[67] Sima, A. A. Encephalopathies: the emerging diabetic complications. Acta Diabetol
(2010). , 47, 279-293.

[68] Hoffman, W. H, Andjelkovic, A. V, Zhang, W, Passmore, G. G, & Sima, A. A. Insulin
and IGF-1 receptors, nitrotyrosin and cerebral neuronal deficits in two young patients with diabetic ketoacidosis and fatal brain edema. Brain Res (2010). , 1343,
168-177.

[69] Mira, A. D, & Ward, H. Encephalopathy following diabetic ketoacidosis in a type 1
diabetes patient. Pract Diab Int (2010). , 27, 76-78.

[70] Guven, A, Cebeci, N, Dursun, A, Aktekin, E, Baumgartner, M, & Fowler, B. Methyl-
malonic acidemia mimicking diabetic ketoacidosis in an infant. Pediatr Diabetes
(2011). May 5. doi:j. x., 1399-5448.

[71] Fritsch, M, Rosenbauer, J, Schober, E, Neu, A, Placzek, K, & Holl, R. W. German
Competence Network Diabetes Mellitus and the DPV Initiative. Predictors of diabetic ketoacidosis in children and adolescents with type 1 diabetes. Experience from a
large multicentre database. Pediatr Diabetes (2011). , 12, 307-312.

[72] Hawkins, K. A, & Pearlson, G. D. Age and gender but not common chronic illnesses
predict odor identification in older African Americans. Am J Geriatr Psychiatry
(2011). , 19, 777-782.

[73] Grassi, M. A, Tikhomirov, A, Ramalingam, S, Below, J. E, Cox, N. J, & Nicolae, D. L.
Genome-wide Meta-analysis for Severe Diabetic Retinopathy". Human Molecular
Genetics (2011). , 20, 2472-2481.

Beta-Cell Function and Dysfunction

Chapter 5

Beta-Cell Function and Failure

Soltani Nepton

Additional information is available at the end of the chapter

1. Introduction

1.1. Beta cells (β-cells)

Beta cells are a type of cell in the pancreas located in the so-called islets of Langerhans. They make up 65-80% of the cells in the islets.

The Islets diameter is about 50 to 300 micrometers. They are composed of several types of cells. At least 70 percent are beta cells, which are localized in the core of the islet. These cells are surrounded by alpha cells that secrete glucagon, smaller numbers of delta cells that secrete somatostatin, and PP cells or F cells that secrete pancreatic polypeptide. All of the cells communicate with each other through extracellular spaces and through gap junctions. This arrangement allows cellular products secreted from one cell type to influence the function of downstream cells. As an example, insulin secreted from beta cells can suppress glucagon secretion.

A neurovascular bundle containing arterioles and sympathetic and parasympathetic nerves enters each islet through the central core of beta cells. The arterioles branch to form capillaries that pass between the cells to the periphery of the islet and then enter the portal venous circulation.

2. Beta cells functions

Insulin is synthesized as preproinsulin in the ribosomes of the rough endoplasmic reticulum in the beta cells (fig 1). Preproinsulin is then cleaved to proinsulin, which is transported to the Golgi apparatus where it is packaged into secretory granules located close to the cell membrane. Proinsulin is cleaved into equimolar amounts of insulin and C-peptide in the secretory granules. The process of insulin secretion involves fusion of the secretory granules with the cell membrane and exocytosis of insulin, C-peptide, and proinsulin

Insulin is a hormone that controls the blood glucose concentration. The liver maintains the base-line glucose level, but the beta cells can respond quickly to spikes in blood glucose by releasing some of its stored insulin while simultaneously producing more. The response time is very quick.

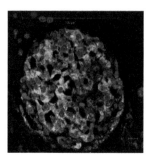

Figure 1 Mouse pancreatic islet as seen by light microscopy. Beta cells can be recognized by the green insulin staining. Glucagon is labeled in red and the nuclei in blue

Apart from insulin, beta cells release C-peptide, a consequence of insulin production, into the bloodstream in equimolar amounts. C-peptide helps to prevent neuropathy and other symptoms of diabetes related to vascular deterioration.Measuring the levels of C-peptide can give a practitioner an idea of the viable beta cell mass.

Beta-cells also produce amylin, also known as IAPP, islet amyloid polypeptide. Amylin functions as part of the endocrine pancreas and contributes to glycemic control. Amylin's metabolic function is now somewhat well characterized as an inhibitor of the appearance of nutrient [especially glucose] in the plasma. Thus, it functions as a synergistic partner to insulin. Whereas insulin regulates long-term food intake, increased amylin decreases food intake in the short term.

GABA (γ amino butyric acid) is produced by pancreatic beta cell. GABA released from beta cells can act on GABA $_A$receptor in the α cells, causing membrane hyperpolarization and hence suppressing glucagon secretion. An impaired insulin-Akt-GABA$_A$ receptors glucagon secretory pathway in the islet may be an underlying mechanism for unsuppressed glucagon secretion, despite hyperglycemia, in diabetic subjects. Some studies demonstrated that beta cells also express GABA $_A$ receptors, forming an autocrine GABA signaling system. However, the role of this autocrine GABA signaling in the regulation of beta cell functions remains largely unknown.

Zinc is needed by over 300 enzyme systems.Some of those are involved with the metabolism of blood sugar and are so important that a lack of zinc, in and of itself, can cause type I or type II diabetes.

Zinc is highly concentrated in the insulin-secreting beta cells of our pancreas. Zinc can keep insulin molecules together in the beta cells.Beta cells must have zinc to function. In fact, beta cells contain their own special zinc transporter called zinc transporter 8 that enables beta cells to take up zinc.Gene alterations in this zinc transporter are now known to cause type II diabetes while type I diabetes is associated with antibodies against this zinc transporter (meaning the immune system knocks out function of beta cells so they can't produce insulin).

Zinc directly influences how insulin is produced and secreted by our beta cells. So the people with zinc deficiency can't store and release insulin.Furthermore, zinc is self-protecting to the beta cells.It has now been shown that zinc directly reduces the inflammatory signals that damage the beta cells, a process that leads to type I diabetes.

3. Mechanisms of insulin secretion from beta cells

The secretion of insulin from pancreatic beta cells is a complex process involving the integration and interaction of multiple external and internal stimuli. Thus, nutrients, hormones, neurotransmitters, and drugs all activate or inhibit insulin secretion. The primary stimulus for insulin release is the beta-cell response to changes in glucose concentration. Normally, glucose induces a biphasic pattern of insulin release. First-phase insulin release occurs within the first few minutes after exposure to an elevated glucose level; this is followed by a more permanent second phase of insulin release. Of particular importance is the observation that first-phase insulin secretion is lost in patients with type 2 diabetes. Thus, molecular mechanisms involved in phasic insulin secretion are important. This processes discussed as follow (fig 2).

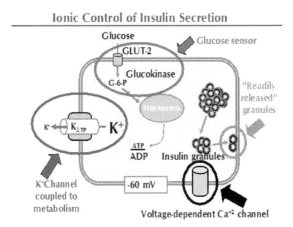

Figure 2. The beta cell structure

A widely accepted sequence of events involved in glucose-induced insulin secretion is as follows:

1. Glucose is transported into beta cells through facilitated diffusion of GLUT2 glucose transporters.

2. Intracellular glucose is metabolized to ATP.

3. Elevation in the ATP/ADP ratio induces closure of cell-surface ATP-sensitive K+ (KATP) channels, leading to cell membrane depolarization.

4. Cell-surface voltage-dependent Ca2+ channels (VDCC) are opened, facilitating extracellular Ca2+ influx into the beta cell.

5. A rise in free cytosolic Ca2+ triggers the exocytosis of insulin.

It is understood that glucose stimulates insulin secretion in the pancreatic beta cell by means of a synergistic interaction between at least two signaling pathways. In the K (ATP) channel-dependent pathway, glucose stimulation increases the entry of extrinsic Ca2+ through voltage-gated channels by closure of the K (ATP) channels and depolarization of the beta cell membrane. The resulting increase in intracellular Ca2+ stimulates insulin exocytosis. While in the GTP-dependent pathway, intracellular Ca2+ is elevated by GTP-dependent proteins and augments the Ca2+-stimulated release. Secretagogues and insulin secretion inhibitors act at intermediate steps of these signaling pathways and influence the process of insulin exocytosis. Several researchers have investigated this intricate mode of known secretagogue action using isolated islets as an *in vitro* model. To quote a few; imidazoline antagonists of alpha 2-adrenoreceptors increase insulin release *in vitro* by inhibiting ATP-sensitive K+ channels in pancreatic beta cells. Some researchers have evaluated the properties of sulphonylurea receptors (SUR) of human islets of Langerhans. They studied the binding affinity of various oral hypoglycaemic agents to the receptor and also tested insulinotropic action of the drugs on intact human islets. This binding potency order was parallel with the insulinotropic potency of the evaluated compounds. Some investigators have shown an insulinotropic effect of Triglitazone (CS-045) and have shown its mode of action to be distinct from glibenclamide (a sulphonylurea drug). A-4166, a derivative of D-phenylalanine, evokes a rapid and short-lived hypoglycaemic action *in vivo*. It has been shown to act via the tolbutamide binding sites14. Some studies showed S21403, a meglitinide analogue to be a novel insulinotropic tool in the treatment of type 2 diabetes, as it affected cationic fluxes and the drugs secretary responses displayed favourable time course of prompt, and not unduly prolonged, activation of beta cells. Some studies demonstrated that tetracaine (an anaesthetic) stimulates insulin secretion by release of intracellular calcium and for the first time elucidated the role of intracellular calcium stores in stimulus-secretion coupling in the pancreatic beta cells. JTT-608, is a nonsulphonylurea oral hypoglycaemic agent which stimulates insulin release at elevated but not low glucose concentrations by evoking PKA-mediated Ca2+ influx.

4. The importance of KATP channels

The KATP channels play an integral role in glucose-stimulated insulin secretion by serving as the transducer of a glucose-generated metabolic signal (ie, ATP) to cell electrical activity (membrane depolarization). Thus, like neurons, beta cells are electrically excitable and capable of generating Ca2+ action potentials that are important in synchronizing islet cell activity and insulin release. In addition to being signal targets for glucose, KATP channels are the targets for sulfonylureas, which are commonly prescribed oral agents in the treatment of type 2 diabetes. The sulfonylureas, like glucose, induce closure of KATP channels and stimulate insulin secretion.

The beta-cell KATP channel is a complex octameric unit of 2 different proteins: the sulfonylurea receptor (SUR-1) and an inward rectifier (Kir6.2). The sulfonylurea receptor belongs to a superfamily of ATP-binding cassette proteins and contains the binding site for sulfonylurea drugs and nucleotides. The inward rectifier represents the K+ conducting pore and is also regulated by ATP. It is interesting that KATP channels are present in other tissues of the body, including heart (SUR-2A/Kir 6.2), smooth muscle (SUR-2B/Kir 6.2), and brain (SUR-1/Kir 6.2). Recently, Mark L. Evans, MD, Yale University Medical School, New Haven, Connecticut, and colleagues have suggested that glucose sensing in the brain during hypoglycemia may be mediated by KATP channels located in brain hypothalamic neurons. Thus, these molecules may also serve as new therapeutic targets for the restoration of impaired hypoglycemia awareness and glucose counterregulation in type 1 diabetes.

5. Voltage-dependent Ca2+ channels: Novel regulators

Extracellular Ca2+ influx through L-type voltage-dependent Ca2+ channels (VDCC) raises free cytoplasmic Ca2+ levels and triggers insulin secretion. The structure of the VDCC is complex and consists of 5 subunits: alpha1, alpha2, beta, gamma, and delta units. The alpha subunit constitutes the ion-conducting pore, whereas the other units serve a regulatory role. Previous work has identified that isoforms of alpha1 subunits interact with exocytotic proteins. More recently, using the yeast hybrid screening method, a novel protein, Kir-GEM, interacting with the beta3 isoform of the VDCC, has been identified by Seino and colleagues. Furthermore, it has been determined that Kir-GEM inhibits alpha ionic activity and prevents cell-surface expression of alpha subunits. The investigators have proposed that in the presence of Ca2+, Kir-GEM binds to the beta isoform, and this interaction interferes in the trafficking or translocation of alpha subunits to the plasma membrane. The relevance of Kir-GEM in insulin secretion was made evident by its attenuation of glucose-stimulated Ca2+ increases and C-peptide secretion in an insulin-secreting cell line.

The potential therapeutic role of Kir-GEM lies in the inhibitory effects on VDCC activity that may serve to protect beta cells from overstimulation and subsequent failure, which is part of the disease etiology of type 2 diabetes.

6. Novel cAMP signaling pathways of insulin release

The incretins are another set of factors that are important hormonal regulators of insulin secretion. The incretins are polypeptide hormones released in the gut after a meal that potentiate insulin secretion in a glucose-dependent manner. Due to their dependence on ambient glucose for action, they are emerging as important new therapeutic agents to promote insulin secretion without accompanying hypoglycemia (a common complication of sulfonylurea treatment).

Unlike sulfonylureas, incretins act by activating Gs (a G-protein that activates adenylyl cyclase) to increase cAMP in beta cells. cAmp, like ATP, is an important signal that regulates insulin release. Typically, the main mechanism of action of cAMP is by activation of an enzyme called protein kinase A (PKA) that, in turn, phosphorylates other substrates to turn on (or off) vital cell functions. Using a biochemical assay called the yeast hybrid screening method to identify and isolate new proteins, some researchers identified a novel protein, cAMP-GEF II, a cAMP sensor (cAMPS) that forms a complex with other intracellular proteins (Rim2 and Rab3) to directly regulate insulin exocytosis. Then, using molecular reagents that antagonize the effects of cAMPS, they observed that incretin-potentiated insulin secretion is attenuated. These results provide a mechanism whereby cAMP can directly promote exocytosis of insulin granules without activation of PKA (ie, a PKA-independent pathway), and thereby provide additional molecular targets for therapeutic intervention.

7. Beta cell dysfunction and apoptosis

Type one diabetes: Islet beta-cells are almost completely destroyed when patients with type 1 diabetes are diagnosed. Type 1 diabetes occurs when the bodies own immune system destroys the beta cells. Some people develop a type of diabetes – called secondary diabetes -- which is similar to type 1 diabetes, but the beta cells are not destroyed by the immune system but by some other factor, such as cystic fibrosis or pancreatic surgery.

Type two diabetes: Defects in insulin action and insulin secretion are both present in type 2 diabetes, and both are believed to be genetically predetermined. In the absence of a defect in beta-cell function, individuals can compensate indefinitely for insulin resistance with appropriate hyperinsulinemia, as observed even in obese populations. Both insulin secretion and insulin action are impaired in type 2 diabetes. However, when allowance is made for the hyperglycaemia and the fact that glucose stimulates insulin secretion, it becomes apparent that the insulin levels in diabetic patients are lower than in healthy controls and inadequate beta-cell function therefore represents a key feature of the disease. Theoretically, the insulin secretory defect could result from either defects of beta-cell function or a reduction in beta-cell mass. Most quantitative estimates indicate that type 2 diabetes associates with either no change or < 30% reduction in beta-cell mass. Moreover, the secretion defect is more severe than can be accounted for solely by the reduction in beta-cell mass. It therefore appears that the insulin secretory defect in type 2 diabetes does not primarily result from insufficient beta-cell mass but rather from an impairment of insulin secretion.

8. Prevention of beta cell dysfunction and apoptosis

Islet beta-cells are almost completely destroyed when patients with type 1 diabetes are diagnosed. To date, insulin substitute therapy is still one of the main treatments. The cure of type 1 diabetes requires beta-cell regeneration from islet cell precursors and prevention of recurring autoimmunity. Therefore, beta-cell replacement, regeneration and proliferation emerge as a new research focus on therapy for type 1 diabetes; however, its application is limited by the shortage of pancreas donors. In-vitro expansion of human cadaveric islet beta cells represents an attractive strategy for generation of abundant beta-like cells. Human beta cells patent a very low proliferation capacity in vivo, and intact isolated islets cultured in suspension do not proliferate, although they remain functional for months. When islets are allowed to attach, limited replication of beta cells can be induced by growth factors or extracellular matrix components before the beta-cell phenotype is lost. Previous accepting of the determinants of tissue mass during adult life is still rudimentary. Insights into this problem may suggest novel approaches for the treatment of neoplastic as well as degenerative diseases. In the case of the pancreas, elucidating the mechanisms that govern β cell mass will be important for the design of regenerative therapy for both type 1 and type 2 diabetes, diseases characterized by an insufficient mass of β cells. It is clear that β cell mass increase during pregnancy and in insulin-resistant states, but evidence on the ability of β cells to regenerate from a severe, diabetogenic injury is conflicting. Whereas autoimmune diabetes is normally irreversible, recent evidence from both humans and rodents suggests that β cell function (i.e., insulin production and the maintenance of glucose homeostasis) can partly recover if autoimmunity is blocked.

Islet beta-cell regeneration and development are controlled by many growth factors, especially insulin-like growth factor-1 (IGF-1). Pancreatic islets produce Igf1 and Igf2, which bind to specific receptors on β-cells. Igf1 has been shown to influence β-cell apoptosis, and both Igf1 and Igf2 increase islet growth; Igf2 does so in a manner additive with fibroblast growth factor 2. Some study showed that IGF-1 can protect beta-cells from the destruction of apoptosis factors and promoting beta-cell survival and proliferation. Interleukin-1beta (IL-1 beta) is a potent pro-inflammatory cytokine that has been shown to inhibit islet beta cell function as well as to activate Fas-mediated apoptosis in a nitric oxide-dependent manner. Furthermore, this cytokine is effective in recruiting lymphocytes that mediate beta cell destruction in type one diabetes. IGF-I has been shown to block IL-1beta actions in vitro.

Glucagon like peptide 1 (GLP-1) is a potent insulin secretagogue released by L-cells of the distal large intestine in response to meal ingestion and, together with glucose-dependent insulinotropic polypeptide (GIP), account for 90% of the incretin effect. Type 2 diabetic patients are characterized by severely impaired β-cell function, reduced plasma GLP-1 response to meal/glucose ingestion that correlates with reduced insulin secretion, and severe β-cell resistance to the stimulatory effect of GLP-1 on insulin secretion. GLP-1 also inhibits glucagon secretion, delays gastric emptying, and promotes weight loss by its appetite-suppressant effect. GLP-1 analogs also stimulate islet neogenesis and β-cell replication and inhibit islet apoptosis. The gluco-incretin hormones GLP-1 and GIP can protect beta-cell against apoptosis induced by cytokines or glucose and free fatty acids. Both hormones bind to specific Gs-coupled receptors, which trigger cAMPformation. In beta-cells, basal cAMP levels controls glucose competence, i.e., the magnitude of the insulin secretion response to a given increase in extracellular glucose concentration. Increases in cAMP levels, for instance as stimulated by GLP-1 or GIP action, potentiate glucose-stimulated insulin secretion by both protein kinase A (PKA)-dependent and independent mechanisms; they also stimulate gene transcription through PKA dependent phosphorylation of the transcription factor CREB. In beta-cells, increased cAMP levels also activate the MAP kinase cascade, leading to rapid phosphorylation of Erk1/2. An activation of the PI3Kinase/Akt pathway is also observed. PI3kinase may be directly activated by the ßγ subunit of Gs, be secondary to transactivation of the EGF receptor by betacellulin, or may follow transcriptional induction of IRS-2 through the PKA/CREB pathway. The IRS- 2/PI3kinase/Akt pathway is known to have anti-apoptotic effects; however, it is unclear why increased expression of IRS-2 leads to activation of its signaling pathway. IRS-2 may be downstream of the insulin (IR) or IGF-1 (IGF-1R) receptors. Studies of mice with beta-cell specific inactivation of either receptor indicated that the insulin receptor was important for compensatory growth of the beta-cells in response to insulin resistance whereas the IGF-1 receptor was involved in the control of glucose competence. Although these properties make GLP-1 an ideal antidiabetic agent, it is rapidly cleaved ($T_{1/2}$ = 1–2 min) by dipeptidyl peptidase-4. GLP-1 enhances beta cell function with an increase in the ability to secrete insulin and restore first phase insulin release. Our pervious study showed that a novel GLP-1 analogue consisting of the fusion of active GLP-1 and IgG heavy chain constant regions (GLP-1/IgG-fc) therapy can enhances beta cell mass. It also could increase insulin secretion. Within the pancreas, GLP-1 expands β-cell mass via promotion of β-cell growth and reduction of β-cell death.

γ-Aminobutyric acid (GABA), a prominent inhibitory neurotransmitter, is present in high concentrations in β-cells of islets of Langerhans. The GABA shunt enzymes, glutamate decarboxylase (GAD) and GABA transaminase (GABA-T) have also been localized in islet β-cells. With the recent demonstration that the 64,000-Mr antigen associated with insulin-dependent diabetes mellitus is GAD, there isincreased interest in understanding the role of GABA in islet functions. Only a small component of β-cell GABA is contained in insulin secretory granules, making it unlikely that GABA, co-released with insulin, is physiologically significant. Our immunohistochemical study of GABA in β-cells of intact islets indicates that GABA is associated with a vesicular compartment distinctly different from insulin secretory granules. Whether this compartment represents a releasable pool of GABA has yet to be determined. GAD in β-cells is associated with a vesicular compartment, similar to the GABA vesicles. In addition, GAD is found in a unique extensive tubular cisternal complex (GAD complex). It is likely that the GABA-GAD vesicles are derived from this GAD-containing complex. Physiological studies on the effect of extracellular GABA on islet hormonal secretion have had variable results. Effects of GABA on insulin, glucagon, and somatostatin secretion have been proposed. The most compelling evidence for GABA regulation of islet hormone secretion comes from studies on somatostatin secretion, where it has an inhibitory effect. Some researchers present new evidence demonstrating the presence of GABAergic nerve cell bodies at the periphery of islets with numerous GABA-containing processes extending into the islet mantle. This close association between GABAergic neurons and islet α- and δ-cells strongly suggests that GABA inhibition of somatostatin and glucagon secretionis mediated by these neurons. Intracellular β-cell GABAA and its metabolismmay have a role in β-cell function. New evidence indicates that GABA shunt activity is involved in regulation of insulin secretion. In addition, GABA or its metabolites may regulate proinsulin synthesis. These new observations provide insight into the complex nature of GABAergic neurons and β-cell GABA in regulation of islet function. Our study showed that GABA exerts has protective and regenerative effects on islet beta cells and reverses diabetes. GABA therapy increased beta cell proliferation and decreased beta cell apoptosis, which in turn increase beta cell mass and induced the reversal of hyperglycemia in the different kind of mice. Our data suggest that GABA exerts has ani-inflammatory effects, and is directly inhibitory to T cells and macrophages.

Magnesium deficiency has recently been proposed as a novel factor implicated in the pathogenesis of the diabetic complications. In our previous study we showed that oral chronic Mg administration could improve islet structure and decrease the blood glucose.

Another potential treatment is the combination of two growth factors called gastrin and epidermal growth factor (EGF), which has been shown to promote beta-cell regeneration in rats.

Many traditional treatments have been recommended in the alternative system of medicine for treatment of diabetes mellitus and regeneration of beta cells such as Garlic, Teucriumpolium, Cinnamon and Psidium guava leaves. Photochemical analysis of those herbs have revealed the presence of flavonoids, which include quercetin and its derivatives. It is concluded that quercetin, a flavonoid with antioxidant properties brings about the regeneration of the pancreatic islets and probably increases insulin release in streptozocin-induced diabetic rats.

Connective tissue growth factor (CTGF), to induce adult β cell mass expansion. Some study showed that CTGF is required for embryonic β cell proliferation3, and that CTGF overexpression in embryonic cells increases β cell proliferation and β cell mass.

The mouse pancreas develops from ventral and dorsal evaginations of the posterior foregut endoderm at embryonic day, a process dependent on the transcription factors Pdx1 and Ptf1. Differentiation of all pancreatic endocrine cell types (α, β, Δ and PP) is dependent on the transcription factor, neurogenin 3 (Ngn3). *Ngn3* expression is controlled by a variety of factors, including the Notch signaling pathway and the transcriptional regulators pancreatic and duodenal homeobox 1 (Pdx1), SRY-box 9 (Sox9) and hepatic nuclear factor 6 (Hnf6). Although β cell neogenesis begins, these early insulin-positive cells do not contribute to mature islets. Instead, endocrine cells that will go on to contribute to the mature islets begin to differentiate period known as the secondary transition. Some transcription factors critically involved in β cell differentiation include NK2 homeobox 2 (Nkx2.2), Nkx6.1, islet 1 (Isl-1), neuronal differentiation 1 (NeuroD1), motor neuron and pancreas homeobox 1(Mnx1), paired box gene 4 (Pax4) and Pdx1.

In adults, physiological stimuli can enhance β cell proliferation during development. Although several factors have been identified that play a role in the regulation of embryonic and neonatal β cell proliferation. One cell cycle regulator that does play a role in embryonic β cell proliferation is the cell cycle inhibitor, p27Kip1. Inactivation of *p27Kip1* during embryogenesis results in an increase in β cell proliferation and subsequently β cell mass. There was no change, however, in early postnatal β cell proliferation, suggesting that p27Kip1 is not crucial to postnatal proliferation.

As mentioned above Pdx1expressed in multipotent pancreatic progenitors in the early stages of pancreas development, but, Pdx1 expression becomes enhanced in insulin-positive cells and is found at only low levels in exocrine cells. This expression pattern is maintained into adulthood and Pdx1 plays a critical rolein maintenance of the mature β cell phenotype. Inactivation of *Pdx1* in embryonic insulin-expressing cells results in a dramatic decrease in β cell proliferation at late gestation, leading to decreased β cell mass at birth and early onset diabetes. Two large Maf (musculoaponeuroticfibrosarcoma oncogene homolog) transcription factors that are closely related to one another, MafA and MafB, are critical for β cell differentiation and embryonic *Pdx1* expression22 and therefore may have an indirect effect on embryonic β cell replication.

Inactivation of the eIF2α endoplasmic reticulum resident kinase, PERK (proteinkinase RNA-like endoplasmic reticulum kinase), specifically in embryonic β cells (PERKΔbeta) results in a 2-fold decrease in β cell proliferation, which persists through postnatal day (P).

Author details

Soltani Nepton

Physiology Department, Faculty of Medicine, Hormozgan University of Medical Science, Iran

References

[1] Beguin P, Nagashima K, Gonoi T, et al. Regulation of Ca2+ channel expression at the cell surface by the small G-protein kir/Gem. Nature. 411:701-706, 2001.

[2] Bhonde R, Shukla RC, Kanitkar M, Shukla R, Banerjee M, Datar S. Isolated islets in diabetes research. Indian J Med Res 125: 425-440, 2007

[3] Butler AE, Janson J, Bonner-Weir S, et al. Decreased B-cell mass in patients with type 2 diabetes. Program and abstracts of the 62nd Scientific Sessions of the American Diabetes Association, 14(18), 2002; San Francisco, California. Poster 1502-P. Diabetes, Volume 51, Supplement 2.

[4] Chang-Chen KJ, Mullur R, Bernal-Mizrachi E. Beta-cell failure as a complication of diabetes. Rev EndocrMetabDisord. 9(4): 329-43, 2008.

[5] Chen ZH, Li T, Chen ZB, Luo B, Sun RP. Prevention of beta cell dysfunction and apoptosis by adenoviral gene transfer of rat insulin-like growth factor 1. Chin Med J. 20;122(18): 2159-64, 2009

[6] Cornu M, Thorens B. GLP-1 protects beta-cells against apoptosis by enhancing the activity of an IGF-2/IGF1-receptor autocrine loop. Islets 1(3): 280-282, 2009

[7]   Cornu M, Yang GY, Jaccard E, Poussin C, Widmann C, Thorens B. Glp-1 Protects Be-
      ta-Cells Against Apoptosis By Increasing The ActivtiyOfAn Igf-2/Igf1-Receptor Au-
      tocrine Loop. Diabetes. 28, 2009

[8]   DeFronzo RA, Abdul-Ghani M. Type 2 Diabetes Can Be Prevented With Early Phar-
      macological Intervention. Diabetes Care. 34(2): S202-S209, 2011

[9]   Evans ML, Keshavarz T, Flanagan DV, et al. ICV brain glibenclamide suppresses
      counterregulatory responses to brain glucopenia in rats: evidence for a role for brain
      KATP channels in hypoglycemia sensing. Program and abstracts of the 62nd Scientif-
      ic Sessions of the American Diabetes Association, 17, 2002; San Francisco, California.
      Abstract 293-OR. Diabetes, Volume 51, Supplement 2.

[10] Fisher TE, Bourque CW. The function of CA(2+) channel subtypes in exocytic secre-
      tion: new perspectives from synaptic and non-synaptic release. ProgBiophysMol Bi-
      ol. 77:269-303, 2001

[11] Giannoukakis N, Mi Z, Rudert WA, Gambotto A, Trucco M, Robbins P. Prevention of
      beta cell dysfunction and apoptosis activation in human islets by adenoviral gene
      transfer of the insulin-like growth factor I. Gene Ther. 7(23):2015-22, 2000.

[12] Gunasekaran U, Hudgens CW, Wright BT, Maulis MF, Gannon M. Differential regu-
      lation of embryonic and adult β cell replication.Cell Cycle. 11(13), 2012

[13] Holst J. State of the art lecture. GLP-1 based therapy of diabetes: facts and expecta-
      tions. Program and abstracts of the 62nd Scientific Sessions of the American Diabetes
      Association; 14(18), 2002, San Francisco, California.

[14] Kashima Y, Shibasaki T, Miki T, Seino S. Importance of the cAMP-GEFII/Rim2 com-
      plex in incretin-potentiated insulin secretion. Program and abstracts of the 62nd Sci-
      entific Sessions of the American Diabetes Association, 14(18), 2002, San Francisco,
      California. 265-OR. Diabetes, Volume 51, Supplement 2.

[15] LeRoith D. Beta-cell dysfunction and insulin resistance in type 2 diabetes: role of
      metabolic and genetic abnormalities. Am J Med, 28(113): 6A:3S-11S, 2002

[16] Mansoori A, Zaheri H, Soltani N, Kharazmi F, Keshavarz M, Kamalinajad M. Effect
      of the administration of Psidium guava leaves on lipid profiles and sensitivity of the
      vascular mesenteric bed to phenylephrine in STZ-induced diabetic rats. JMD, 2(1):
      138-145, 2012

[17] Mikhailov MV, Mikhailova EA, Ashcroft SJ. Structure-function relationships in the
      beta-cell K (ATP) channel.BiochemSoc Trans. 30(2):323-7, 2002

[18] Miki T, Liss B, Minami K, et al. KATP channels in the maintenance of glucose homeo-
      stasis. Program and abstracts of the 62nd Scientific Sessions of the American Diabetes
      Association, 14(18), 2002, San Francisco, California. Poster 1492-P. Diabetes, Volume
      51, Supplement 2.

[19] Mirghazanfari SM, Keshavarz M, Nabavizadeh F, Soltani N, Kamalinejad M. 2010.
      The effect of Teucriumpolium L. Extracts on insulin release from in situ isolated per-

fused rat pancrease in newly modified isolation method: the role of Ca and K channels. Iranian Biomedical Journal. 14(4):178-185

[20] Russ HA, Sintov E, Anker-Kitai L, Friedman O, Lenz A, Toren G, Farhy C, Pasmanik-
Chor M, Oron-Karni V, Ravassard P, Efrat S. Insulin-Producing Cells Generated from
Dedifferentiated Human Pancreatic Beta Cells Expanded In Vitro. PLoS ONE 6(9):
e25566, 2011

[21] Seino S. Plenary Lecture: Molecular mechanisms of insulin secretion. Program and
abstracts of the 62nd Scientific Sessions of the American Diabetes Association, 14(18),
2002, San Francisco, California. Diabetes, Volume 51, Supplement 2.

[22] Soltani N, Keshavarz M, Dehpour AR. 2007. Effect of oral magnesium sulfate administration on blood pressure and lipid profile in streptozocin diabetic rat.Eur J Pharmacol. 560(2-3):201-5

[23] Soltani N, Kumar M, Glinka Y, Prud'homme GJ, Wang Q. 2007. Gene therapy of diabetes using a novel GLP-1/IgG1-Fc fusion construct normalizes glucose levels in
db/db mice.Gene Ther. 14(2):162-72

[24] Soltani N, Qiu H, Aleksic M, Glinka Y, Zhao F, Liu R, Li Y, Zhang N, Chakrabarti R,
Ng T, Jin T, Zhang H, Lu WY, Feng ZP, Prud'homme GJ, Wang Q. GABA exerts protective and regenerative effects on islet beta cells and reverses diabetes. ProcNatlA-
cadSci U S A. Jun 27, 2011

Chapter 6

Beta Cell Function After Islet Transplantation

Morihito Takita, Nigar Seven, Marlon F. Levy and
Bashoo Naziruddin

Additional information is available at the end of the chapter

1. Introduction

1.1. Islet cell transplantation for type 1 diabetes

The transplantation of pancreatic islets of Langerhans is a promising treatment for "brittle" type 1 diabetics, because it is a minimally invasive procedure that replenishes the beta cell mass lost due to autoimmunity. This procedure also provides an opportunity for a "cure" from diabetes based on the achievement of freedom from dependence on exogenous insulin and severe hypoglycemic events. Although islet transplants had been attempted for several decades, they achieved minimum success in terms of post-transplant graft function. The publication of the Edmonton Protocol [1] documenting consistent achievement of insulin independence after islet transplantation, has led to a dramatic increase not only in the number of procedures performed worldwide but also in other related areas in the field of islet transplantation. Breakthroughs have been made in the area of pancreas procurement and preservation with study into ductal preservation, the two layer method, and the type of preservation solution used. Furthermore, there has been much progress in the islet isolation process by bringing standards up to cGMP qualifications, optimization of collagenase enzymes, and using iodixanol for continuous density gradient purification [2]. Some of the hurdles facing further success in this treatment are:

i.   lack of suitable donor pancreases;

ii.   difficulties in isolating high quality islets on a consistent basis;

iii.   improving the engraftment of transplanted islets;

iv.   development of an islet-friendly immunosuppression and

v.   improving long-term survival of transplanted islets.

1.2. Post-transplant outcome

According to a recent report from the Collaborative Islet Transplant Registry, 677 patients have received either an islet transplant alone (ITA) or islets-after-kidney (IAK) transplants [3]. There has been a remarkable improvement in the post-transplant graft function in recent times. Prior to the publication of Edmonton protocol, the achievement of insulin-independent status by islet transplant recipients was <10%. Patients treated initially under the Edmonton protocol showed remarkable achievement of 82% insulin-independent status at one year post-transplant. However, this result proved to be unsustainable when the five year insulin-independence rates fell to 12.5% at the same center [4]. This data resulted in skepticism on the use of allogeneic islet transplantation as a reliable treatment for long-term success. With the introduction of thymoglobulin at induction phase and the combination of prograf, rapamycin and/or mycophenolate mofetil as maintenance immunosuppressive agents, the islet transplant survival rate has significantly improved to 50% at five year post-transplant [5]. Control of inflammatory reaction during peri-transplant period with the use of TNF-α blockers also played a key role in this improvement. These remarkable results necessitated comparison with whole pancreas transplantation which is considered as an established clinical procedure. Although whole organ treatment achieved high levels of graft survival in the years 1994-1997, the islet survival rate at five years has reached around fifty percent in 2010-2011, comparable to the level of whole pancreas graft success [5]. Moreover, islet cell transplantation seems to confer significantly better glycemic control than maximal medical therapy, and essentially eliminates hypoglycemic unawareness. These results have brought back the enthusiasm in this field.

2. Molecular mechanism of beta cell dysfunction

2.1. Early events after islet transplantation

The liver is the most commonly used site for transplantation of islets. Data supporting the use of this transplant site came from autologous islet transplants in patients with chronic pancreatitis, which showed that islets can function inside the liver for several years. There are several drawbacks associated with the liver as a host site for islets. Major factors affecting islet function include hypoxia, drug toxicity and instant blood-mediated inflammatory reaction (IBMIR). Together, these events may lead to loss of up to 75% of islet transplant mass. IBMIR is primarily a response of innate immune system to isolated islets. Major characteristics of IBMIR include activation of coagulation and complement cascades and infiltration of inflammatory cells. Several approaches are adopted to minimize the deleterious effects of IBMIR which include infusion of low molecular weight dextran sulfate and also inclusion of anti-inflammatory molecules during the infusion of islets. Besides the innate immune response, islets transplanted into liver may experience low oxygen tension. Activation of resident Kupffer cells may pose additional risk to islet survival. In addition, high concentrations of immunosuppressive drugs in the portal vein are likely to exert toxic effect on the transplanted islet mass [6].

2.2. Alloimmunity

The exposure of body to allogeneic tissues via organ/cell transplantation, blood transfusions, pregnancy can cause development of anti-human leukocyte antigen (HLA) antibodies [7]. These *de novo* HLA antibodies have been shown to play a significant role in the early graft loss after solid organ transplantation [8]. Currently, HLA matching between the recipients and donors is not performed before islet cell transplantation. Moreover, to achieve and/or maintain insulin independence and good metabolic control in an islet recipient, multiple islet infusions from multiple donors and high doses of immunosuppressants are generally required. The requirement of multi-donor infusions and reduction or weaning of immunosuppressants due to significant adverse effects could cause patients eventually to develop HLA antibodies against islet graft.

The issue of sensitization of alloantigens after islet cell transplantation has been raised by the Edmonton group in 2007 [9]. 98 islet transplant recipients were screened for HLA antibodies by flow-based methods. Twenty-nine patients (31%) represented *de novo* donor specific antibodies following islet transplantation. Among 14 recipients who discontinued immunosuppression, 10 recipients (71%) were largely sensitized with panel reactive antibody ≥50%. On the other hand, only 11 of 69 (16%) recipients who continued immunosuppression became broadly sensitized posttransplant. This study suggested that development of HLA antibodies after islet transplantation is concerning and withdrawal of immunosuppression completely following failed islet transplantation raises the risk for broad sensitization. Along with the report of Edmonton group, there are several studies that have demonstrated that islet alone transplant recipients develop donor-specific and/or nondonor-specific HLA antibodies, especially following discontinuation of immunosuppression [10-13].

In contrast, in the report of Geneva group it was shown that multiple islet infusions did not act as a risk factor for appearance of anti-HLA antibodies [14]. The group claimed that transplantation of islets in liver might cause less immunogenicity. After combined kidney-islet transplantation and continued immunosuppression even with failed islet graft function, patients had a low risk for sensitization as long as their kidney remained functional.

It has been known that islets express mainly HLA class I antigens on their surfaces. Previous reports demonstrated that patients develop antibodies posttransplant not only against HLA class I antigens, but also against HLA class II antigens [9]. Jackson et al. showed that there would be an induction of HLA class II expression on human islets under inflammatory conditions, which in return may be a possible cause of allosensitization [15]. For this aim, the group conducted an experiment in which they had two groups of isolated human islets; group 1 was control group and cultured at 37°C, whereas group 2 was cultured in the same condition and treated with tumor necrosis factor alpha (TNF-α) and interferon gamma (INF-γ). Presence of HLA class II on islet surface was analyzed by real-time polymerase chain reaction (PCR), immunofluorescence and flow cytometry. Expression of class II transactivator, HLA-DR-α and HLA-DR-β1 increased maximum 9.38, 18.95 and 46.5 fold respectively in group 2 compared to control group after 24 hours of incubation with TNF-α and INF-γ which is shown by real-time PCR analysis. Fluorescent imaging and flow cytometric analysis confirmed the significant increase in the expression of HLA class II expression both on islet α and β cells after cytokine treatment. Inflammatory conditions shortly after islet transplantation up-regulates HLA class II antigens on islet surfaces that trigger alloimmunity. Thus, protocols which provide adequate and efficient control of inflammation after islet transplantation should be considered to improve islet transplant outcome.

Collaborative Islet Transplant Registry reported the sensitization rates against HLA class I antigens pre- and posttransplant in islet alone recipients in 2011 [16]. Data is collected from 303 islet alone recipients between January 1999 and December 2008. Panel reactive antibody (PRA) pretransplant and PRA at 6 months and yearly posttransplant correlated to measures of islet graft failure. Pretransplant PRA showed not to be a predictor of islet graft failure; whereas there was 3.6 fold increased hazard ratio for graft failure when the recipient developed PRA≥20% post-transplant. Each additional islet infusion increased the cumulative number of mismatched HLA alleles from a median of 3 to 9; respectively for one infusion and for 3 infusions. Significantly higher rate of PRA ≥ 20% was observed in recipients who had complete graft loss with discontinued immunosuppression compared to recipients who had functioning grafts with continuing immunosuppression. Development of *de novo* HLA class I antibodies is less pronounced in recipients with exposure to repeat HLA class I mismatched than increased class I mismatch. Reducing the number of islet donors used for each patient and repeating HLA I mismatches with consequent islet transplantation without presence of donor specific anti-HLA antibodies are vital factors to decrease the risk of allosensitization.

Currently, there is no clearly defined monitoring tool for alloimmunity in islet cell transplantation, but researchers have proposed many experimental tools to assess alloreactivity in islet transplanted patients. Alloantibodies, soluble CD30 level, cytotoxic lymphocyte gene expression and microparticles in peripheral blood are the markers which were shown to detect allogeneic rejection after islet transplantation. Monitoring panel reactive antibody in immunosuppressed recipients had little clinical value to assess islet graft survival [16, 17].

Team	Approach	Outcome	References
Edmonton group	Alloantibodies	Pretransplant HLA antibodies reduce graft survival after islet transplantation.	[9]
CITR report	Alloantibodies	Monitoring PRA in immunosuppressed patients had little clinical value for islet graft survival.	[16]
Minnesota group	Soluble CD30	No correlation between sCD30 levels and graft function at 1 year was found. A greater reduction in sCD30 levels posttransplant was associated with full graft function.	[18]
Miami group	Cytotoxic lymphocyte (CL) gene expression	Increased CL gene levels could predict islet allograft loss.	[19]
GRAGIL group	Microparticles	MPs and C-peptide showed opposite pattern. MPs levels in peripheral blood increase with acute rejection of islet allograft.	[20]

Table 1. Immunologic tools to assess alloimmunity after islet cell transplantation

Soluble CD30 (sCD30) is a cell membrane protein of tumor necrosis factor receptor family. sCD30 is released into blood with the activation of CD30 + T cells, leading to speculation that it may act as a marker for immune system activation [21]. Although it has been shown to be predictive for acute rejection in lung, kidney, and heart transplantation [22-24], there are not many reports about the role of sCD30 in the prediction of early graft loss following islet transplantation. In the study of Hire et al., 19 allograft islet recipients treated with three different immunosuppression inductions were evaluated retrospectively for the serum sCD30 levels [18]. Pretransplant, early posttransplant day (day 4–7), one month posttransplant, late posttransplant (day 90–120) sCD30 levels were measured and correlated with islet graft outcomes at 1 year. No correlation between sCD30 levels at any time point and graft function at 1 year was found. However, a greater reduction in SCD30 levels posttransplant was associated with full graft function. Therefore, sCD30 may be of value for immune monitoring of islet allografts.

Cytotoxic lymphocyte (CL) genes granzyme, Fas ligand and perforin may play an active role in the course of acute allograft rejection. University of Miami group studied 13 islet transplant recipients treated with steroid-free immunosuppressive regimen in order to demonstrate whether CL gene expression could be a predictor of allogeneic rejection [19]. All patients attained insulin independence; however, 8 of them restarted insulin therapy. Real-time PCR was used to assess CL gene mRNA levels. The group demonstrated that recipients who restarted insulin therapy had a significant elevation of CL gene mRNA levels and the most reliable measure of ongoing graft loss was granzyme B. Hence, increased blood CL gene levels might be a potential marker to predict islet allograft loss.

Microparticles (MP) are plasma membrane fragments of apoptotic cells in peripheral blood. The quantity of microparticles is correlated with the degree of cell death, so they are considered to be indicators of apoptosis. Kessler et al. demonstrated the elevation of microparticles in peripheral blood at the time of acute rejection following intraportal islet transplantation with a case report [25]. Loss of islet graft function without the presence of GAD65, IA2 or anti-HLA antibodies brought up the diagnosis of acute cellular rejection. With a successful steroid bolus therapy, MPs level declined and the patient regained islet function. In 2011, Toti et al. [20] demonstrated from three islet transplant recipients that in the case of rejection, C-peptide and MPs levels exhibited opposite pattern and a decline in C-peptide was related with increased insulin needs. This data suggested an increment in MPs level might indicate allogeneic rejection. Thus, MPs level in peripheral blood might be a useful tool to monitor allogeneic rejection after islet transplantation.

2.3. Autoimmune recurrence

Type 1 diabetes is an autoimmune disease in which pancreatic beta cells are destroyed through a T-cell mediated mechanism in genetically susceptible individuals [26]. Autoantibodies against pancreatic islets comprise anti-glutamate decarboxylase 65 (GAD65), islet cell autoantibody (ICA), anti-insulin autoantibody (IAA), anti-tyrosine phosphatase autoantibody (IA-2) and against zinc transporter ZnT8. Antibodies present in serum against these pancreatic islet antigens are commonly used to predict and or diagnose the disease in clinical practice. For successful islet cell replacement, it is crucial to prevent recurrent destruction of beta cells through existing autoimmune destruction. The graft failure due to recurrent autoimmunity in a pancreas segment transplanted between identical twins was proven with the demonstration of insulitis in the transplanted tissue [27]. Islet specific T cells seem to have a basic role in the process of autoimmune destruction of beta cells [28].

To investigate T-cell allo- and autoreactivities in peripheral blood following islet transplantation, Roep et al. examined 7 islet allograft recipients [29]. They showed that three patients who got thymoglobulin for induction immunosuppression and retained full islet function for more than 1 year exhibited minor autoreactivites but no alloreactivities. Three patients who did not get thymoglobulin had rapid decline (<3 weeks) in islet function and showed alloreactivities; but one out of these three patients had rapid increase in autoreactivity to several islet autoantigens prior to alloreactivity. One recipient who did not receive thymoglobulin exhibited hyperautoreacivity with no detectable alloreaactivity and developed delayed loss of islet graft function consequently (<33 weeks); which indicated that autoimmune recurrence might be the cause of chronic islet graft dysfunction. In this study, because of the excellent outcomes in thymoglobulin group, the authors evaluated allo- and autoimmunity again in a bigger sample sized group in 2008 [30]. 21 islet recipients under thymoglobulin induction and tacrolimus plus mycophenolate mofetil maintenance immunosuppressive regimen were studied. Immunity against allo- and autoantigens were checked at pretransplant and at 1 year posttransplant. The analyses showed that existence of cellular autoimmunity pretransplant and posttransplant was related with delayed insulin independence and lower levels of circulating C-peptide during the first year posttransplant. Seven out of eight patients with no previous T-cell autoreactivity achieved insulin independence; whereas none of the four patients with autoantibodies against GAD and IA-2 before transplantation became insulin independent. Cellular alloreactivity and autoantibody levels did not show significant involvement with the outcome. Based on these findings, the authors commented that thymoglobulin may cope sufficiently with alloimmunity, but insufficient to control islet autoreactivity in an early period. The issue of autoimmunity remains unaddressed and needs further investigation.

Team	Approach	Outcome	References
Roep et al.	Autoantibodies	Autoandibodies increased due to autoimmune activity, but did not indicate loss of graft function.	[29]
Roep et al.	T-cell autoreactivity in peripheral blood	Pre- and posttransplant cellular autoimmunity were associated with delayed insulin independence. Autoantibody levels did not affect islet allograft outcome.	[30]
Matsumoto et al.	GAD65 specific global immune assay	Broad repertoire of islet antigen-specific T cells secreting various cytokines were related with chronic graft failure.	[31]

Table 2. Immunologic tools to assess autoimmunity after islet cell transplantation

Autoimmunity recurrence might be assessed by monitoring islet specific autoantibodies and T-cell autoreactivity. But the association between autoantibodies and insulin independence and islet graft outcome are variable; increase in autoantibody levels were shown due to autoimmune activity but did not indicate loss of islet graft function [29, 32]. Assays that measure anti-islet cellular autoimmunity before and after islet transplantation demonstrated that pre-and posttransplant cellular autoimmunity were related with delayed insulin independence and lower levels of circulating C-peptide during the first year posttransplant [30]. Nonetheless, in this study islet allograft outcome did not seem to be affected by autoantibody levels or cellular alloreactivity.

Matsumoto et al. have reported on a global immune assay specific for GAD65 (EpiMax) in order to analyze the property of autoreactive T-cell responses [31]. Five type 1 diabetic patients were studied 1 year after allogeneic islet transplantation. All patients achieved insulin independence at 1 year. Three out of five patients maintained long-term insulin independence and EpiMax affirmed minimum T-cell responses in these patients. In contrast, the two patients who developed chronic graft failure and lost insulin independence showed broad repertoire of GAD65 specific T-cells secreting various types of cytokines, including IL-5, IL-13, IL-17, TNF- alpha, and IFN-gamma. In addition to those observations, IFN-γ and IL-13 expressing CD4+ T cells and IFN-γ expressing CD8+ T cells were encountered in the other two failed patients. These findings suggested that broad repertoire of islet antigenspecific T cells which secrete variable types of cytokines were related with chronic graft failure, preventing islet recipients from maintaining long-term insulin independence.

Immunosuppression

Following transplantation of islets, administration of immunosuppression is essential to maintain graft function. However, most of the immunosuppressive drugs also have adverse effects on beta cell function. Careful selection of immunosuppressive regimen is critical for prolonged function of transplanted islets.

2.3.1. Early period of islet cell transplantation

Corticosteroid was a widely used agent as maintenance immunosuppression in the pioneering days of islet cell transplantation in 1990's (Table 3). During this decade, majority of islet cell transplants were after or performed simultaneously with kidney transplantation. Corticosteroid has antiinflammatory as well as immunosuppressive effects by direct or indirect actions on various leukocytes, including T lymphocytes, monocytes and macrophages, through glucocorticoid receptor [33, 34]. However, steroid therapy leads to β cell dysfunction and insulin resistance. [35, 36] Deterioration of insulin secretion from β cell by steroid treatment has been reported, caused by enhanced α-adrenergic receptor signaling [37], β cell apoptosis [38] and activated K^+ channel [39]. Insulin resistance in liver, adipose tissue and skeletal muscle by long-term steroid administration are well known clinically and in basic studies [40-42]. Thus, steroid use for the purpose of maintenance immunosuppression has been averted in the recent decade of islet transplantation (Table 3).

The calcineurin inhibitors (CNIs) have been major players in maintenance immunosuppression of islet cell transplantation. Cyclosporine A and tacrolimus are currently available CNIs in clinic. They inhibit calcineurin, a serine-threonine phosphatase, which is responsible for dephosphorylation of nuclear factor for activated T cells (NF-AT), which in turn results in inactivation of the transcription of cytokine genes. However, CNIs might have β cell toxicity since calcineurin is expressed in β cell and regulates β cell growth as well as function [43, 44].

Azathioprine is a purine analog, serving as a blocker of de novo pathway in purine synthesis in actively proliferative cells such as T cells and B cells [45]. Currently this drug is used for immunosuppression in allogeneic transplantation and autoimmune disease like rheumatoid arthritis as well as therapy in hematologic malignancies [46]. Azathioprine may also prevent the onset of diabetes [47, 48] and no major β cell toxicity of azathioprine has been reported.

2.3.2. Edmonton protocol

Remarkable success in islet transplant survival was achieved by the University of Alberta group using steroid-free immunosuppression regimen that included daclizumab, tacrolimus and sirolimus, resulting in that all 7 recipients achieving insulin independence [1]. The benefit of Edmonton protocol is to eliminate the risk of steroid-induced β cell toxicity as well as insulin resistance and increasing the dose of transplanted islets. However, the protocol uses tacrolimus that has the effect of β cell deterioration.

Publication year	Pts no.	Induction therapy	Maintenance therapy			Transplant type	Donor no.*	Major outcomes	Refs
			Steroid	CNIs	Other				
1990	9			✓ Tac		Islet after liver transplant	M/S	5 pts achieved II	[49]
1991	3		✓ Pred	✓ CsA	✓ Aza	ITA	M/S	Rejected 2 weeks after ITA	[50]
	3	✓ mALG	✓ Pred	✓ CsA	✓ Aza	IAK	S	Partial function**	
	3	✓ mALG	✓ Pred	✓ CsA	✓ Aza	IAK	M	II for 7, 14 and 121 days	
1991	4	✓ ATG (3 pts)	✓ Pred	✓ CsA	✓ Aza	IAK	M/S	1 pt achieved II	[51]
	2	✓ ATG	✓ Pred	✓ CsA	✓ Aza	SIK	M/S		
1992	10			✓ Tac		Simultaneous Islet-Liver transplant	S	6 pts achieved II	[52]

Publication year	Pts no.	Induction therapy	Maintenance therapy			Transplant type	Donor no.*	Major outcomes	Refs
	4		✓Pred ✓Tac			Simultaneous Islet-Liver transplant	S	Partial function**	
	7		✓Pred ✓Tac			SIK	M	Partial function**	
1993	2	✓mALG ✓15-DSG	✓Pred ✓CsA ✓Aza			SIK	S	1 pt achieved II	[53]
1997	6		✓mPred ✓Tac			Simultaneous Islet-Liver-Bone marrow transplant	S	3 pts achieved II	[54]
1997	8	✓OKT3	✓mPred ✓CsA ✓Aza			IAK (7 pts) or SIK (1 pt)	M/S	2 pts achieved II	[55]
1997	20	✓ATG	✓Pred ✓CsA ✓Aza			IAK (7 pts) or SIK (13 pt)	M/S	7 pts achieved II	[56]
1997	3	✓ATG	✓Pred ✓CsA ✓MMF			SIK (2 pts) or IAK (1 pt)	M/S	Partial function**	[57]
1998	7	✓ATG (3pts)	✓Pred ✓CsA ✓Aza			IAK	M	2 pts achieved II	[58]
1999	12	✓ATG	✓Pred ✓CsA ✓Aza			IAK (12 pts) or SIK (12pts)	M/S	Partial function**	[59]

Table 3. Immunosuppression protocols in clinical islet transplants published in 1990's. *M: Multiple donor transplants, S: Single donor transplant. ** Not achieved II, but positive C-peptide or decreased insulin requirement was confirmed. Abbreviations; 15-DSG: 15-deoxyspergualin, ATG: antithymocyte globulin, Aza: azathioprine, CNIs: Calcineurin inhibitors, CsA: Cyclosporine A, IAK: Islet after kidney transplantation, II: Insulin Independence, ITA: Islet transplantation alone, mALG: Minnesota antilymphoblast globulin, MMF: mycophenolic mofetil, mPred: methylprednisolone, Pred: Prednisone, SIK: Simultaneous islet kidney transplantation, Tac: Tacrolimus.

Publication year	Pts no.	Induction therapy	Maintenance therapy			Transplant type	Donor no.*	Major outcomes	Refs
			Steroid	CNIs	Other				
2000	13	✓ATG or ✓Bas	✓Pred	✓CsA	✓Aza or ✓MMF	SIK, IAK or Islet after lung transplant	M/S	2 pts achieved II	[60]
2000	7	✓Dac		✓Tac	✓Sir	ITA	M	100% II	[1]
2001	2	✓ATG or ✓Bas	✓Pred	✓CsA	✓MMF	SIK (5 pts) or IAK (2 pts)	M/S	Partial function**	[61]

Publi-cation year	Pts no.	Induction therapy	Maintenance therapy			Transplant type	Donor no.*	Major outcomes	Refs
2001	10	✓ Bas	✓ Pred	✓ CsA	✓ MMF	IAK	M/S	2 pts achieved II	[62]
2003	6	✓ Dac		✓ Tac	✓ Sir	ITA	M/S	3 pts achieved II	[63]
2004	6	✓ OKT3γ1		✓ Tac	✓ Sir	ITA	S	4 pts achieved II	[64]
2004	13	✓ Dac		✓ Tac	✓ Sir	ITA (9 pts) or IAK (4 pts)	M	11 pts achieved II	[65]
2004	10	✓ Dac		✓ Tac	✓ Sir	ITA	M/S	5 pts achieved II	[66]
2004	6	✓ Dac		✓ Tac	✓ Sir	SIK	M	5 pts achieved II	[67]
2005	8	✓ ATG ✓ Dac ✓ Eta		✓ Tac	✓ MMF ✓ Sir	ITA	S	100% II after single infusion	[68]
2005	16	✓ Dac ✓ Inf (8pts)		✓ Tac	✓ Sir	ITA	M/S	14 pts achieved II	[69]
2005	22	✓ Dac/ ✓ Bas		✓ Tac/ ✓ CsA	✓ Sir/ ✓ Eve	IAK or ITA	M/S	15 pts achieved II	[70]
2005	65	✓ Dac		✓ Tac	✓ Sir	ITA	M/S	44 pts achieved II	[4]
2005	10	✓ ATG or ✓ Bas		✓ Tac	✓ Sir or ✓ MMF	ITA	M/S	100% II	[71]
2006	8	✓ Dac		✓ Tac	✓ Sir	IAK	M/S	100% II	[72]
2006	6	✓ Dac		✓ Tac	✓ Sir	ITA	M	3 pts achieved II	[73]
2006	36	✓ Dac		✓ Tac	✓ Sir	ITA	M/S	16 pts achieved II	[74]
2007	11	✓ Dac		✓ Tac	✓ Sir or ✓ MMF plus ✓ Exe		M/S	8 pts achieved II	[75]
2007	10	✓ Dac		✓ Tac	✓ Sir	ITA	M/S	6 pts achieved II	[76]
2007	19	✓ Dac		✓ Tac	✓ Sir or ✓ MMF	ITA	M/S	16 pts achieved II	[77]

Publication year	Pts no.	Induction therapy	Maintenance therapy			Transplant type	Donor no.*	Major outcomes	Refs
2008	5	✓ATG		✓Tac	✓Sir	ITA	M	3 pts achieved II	[78]
	5	✓ATG			✓Sir	ITA	M	Partial function**	
2008	13	✓Dac		✓Tac	✓Sir	SIK	M/S	7 pts achieved II	[79]
2008	7	✓Dac ✓Inf ✓Eta	✓Pred (2 pts) or mPred (1 pt)	✓Tac	✓Sir ✓MMF (2 pts)	IAK	M/S	6 pts achieved II	[80]
2008	6	✓ATG ✓Eta		✓CyA	✓Eve →MMF	ITA	M/S	5 pts achieved II	[81]
2008	4	✓Dac		✓Tac	✓Sir	ITA	M	100% II	[82]
	6	✓Dac ✓Eta		✓Tac	✓Sir ✓Exe	ITA	M/S	100% II	
2008	3	✓Ale		✓Tac	✓Sir ✓MPA	ITA	M/S	2 pts achieved II	[83]
2008	6	✓Dac ✓Inf		✓Tac	✓Sir	Islet transplant with Bone marrow	S	3 pts achieved II	[84]
2009	14	✓Dac		✓Tac	✓Sir	ITA	M	100% II	[85]
2009	15	✓Dac or ✓Bas		✓Tac	✓Sir	IAK	M/S	100 pts achieved II	[86]
2010	8	✓ATG			✓Sir ✓MMF ✓Efa	ITA	M/S	100% II	[87]
2010	8	✓Dac		✓Tac	✓Sir	ITA	M/S	100% II	[88]
	4	✓Dac		✓Tac	✓Sir ✓Efa	ITA	S	100% II after single infusion	
2010	5	✓ATG ✓Bela			✓Sir or ✓MMF	ITA	M/S	100% II after single infusion	[89]
	5	✓ATG ✓Efa			✓Sir or ✓MMF	ITA	M/S	100% II after single infusion	
2011	3	✓ATG ✓Eta ✓Ana		✓Tac	✓MMF	ITA	M/S	100% II after single infusion	[90]
	3	✓Dac		✓Tac	✓Sir	ITA	M	100% II	

Publi-cation year	Pts no.	Induction therapy	Maintenance therapy	Transplant type	Donor no.*	Major outcomes	Refs
2011	4			ITA**	M/S	Partial function***	[91]

Table 4. Immunosuppression protocols in clinical islet transplants published after 2000. *M: Multiple donor transplants, S: Single donor transplant. **Microencapsulated islets transplanted. *** Not achieved II, but positive C-peptide or decreased insulin requirement was confirmed. Abbreviations; Ale: Alemtuzumab, ATG: antithymocyte globulin, Aza: azathioprine, Ana: anakinra, Bas: basiliximab, Bela: belatacept, CNIs: Calcineurin inhibitors, CsA: Cyclosporine A, Dac: daclizumab, Efa: efalizumab, Eta: etanercept, Eve: everolimus, Exe: exenatide, IAK: islet after kidney transplantation, II: insulin independence, Inf: infliximab, ITA: islet transplantation alone, mALG: Minnesota antilymphoblast globulin, MMF: mycophenolic mofetil, MPA: mycophenolic acid, mPred: methylprednisolone, Pred: prednisone, SIK: simultaneous islet kidney transplantation, Sir: sirolimus, Tac: tacrolimus

Sirolimus is an inhibitor of mammalian target of rapamycin (mTOR), which plays an important role in cell cycle from late G1 to S phase in T cells [92]. The effect of sirolimus in β cell function is still unclear; impaired β cell proliferation and islet graft function by sirolimus has been reported [93-95] while Melzi et al found no significant adverse effect of sirolimus in islet engraftment [96]. Gao et al reported sirolimus and daclizumab did not show any individual or synergistic negative effects on islet proliferation [97]. However, insulin independence in Edmonton protocol was not sustained for a long-term resulting in 12.5% at 5 year after islet transplant [4].

2.3.3. Newer immunosuppression protocols

Recent clinical trials implementing monoclonal antibodies such as basiliximab (anti-IL-2 receptor)[70], efalizumab (anti-LFA-1)[89], alemtuzumab (anti-CD52)[83] have shown high rate of insulin independence after transplant. These monoclonal antibodies are produced as molecular targeting agents and considered as less likely to have direct effects on β cell function.

Currently major islet transplant centers are increasingly adopting stronger induction immunosuppression comprised of T cell depletion using anti-thymocyte globulin, alemtuzumab or OKT3γ1 (anti-CD3) plus anti-TNF-α treatment. This has resulted in significantly improved long-term maintenance of insulin independence [3, 5].

In maintenance immunosuppression, tacrolimus is still a key medication; although, there is controversy on the use of tacrolimus and its effect to islet graft function as described above (See § 2.5.1). Mycophenolate mofetil (MMF) is also used for maintenance immunosuppression, inhibiting proliferation of T and B cells and promoting apoptosis of activated T cells [98, 99]. Gallo et al recently showed that MMF was able to reduce survival of β cells, impair glucose-stimulated insulin secretion and β cell proliferation [100]. Posselt et al reported excellent islet transplant outcome using CNI-free immunosuppression that included belatacept [89], which is a fusion protein with Fc fragment of a human IgG linked to cytotoxic T lymphocyte-associated antigen 4 (CTLA-4) that allows costimulation blockade of CD80 and CD86 on antigen presenting cells [101]. Overall islet investigators have continued to make efforts to find effective immunosuppression with less effect on β cell function while enhancing β cell function such as exenatide which is a glucagon-like peptide-1 (GLP-1) analog [75].

2.4. Islet encapsulation

The islet encapsulation aims to eliminate or reduce the dose of immunosuppression, which is a major obstacle in current islet transplantation, by isolating islets from blood flow and avoiding direct interaction with antibodies and immune cells such as lymphocytes and macrophages. However, few clinical trials using encapsulation technique have been reported [91, 102]. The University of Peruga group demonstrated the efficacy of microencapsulated human islets with sodium alginate in 4 type 1 diabetic patients, who were able to reduce HbA1c level and the amounts of exogenous insulin injection [91]. Elliot RB et al. showed a case report on xenotransplantation using alginate-encapsulated porcine islets, also allowing reduction of insulin dose [102]. In both reports, islet recipients did not use any immunosuppressants although insulin independence was not achieved, suggesting the advantage and limitation of current encapsulation strategy (Figure 1).

There are several methods of islet encapsulation; macrocapsular devices, microencapsulation and surface modification. A macrocapsular device that is composed of polytetrafluoroethylene membrane enabled delayed onset of diabetes in mice model [103]. Microencapsulation of islets has been prepared using various materials such as alginate, agarose and collagen [104-106]. An issue of microencapsulation is the enlargement of the size of islet mass; microencapsulation of an islet can increase the size by as much as 3 to 5 folds of the original islet. Alternatively, surface modification of islets is a strategy to reduce the tissue volume. Polyethylene glycol (PEG) is a hydrogel polymer and can be used for conformal coating to encapsulate islets in the process of polymerization [107]. PEGylation, i.e. PEG conjugation at the islet surface, is the another way of islet encapsulation without significant increase in tissue size [108]. Recently, PEGylation attached with biologically active agents of heparin, activated protein C, urokinase or thrombomodulin has been developed to prevent the local coagulation immediately after islet infusion [109-112]. These techniques were recently developed and the sustainability of PEGylation needs to be proven.

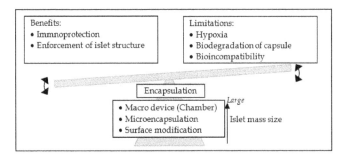

Figure 1. Benefits and current limitations of islet encapsulation.

3. Clinical assessment of beta cell function

Monitoring graft function is a major concern in clinical management of islet recipients since islet graft dysfunction in both acute phase after transplant and chronic phase is an obstacle to its widespread use as a standard care for type 1 diabetes. Furthermore, isolated islets are transplanted via the portal vein into the liver, making it difficult to employ biopsy examination of engrafted islets. Hence, several methodologies to predict islet graft function indirectly have been proposed. In this section, indices currently available for clinical assessment of islet graft function are discussed (Table 5).

3.1. Blood tests and clinical indices

3.1.1. Glucose tolerance/stimulation test

Glucose tolerance test (GTT) is a basic assessment method to diagnose diabetes although glucose stimulation; in itself has risk of artificial hyperglycemia for type 1 diabetic patients. Baidal et al reported that acute insulin/C-peptide release, mixed meal stimulation index, time-to-peak C-peptide, 90min glucose level and area under the curve of glucose values could predict islet dysfunction [113]. Arginine stimulation test is also useful for the evaluation of islet graft function. Glucose-potentiation slope and the maximal response in arginine stimulation test were significantly associated with β cell secretory capacity in a report from University of Pennsylvania group [114].

3.1.2. HYPO score and LI

Hypoglycemic (HYPO) score and lability index (LI) are calculated based on patients' journals of self-monitoring blood glucose (SMBG) for a month, providing a link to graft function through the quality of glycemic control [115]. These assessment tools are beneficial since a major endpoint of clinical allogeneic islet transplantation is to prevent hypoglycemic events; however, HYPO and LI calculations require a number of glucose measurements and hence are only calculated on a monthly or yearly basis using a complex scoring system.

3.1.3. SUITO index

A simple evaluation method using fasting blood glucose and C-peptide levels has been proposed, called secretory unit of islet transplant objects (SUITO) index [116]. The SUITO index was originally developed using the concept of the homeostasis model assessment for insulin secretion (HOMA-β) model, where healthy person has 100 of SUITO index. The calculation uses serum C-peptide levels instead of insulin levels, since islet recipient may be administering exogenous insulin during graft dysfunction and overlapped measurement of endogenous and exogenous insulin amounts are avoided [117]. SUITO index can provide reference value for insulin independence and elimination of hypoglycemia [118]. In addition, SUITO index allows extensive link to quality of life in islet recipients [119].

3.1.4. C-peptide/glucose ratio and C-peptide/glucose*creatinine ratio

C-peptide per glucose ratio (CP/G) is also a simple technique to predict islet graft function using blood glucose and C-peptide, similar to the SUITO index [120]. To correct islet graft function in patients with renal dysfunction, C-peptide/glucose*creatinine ratio has also been proposed. University of Miami group showed that CP/G correlated with 90min glucose level and β score [120].

3.1.5. β score

This scoring system uses data on fasting blood glucose, HbA1c, stimulated C-peptide, and absence of insulin or oral diabetic medication, that cover multiple aspect of glycemic control in islet recipients [121]. Correlation between β score and 90 min glucose level after mixed meal tolerance test has also been reported.

3.1.6. TEF

Transplant estimated function (TEF) is calculated by a formula using daily exogenous insulin requirements and HbA1c, that are routinely measured at clinic, eliminating glucose stimulation test when compared to β score [122]. TEF correlated well with β score and insulin response to arginine stimulation test.

3.1.7. TFIM model

Transplanted functional islet mass (TFIM) model is a recently proposed index that is aimed to guide the decision to use a specific islet preparation [123]. TFIM model is composed of transplanted islet volume, increment of insulin secretion, cold ischemia time and exocrine tissue volume transplanted, and can predict islet graft function.

3.2. Clinical image study

Functional mass of transplanted islets can be observed by the combination of the radioisotope-labeled grafts using 18F-fluorodeoxyglucose ([18F]FDG) and positron emission tomography with computed tomography (PET/CT) [124, 125]. Although this technique is only applicable to capture early phase of transplantation up to 60 min after transplant, islet graft loss as well as transplanted islet distribution in the liver can be observed. Nano-iron particle also visualizes engrafted islet mass using magnetic resonance imaging (MRI) and allows longer follow-up when compared to PET/CT technique [126, 127].

Method	Variables required	Advantage	Disadvantage	Reference
GTT	A series of glucose or C-peptide values during glucose stimulation	Widely available method in clinic	The risk of hyperglycemia Repeated blood collection	[113, 114]
HYPO score and LI	Detailed self-recorded journal of glucose levels and hypoglycemic episodes	Direct evaluation of hypoglycemia that is a major outcome in islet transplantation	Number of records for monthly basis are required Complex calculation for LI	[115]
SUITO index	Fasting serum C-peptide and glucose level	Simple calculation Easy prediction of graft function corresponding to insulin independence.	Limited application to other species	[118, 119]
CP/G	Fasting serum C-peptide and glucose level	Simple calculation	Limited information on extended outcomes of hypoglycemia	[120]
β score	Fasting glucose, HbA1c, Daily insulin dose, Stimulated C-peptide	To capture multiple aspects of glycemic control	Composite scoring system requiring 4 variables including the results from glucose stimulation test	[121]
TEF	A series of records on HbA1c and daily insulin amounts	To eliminate glucose stimulation test compared to β score Calculation using variables that can be collected in standard diabetes care	Adjustment of coefficients by individual patient	[122, 128]
TFIM Model	Volume of transplanted islets, increment of insulin secretion, cold ischemia time and volume of transplanted exocrine tissue	To follow graft function using isolation results	Validated using data on islet after kidney transplantation	[123]
Radiologic imaging technique; PET/CT	Radioisotope-labeled islets PET/CT machine	To allow evaluation of islet graft mass and the distribution in the liver	The measurement only applicable for early phase of transplantation due to half-time of radioisotope Labeling procedure required	[124, 125]
Radiologic imaging technique; MRI	Iron-nanoparticle labeled islets MRI machine	To allow longitudinal follow up of islet mass	Labeling procedure required Iron overload	[126, 127]

Table 5. Clinical assessment of β cell function

3.3. Autologous Islet Transplantation

Patients with refractory chronic pancreatitis undergo total or partial pancreatectomy to alleviate pain and also autologous islet transplantation to retain pancreatic endocrine function after surgery. Islets isolated from pancreas are infused intraportally into the liver. Assessment of beta cell function in such autologous islet transplant patients typically follows the methods described for allogeneic islet transplantation. For example, the SUITO index can be applicable to autologous islet transplantation and was founded as an excellent predictor of insulin independence [129]. However, no immune response against infused islets is expected in these patients. Post-transplant function of autologous islets has been shown to be much better than in allogeneic combination; β cell mass more than 10,000 IEQ/kg of islet yield is considered for a factor of insulin independence in allogeneic transplants while islet yield over 5,000 IEQ/kg is the successful factor in autologous transplantation [130]. After achievement of insulin independent status, patients receiving autologous islets have better long term survival of graft. Most patients also achieve significant relief from pain and improve their quality of life.

4. Conclusion

Islet transplantation has been shown to be a very promising treatment that could result in freedom from requirement of exogenous insulin in type 1 diabetic patients. One of the major advantages of islet transplantation is the minimally invasive nature of the procedure when compared to whole organ pancreas transplantation. Despite its wide spread use at several major transplant centers, the volume of patients receiving islet transplants remain low when compared to the number of "brittle" type 1 diabetic patients eligible for this procedure. Recently impressive gains have been made in the improvement of post-transplant islet function. This is primarily due to the use of T-cell depleting immunosuppression during induction phase after transplant followed by use of tacrolimus, rapamycin and or mycophenolic mofetil during the maintenance phase. In addition several advances made in donor selection, pancreas procurement, enzymatic digestion, islet purification and islet culture seem to have contributed to this success. Recent completion of a large scale phase III clinical trial sponsored by the NIH has given hope that soon this procedure may be approved for clinical use. In light of these advances, there is optimism that the remaining hurdles could be overcome to improve the long term function of the transplanted islets.

Acknowledgements

This work was supported by grants from the National Institute of Diabetes and Digestive and Kidney Diseases (1R21DK090513-01 to M.F.L.), the Juvenile Diabetes Research Foundation (#5-2010-668 to B.N. and #3-2011-447 to M.T.) and by the Baylor Health Care System Foundation.

Author details

Morihito Takita[1], Nigar Seven[1], Marlon F. Levy[2] and Bashoo Naziruddin[2*]

*Address all correspondence to: BashooN@Baylorhealth.edu

1 Baylor Research Institute, Islet Cell Laboratory, Dallas, USA

2 Baylor Simmons Transplant Institute, Dallas, USA

References

[1] Shapiro, A. M., Lakey, J. R., Ryan, E. A., Korbutt, G. S., Toth, E., Warnock, G. L., et al. (2000). Islet transplantation in seven patients with type 1 diabetes mellitus using a glucocorticoid-free immunosuppressive regimen. *N Engl J Med*, 343(4), 230-8.

[2] Matsumoto, S. (2010). Islet cell transplantation for Type 1 diabetes. *J Diabetes*, 2(1), 16-22.

[3] Barton, F. B., Rickels, M. R., Alejandro, R., Hering, B. J., Wease, S., Naziruddin, B., et al. (2012). Improvement in outcomes of clinical islet transplantation: 1999-2010. *Diabetes Care*, 35(7), 1436-45.

[4] Ryan, E. A., Paty, B. W., Senior, P. A., Bigam, D., Alfadhli, E., Kneteman, N. M., et al. (2005). Five-year follow-up after clinical islet transplantation. *Diabetes*, 54(7), 2060-9.

[5] Bellin, MD, Barton, F. B., Heitman, A., Harmon, J. V., Kandaswamy, R., Balamurugan, A. N., et al. (2012). Potent induction immunotherapy promotes long-term insulin independence after islet transplantation in type 1 diabetes. *Am J Transplant*, 12(6), 1576-83.

[6] Carlsson, P. O. (2011). Influence of microenvironment on engraftment of transplanted β-cells. *Ups J Med Sci*, 116(1), 1-7.

[7] Terasaki, P. I., & Cai, J. (2005). Humoral theory of transplantation: further evidence. *Curr Opin Immunol*, 17(5), 541-5.

[8] Terasaki, P. I. (2003). Humoral theory of transplantation. *Am J Transplant*, 3(6), 665-73.

[9] Campbell, P. M., Senior, P. A., Salam, A., Labranche, K., Bigam, D. L., Kneteman, N. M., et al. (2007). High risk of sensitization after failed islet transplantation. *Am J Transplant*, 7(10), 2311-7.

[10] Rickels, M. R., Kamoun, M., Kearns, J., Markmann, J. F., & Naji, A. (2007). Evidence for allograft rejection in an islet transplant recipient and effect on beta-cell secretory capacity. *J Clin Endocrinol Metab*, 92(7), 2410-4.

[11] Campbell, P. M., Salam, A., Ryan, E. A., Senior, P., Paty, B. W., Bigam, D., et al. (2007). Pretransplant HLA antibodies are associated with reduced graft survival after clinical islet transplantation. *Am J Transplant*, 7(5), 1242-8.

[12] Mohanakumar, T., Narayanan, K., Desai, N., Ramachandran, S., Shenoy, S., Jendri-sak, M., et al. (2006). A significant role for histocompatibility in human islet trans-plantation. *Transplantation*, 82(2), 180-7.

[13] Kessler, L., Parissiadis, A., Bayle, F., Moreau, F., Pinget, M., Froelich, N., et al. (2009). Evidence for humoral rejection of a pancreatic islet graft and rescue with rituximab and IV immunoglobulin therapy. *Am J Transplant*, 9(8), 1961-6.

[14] Ferrari-Lacraz, S., Berney, T., Morel, P., Marangon, N., Hadaya, K., Demuylder-Mis-chler, S., et al. (2008). Low risk of anti-human leukocyte antigen antibody sensitiza-tion after combined kidney and islet transplantation. *Transplantation*, 86(2), 357-9.

[15] Jackson, A. M., Connolly, J. E., Matsumoto, S., Noguchi, H., Onaca, N., Levy, M. F., et al. (2009). Evidence for Induced Expression of HLA Class II on Human Islets: Possi-ble Mechanism for HLA Sensitization in Transplant Recipients. *Transplantation*, 87(4), 500-6.

[16] Naziruddin, B., Wease, S., Stablein, D., Barton, F. B., Berney, T., Rickels, M. R., et al. (2012). HLA Class I Sensitization in Islet Transplant Recipients- Report from the Col-laborative Islet Transplant Registry. *Cell Transplant*, 21(5), 901-908.

[17] Cardani, R., Pileggi, A., Ricordi, C., Gomez, C., Baidal, D. A., Ponte, G. G., et al. (2007). Allosensitization of islet allograft recipients. *Transplantation*, 84(11), 1413-27.

[18] Hire, K., Hering, B., & Bansal-Pakala, P. (2010). Relative reductions in soluble CD30 levels post-transplant predict acute graft function in islet allograft recipients receiv-ing three different immunosuppression protocols. *Transpl Immunol*, 23(4), 209-14.

[19] Han, D., Xu, X., Baidal, D., Leith, J., Ricordi, C., Alejandro, R., et al. (2004). Assess-ment of cytotoxic lymphocyte gene expression in the peripheral blood of human islet allograft recipients: elevation precedes clinical evidence of rejection. *Diabetes*, 53(9), 2281-90.

[20] Toti, F., Bayle, F., Berney, T., Egelhofer, H., Richard, MJ, Greget, M., et al. (2011). Studies of circulating microparticle release in peripheral blood after pancreatic islet transplantation. *Transplant Proc*, 43(9), 3241-5.

[21] Del Prete, G., De Carli, M., D'Elios, MM, Daniel, K. C., Almerigogna, F., Alderson, M., et al. (1995). CD30-mediated signaling promotes the development of human T helper type 2-like T cells. *J Exp Med*, 182(6), 1655-61.

[22] Platt, R. E., Wu, K. S., Poole, K., Newstead, C. G., & Clark, B. (2009). Soluble CD30 as a prognostic factor for outcome following renal transplantation. *J Clin Pathol*, 62(7), 662-3.

[23] Shah, A. S., Leffell, M. S., Lucas, D., & Zachary, A. A. (2009). Elevated pretransplanta-tion soluble CD30 is associated with decreased early allograft function after human lung transplantation. *Hum Immunol*, 70(2), 101-3.

[24] Spiridon, C., Hunt, J., Mack, M., Rosenthal, J., Anderson, A., Eichhorn, E., et al. (2006). Evaluation of soluble CD30 as an immunologic marker in heart transplant re-cipients. *Transplant Proc*, 38(10), 3689-91.

[25] Kessler, L., Toti, F., Egelhofer, H., Richard, MJ, Greget, M. N. K., Moreau, F., et al. (2011). Acute cellular rejection of a pancreatic islet graft and rescue by steroid thera-py: study of microparticles release in peripheral blood. In , 151.

[26] Kolb, H., Kolb-Bachofen, V., & Roep, B. O. (1995). Autoimmune versus inflammatory type I diabetes: a controversy? *Immunol Today*, 16(4), 170-2.

[27] Sutherland, D. E., Goetz, F. C., & Sibley, R. K. (1989). Recurrence of disease in pan-creas transplants. *Diabetes*, 38, 1, 85-7.

[28] Roep, B. O. (2003). The role of T-cells in the pathogenesis of Type 1 diabetes: from cause to cure. *Diabetologia*, 46(3), 305-21.

[29] Roep, B. O., Stobbe, I., Duinkerken, G., van Rood, J. J., Lernmark, A., Keymeulen, B., et al. (1999). Auto- and alloimmune reactivity to human islet allografts transplanted into type 1 diabetic patients. *Diabetes*, 48(3), 484-90.

[30] Huurman, V. A., Hilbrands, R., Pinkse, G. G., Gillard, P., Duinkerken, G., van de Linde, P., et al. (2008). Cellular islet autoimmunity associates with clinical outcome of islet cell transplantation. *PLoS One*, 3(6), e2435.

[31] Matsumoto, S., Chujo, D., Shimoda, M., Takita, M., Sugimoto, K., Itoh, T., et al. (2011). Analysis of long-term insulin independence cases after allogeneic islet trans-plantation. *Am J Transplant*, 11(2), 175-176.

[32] Braghi, S., Bonifacio, E., Secchi, A., Di Carlo, V., Pozza, G., & Bosi, E. (2000). Modula-tion of humoral islet autoimmunity by pancreas allotransplantation influences allog-raft outcome in patients with type 1 diabetes. *Diabetes*, 49(2), 218-24.

[33] Ashwell, J. D., Lu, F. W., & Vacchio, M. S. (2000). Glucocorticoids in T cell develop-ment and function*. *Annu Rev Immunol*, 18, 309-45.

[34] Mc Ewen, B. S., Biron, C. A., Brunson, K. W., Bulloch, K., Chambers, W. H., Dhabhar, F. S., et al. (1997). The role of adrenocorticoids as modulators of immune function in health and disease: neural, endocrine and immune interactions. *Brain Res Brain Res Rev*, 23(1-2), 79-133.

[35] Daneman, D. (2006). Type 1 diabetes. *Lancet*, 367(9513), 847-58.

[36] Association, A. D. (2012). Diagnosis and classification of diabetes mellitus. *Diabetes Care*, 35(1), S64-71.

[37] Davani, B., Portwood, N., Bryzgalova, G., Reimer, M. K., Heiden, T., Ostenson, C. G., et al. (2004). Aged transgenic mice with increased glucocorticoid sensitivity in pancreatic beta-cells develop diabetes. *Diabetes*, 53(1), S51-9.

[38] Ranta, F., Avram, D., Berchtold, S., Düfer, M., Drews, G., Lang, F., et al. (2006). Dexamethasone induces cell death in insulin-secreting cells, an effect reversed by exendin-4. *Diabetes*, 55(5), 1380-90.

[39] Ullrich, S., Berchtold, S., Ranta, F., Seebohm, G., Henke, G., Lupescu, A., et al. (2005). Serum- and glucocorticoid-inducible kinase 1 (SGK1) mediates glucocorticoid-induced inhibition of insulin secretion. *Diabetes*, 54(4), 1090-9.

[40] Vegiopoulos, A., & Herzig, S. (2007). Glucocorticoids, metabolism and metabolic diseases. Mol Cell Endocrinol; , 275(1-2), 43-61.

[41] Walker, B. R. (2007). Glucocorticoids and cardiovascular disease. *Eur J Endocrinol*, 157(5), 545-59.

[42] Schäcke, H., Döcke, W. D., & Asadullah, K. (2002). Mechanisms involved in the side effects of glucocorticoids. *Pharmacol Ther*, 96(1), 23-43.

[43] Heit, J. J., Apelqvist, A. A., Gu, X., Winslow, M. M., Neilson, J. R., Crabtree, G. R., et al. (2006). Calcineurin/NFAT signalling regulates pancreatic beta-cell growth and function. *Nature*, 443(7109), 345-9.

[44] Soleimanpour, S. A., Crutchlow, M. F., Ferrari, A. M., Raum, J. C., Groff, D. N., Rankin, M. M., et al. (2010). Calcineurin signaling regulates human islet {beta}-cell survival. *J Biol Chem*, 285(51), 40050-9.

[45] Elion, G. B. (1993). The George Hitchings and Gertrude Elion Lecture. *The pharmacology of azathioprine. Ann N Y Acad Sci*, 685, 400-7.

[46] Maltzman, J. S., & Koretzky, G. A. (2003). Azathioprine: old drug, new actions. *J Clin Invest*, 111(8), 1122-4.

[47] Calafiore, R., Basta, G., Falorni, A., Pietropaolo, M., Picchio, M. L., Calcinaro, F., et al. (1993). Preventive effects of azathioprine (AZA) on the onset of diabetes mellitus in NOD mice. *J Endocrinol Invest*, 16(11), 869-73.

[48] Harrison, L. C., Colman, P. G., Dean, B., Baxter, R., & Martin, F. I. (1985). Increase in remission rate in newly diagnosed type I diabetic subjects treated with azathioprine. *Diabetes*, 34(12), 1306-8.

[49] Tzakis, A. G., Ricordi, C., Alejandro, R., Zeng, Y., Fung, J. J., Todo, S., et al. (1990). Pancreatic islet transplantation after upper abdominal exenteration and liver replacement. *Lancet*, 336(8712), 402-5.

[50] Scharp, D. W., Lacy, P. E., Santiago, J. V., Mc Cullough, C. S., Weide, L. G., Boyle, P. J., et al. (1991). Results of our first nine intraportal islet allografts in type 1, insulin-dependent diabetic patients. *Transplantation*, 51(1), 76-85.

[51] Socci, C., Falqui, L., Davalli, A. M., Ricordi, C., Braghi, S., Bertuzzi, F., et al. (1991). Fresh human islet transplantation to replace pancreatic endocrine function in type 1 diabetic patients. *Report of six cases. Acta Diabetol*, 28(2), 151-7.

[52] Ricordi, C., Tzakis, A. G., Carroll, P. B., Zeng, Y. J., Rilo, H. L., Alejandro, R., et al. (1992). Human islet isolation and allotransplantation in 22 consecutive cases. *Transplantation*, 53(2), 407-14.

[53] Gores, P. F., Najarian, J. S., Stephanian, E., Lloveras, J. J., Kelley, S. L., & Sutherland, D. E. (1993). Insulin independence in type I diabetes after transplantation of unpurified islets from single donor with 15-deoxyspergualin. *Lancet*, 341(8836), 19-21.

[54] Ricordi, C., Alejandro, R., Angelico, M. C., Fernandez, L. A., Nery, J., Webb, M., et al. (1997). Human islet allografts in patients with type 2 diabetes undergoing liver transplantation. *Transplantation*, 63(3), 473-5.

[55] Alejandro, R., Lehmann, R., Ricordi, C., Kenyon, N. S., Angelico, M. C., Burke, G., et al. (1997). Long-term function (6 years) of islet allografts in type 1 diabetes. *Diabetes*, 46(12), 1983-9.

[56] Secchi, A., Socci, C., Maffi, P., Taglietti, M. V., Falqui, L., Bertuzzi, F., et al. (1997). Islet transplantation in IDDM patients. *Diabetologia*, 40(2), 225-31.

[57] Tibell, A., Brendel, M., Wadström, J., Brandhorst, D., Brandhorst, H., Eckhard, M., et al. (1997). Early experience with a long-distance collaborative human islet transplant programme. *Transplant Proc*, 29(7), 3124-5.

[58] Keymeulen, B., Ling, Z., Gorus, F. K., Delvaux, G., Bouwens, L., Grupping, A., et al. (1998). Implantation of standardized beta-cell grafts in a liver segment of IDDM patients: graft and recipients characteristics in two cases of insulin-independence under maintenance immunosuppression for prior kidney graft. *Diabetologia*, 41(4), 452-9.

[59] Bretzel, R. G., Brandhorst, D., Brandhorst, H., Eckhard, M., Ernst, W., Friemann, S., et al. (1999). Improved survival of intraportal pancreatic islet cell allografts in patients with type-1 diabetes mellitus by refined peritransplant management. *J Mol Med (Berl)*, 77(1), 140-3.

[60] Oberholzer, J., Triponez, F., Mage, R., Andereggen, E., Bühler, L., Crétin, N., et al. (2000). Human islet transplantation: lessons from 13 autologous and 13 allogeneic transplantations. *Transplantation*, 69(6), 1115-23.

[61] Tibell, A., Bolinder, J., Hagström-Toft, E., Tollemar, J., Brendel, M., Eckhard, M., et al. (2001). Experience with human islet transplantation in Sweden. *Transplant Proc*, 33(4), 2535-6.

[62] Benhamou, P. Y., Oberholzer, J., Toso, C., Kessler, L., Penfornis, A., Bayle, F., et al. (2001). Human islet transplantation network for the treatment of Type I diabetes: first data from the Swiss-French GRAGIL consortium (1999-2000). Groupe de Recherche Rhin Rhjne Alpes Genève pour la transplantation d'Ilots de Langerhans. *Diabetologia*, 44(7), 859-64.

[63] Hirshberg, B., Rother, K. I., Digon, B. J., Lee, J., Gaglia, J. L., Hines, K., et al. (2003). Benefits and risks of solitary islet transplantation for type 1 diabetes using steroid-sparing immunosuppression: the National Institutes of Health experience. *Diabetes Care*, 26(12), 3288-95.

[64] Hering, B. J., Kandaswamy, R., Harmon, J. V., Ansite, JD, Clemmings, S. M., Sakai, T., et al. (2004). Transplantation of cultured islets from two-layer preserved pancreases in type 1 diabetes with anti-CD3 antibody. *Am J Transplant*, 4(3), 390-401.

[65] Frank, A., Deng, S., Huang, X., Velidedeoglu, E., Bae, Y. S., Liu, C., et al. (2004). Transplantation for type I diabetes: comparison of vascularized whole-organ pancreas with isolated pancreatic islets. Ann Surg discussion 640-3., 240(4), 631-40.

[66] Goss, J. A., Goodpastor, S. E., Brunicardi, F. C., Barth, M. H., Soltes, G. D., Garber, A. J., et al. (2004). Development of a human pancreatic islet-transplant program through a collaborative relationship with a remote islet-isolation center. *Transplantation*, 77(3), 462-6.

[67] Lehmann, R., Weber, M., Berthold, P., Züllig, R., Pfammatter, T., Moritz, W., et al. (2004). Successful simultaneous islet-kidney transplantation using a steroid-free immunosuppression: two-year follow-up. *Am J Transplant*, 4(7), 1117-23.

[68] Hering, B. J., Kandaswamy, R., Ansite, Eckman. P. M., Nakano, M., Sawada, T., et al. (2005). Single-donor, marginal-dose islet transplantation in patients with type 1 diabetes. *JAMA*, 293(7), 830-5.

[69] Froud, T., Ricordi, C., Baidal, D. A., Hafiz, M. M., Ponte, G., Cure, P., et al. (2005). Islet transplantation in type 1 diabetes mellitus using cultured islets and steroid-free immunosuppression: Miami experience. *Am J Transplant*, 5(8), 2037-46.

[70] Kempf, M. C., Andres, A., Morel, P., Benhamou, P. Y., Bayle, F., Kessler, L., et al. (2005). Logistics and transplant coordination activity in the GRAGIL Swiss-French multicenter network of islet transplantation. *Transplantation*, 79(9), 1200-5.

[71] Warnock, G. L., Meloche, R. M., Thompson, D., Shapiro, R. J., Fung, M., Ao, Z., et al. (2005). Improved human pancreatic islet isolation for a prospective cohort study of islet transplantation vs best medical therapy in type 1 diabetes mellitus. *Arch Surg*, 140(8), 735-44.

[72] Toso, C., Baertschiger, R., Morel, P., Bosco, D., Armanet, M., Wojtusciszyn, A., et al. (2006). Sequential kidney/islet transplantation: efficacy and safety assessment of a steroid-free immunosuppression protocol. *Am J Transplant*, 6(5 Pt 1), 1049-1058.

[73] O'Connell, P. J., Hawthorne, W. J., Holmes-Walker, D. J., Nankivell, B. J., Gunton, J. E., Patel, A. T., et al. (2006). Clinical islet transplantation in type 1 diabetes mellitus: results of Australia's first trial. *Med J Aust*, 184(5), 221-5.

[74] Shapiro, A. M., Ricordi, C., Hering, B. J., Auchincloss, H., Lindblad, R., Robertson, R. P., et al. (2006). International trial of the Edmonton protocol for islet transplantation. *N Engl J Med*, 355(13), 1318-30.

[75] Ghofaili, K. A., Fung, M., Ao, Z., Meloche, M., Shapiro, R. J., Warnock, G. L., et al. (2007). Effect of exenatide on beta cell function after islet transplantation in type 1 diabetes. *Transplantation*, 83(1), 24-8.

[76] Badet, L., Benhamou, P. Y., Wojtusciszyn, A., Baertschiger, R., Milliat-Guittard, L., Kessler, L., et al. (2007). Expectations and strategies regarding islet transplantation: metabolic data from the GRAGIL 2 trial. *Transplantation*, 84(1), 89-96.

[77] Maffi, P., Bertuzzi, F., De Taddeo, F., Magistretti, P., Nano, R., Fiorina, P., et al. (2007). Kidney function after islet transplant alone in type 1 diabetes: impact of immunosuppressive therapy on progression of diabetic nephropathy. *Diabetes Care*, 30(5), 1150-5.

[78] Gillard, P., Ling, Z., Mathieu, C., Crenier, L., Lannoo, M., Maes, B., et al. (2008). Comparison of sirolimus alone with sirolimus plus tacrolimus in type 1 diabetic recipients of cultured islet cell grafts. *Transplantation*, 85(2), 256-63.

[79] Gerber, P. A., Pavlicek, V., Demartines, N., Zuellig, R., Pfammatter, T., Wüthrich, R., et al. (2008). Simultaneous islet-kidney vs pancreas-kidney transplantation in type 1 diabetes mellitus: a 5 year single centre follow-up. *Diabetologia*, 51(1), 110-9.

[80] Cure, P., Pileggi, A., Froud, T., Messinger, S., Faradji, RN, Baidal, D. A., et al. (2008). Improved metabolic control and quality of life in seven patients with type 1 diabetes following islet after kidney transplantation. *Transplantation*, 85(6), 801-12.

[81] Bellin, M. D., Kandaswamy, R., Parkey, J., Zhang, H. J., Liu, B., Ihm, S. H., et al. (2008). Prolonged insulin independence after islet allotransplants in recipients with type 1 diabetes. *Am J Transplant*, 8(11), 2463-70.

[82] Gangemi, A., Salehi, P., Hatipoglu, B., Martellotto, J., Barbaro, B., Kuechle, J. B., et al. (2008). Islet transplantation for brittle type 1 diabetes: the UIC protocol. *Am J Transplant*, 8(6), 1250-61.

[83] Froud, T., Baidal, D. A., Faradji, R., Cure, P., Mineo, D., Selvaggi, G., et al. (2008). Islet transplantation with alemtuzumab induction and calcineurin-free maintenance immunosuppression results in improved short- and long-term outcomes. *Transplantation*, 86(12), 1695-701.

[84] Mineo, D., Ricordi, C., Xu, X., Pileggi, A., Garcia-Morales, R., Khan, A., et al. (2008). Combined islet and hematopoietic stem cell allotransplantation: a clinical pilot trial to induce chimerism and graft tolerance. *Am J Transplant*, 8(6), 1262-74.

[85] Vantyghem, M. C., Kerr-Conte, J., Arnalsteen, L., Sergent, G., Defrance, F., Gmyr, V., et al. (2009). Primary graft function, metabolic control, and graft survival after islet transplantation. *Diabetes Care*, 32(8), 1473-8.

[86] Borot, S., Niclauss, N., Wojtusciszyn, A., Brault, C., Demuylder-Mischler, S., Müller, Y., et al. (2011). Impact of the number of infusions on 2-year results of islet-after-kidney transplantation in the GRAGIL network. *Transplantation*, 92(9), 1031-8.

[87] Posselt, A. M., Bellin, M. D., Tavakol, M., Szot, G. L., Frassetto, L. A., Masharani, U., et al. (2010). Islet transplantation in type 1 diabetics using an immunosuppressive protocol based on the anti-LFA-1 antibody efalizumab. *Am J Transplant*, 10(8), 1870-80.

[88] Turgeon, N. A., Avila, J. G., Cano, J. A., Hutchinson, J. J., Badell, I. R., Page, A. J., et al. (2010). Experience with a novel efalizumab-based immunosuppressive regimen to facilitate single donor islet cell transplantation. *Am J Transplant*, 10(9), 2082-91.

[89] Posselt, A. M., Szot, G. L., Frassetto, L. A., Masharani, U., Tavakol, M., Amin, R., et al. (2010). Islet transplantation in type 1 diabetic patients using calcineurin inhibitor-free immunosuppressive protocols based on T-cell adhesion or costimulation blockade. *Transplantation*, 90(12), 1595-601.

[90] Matsumoto, S., Takita, M., Chaussabel, D., Noguchi, H., Shimoda, M., Sugimoto, K., et al. (2011). Improving Efficacy of Clinical Islet Transplantation with Iodixanol Based Islet Purification, Thymoglobulin Induction and Blockage of IL-1-beta and TNF-alpha. Cell. *Transplant*, 20(10), 1641-1647.

[91] Basta, G., Montanucci, P., Luca, G., Boselli, C., Noya, G., Barbaro, B., et al. (2011). Long-term metabolic and immunological follow-up of nonimmunosuppressed patients with type 1 diabetes treated with microencapsulated islet allografts: four cases. *Diabetes Care*, 34(11), 2406-9.

[92] Raught, B., Gingras, A. C., & Sonenberg, N. (2001). The target of rapamycin (TOR) proteins. *Proc Natl Acad Sci U S A*, 98(13), 7037-44.

[93] Niclauss, N., Bosco, D., Morel, P., Giovannoni, L., Berney, T., & Parnaud, G. (2011). Rapamycin impairs proliferation of transplanted islet β cells. *Transplantation*, 91(7), 714-22.

[94] Zhang, N., Su, D., Qu, S., Tse, T., Bottino, R., Balamurugan, A. N., et al. (2006). Sirolimus is associated with reduced islet engraftment and impaired beta-cell function. *Diabetes*, 55(9), 2429-36.

[95] Tanemura, M., Ohmura, Y., Deguchi, T., Machida, T., Tsukamoto, R., Wada, H., et al. (2012). Rapamycin causes upregulation of autophagy and impairs islets function both in vitro and in vivo. *Am J Transplant*, 12(1), 102-14.

[96] Melzi, R., Maffi, P., Nano, R., Sordi, V., Mercalli, A., Scavini, M., et al. (2009). Rapamycin does not adversely affect intrahepatic islet engraftment in mice and improves early islet engraftment in humans. *Islets*, 1(1), 42-9.

[97] Gao, R., Ustinov, J., Korsgren, O., & Otonkoski, T. (2007). Effects of immunosuppressive drugs on in vitro neogenesis of human islets: mycophenolate mofetil inhibits the proliferation of ductal cells. *Am J Transplant*, 7(4), 1021-6.

[98] Allison, A. C., & Eugui, E. M. (2005). Mechanisms of action of mycophenolate mofetil in preventing acute and chronic allograft rejection. *Transplantation*, 80(2), S181-90.

[99] Cohn, R. G., Mirkovich, A., Dunlap, B., Burton, P., Chiu, S. H., Eugui, E., et al. (1999). Mycophenolic acid increases apoptosis, lysosomes and lipid droplets in human lymphoid and monocytic cell lines. *Transplantation*, 68(3), 411-8.

[100] Gallo, R., Natale, M., Vendrame, F., Boggi, U., Filipponi, F., Marchetti, P., et al. (2012). In vitro effects of mycophenolic acid on survival, function, and gene expression of pancreatic beta-cells. *Acta Diabetol.*

[101] Vincenti, F., Dritselis, A., & Kirkpatrick, P. (2011). Belatacept. *Nat Rev Drug Discov*, 10(9), 655-6.

[102] Elliott, R. B., Escobar, L., Tan, P. L., Muzina, M., Zwain, S., & Buchanan, C. (2007). Live encapsulated porcine islets from a type 1 diabetic patient 9.5 yr after xenotransplantation. *Xenotransplantation*, 14(2), 157-61.

[103] Lee, S. H., Hao, E., Savinov, A. Y., Geron, I., Strongin, A. Y., & Itkin-Ansari, P. (2009). Human beta-cell precursors mature into functional insulin-producing cells in an immunoisolation device: implications for diabetes cell therapies. *Transplantation*, 87(7), 983-91.

[104] Siebers, U., Horcher, A., Bretzel, R. G., Federlin, K., & Zekorn, T. (1997). Alginate-based microcapsules for immunoprotected islet transplantation. *Ann N Y Acad Sci*, 831, 304-12.

[105] Kobayashi, T., Aomatsu, Y., Iwata, H., Kin, T., Kanehiro, H., Hisanaga, M., et al. (2003). Indefinite islet protection from autoimmune destruction in nonobese diabetic mice by agarose microencapsulation without immunosuppression. *Transplantation*, 75(5), 619-25.

[106] Lee, B. R., Hwang, J. W., Choi, Y. Y., Wong, S. F., Hwang, Y. H., Lee, D. Y., et al. (2012). In situ formation and collagen-alginate composite encapsulation of pancreatic islet spheroids. *Biomaterials*, 33(3), 837-45.

[107] Cruise, G. M., Scharp, D. S., & Hubbell, J. A. (1998). Characterization of permeability and network structure of interfacially photopolymerized poly(ethylene glycol) diacrylate hydrogels. *Biomaterials*, 19(14), 1287-94.

[108] Lee, D. Y., Lee, S., Nam, J. H., & Byun, Y. (2006). Minimization of immunosuppressive therapy after islet transplantation: combined action of heme oxygenase-1 and PEGylation to islet. *Am J Transplant*, 6(8), 1820-8.

[109] Cabric, S., Sanchez, J., Lundgren, T., Foss, A., Felldin, M., Källen, R., et al. (2007). Islet surface heparinization prevents the instant blood-mediated inflammatory reaction in islet transplantation. *Diabetes*, 56(8), 2008-15.

[110] Contreras, J. L., Eckstein, C., Smyth, C. A., Bilbao, G., Vilatoba, M., Ringland, S. E., et al. (2004). Activated protein C preserves functional islet mass after intraportal transplantation: a novel link between endothelial cell activation, thrombosis, inflammation, and islet cell death. *Diabetes*, 53(11), 2804-14.

[111] Stabler, C. L., Sun, X. L., Cui, W., Wilson, J. T., Haller, CA, & Chaikof, E. L. (2007). Surface re-engineering of pancreatic islets with recombinant azido-thrombomodulin. *Bioconjug Chem*, 18(6), 1713-5.

[112] Totani, T., Teramura, Y., & Iwata, H. (2008). Immobilization of urokinase on the islet surface by amphiphilic poly(vinyl alcohol) that carries alkyl side chains. *Biomaterials*, 29(19), 2878-83.

[113] Baidal, D. A., Faradji, R. N., Messinger, S., Froud, T., Monroy, K., Ricordi, C., et al. (2009). Early metabolic markers of islet allograft dysfunction. *Transplantation*, 87(5), 689-97.

[114] Rickels, M. R., Schutta, M. H., Markmann, J. F., Barker, C. F., Naji, A., & Teff, K. L. (2005). {beta}-Cell function following human islet transplantation for type 1 diabetes. *Diabetes*, 54(1), 100-6.

[115] Ryan, E. A., Shandro, T., Green, K., Paty, B. W., Senior, P. A., Bigam, D., et al. (2004). Assessment of the severity of hypoglycemia and glycemic lability in type 1 diabetic subjects undergoing islet transplantation. *Diabetes*, 53(4), 955-62.

[116] Matsumoto, S., Noguchi, H., Hatanaka, N., Shimoda, M., Kobayashi, N., Jackson, A., et al. (2009). SUITO index for evaluation of efficacy of single donor islet transplantation. *Cell Transplant*, 18(5), 557-62.

[117] Yamada, Y., Fukuda, K., Fujimoto, S., Hosokawa, M., Tsukiyama, K., Nagashima, K., et al. (2006). SUIT, secretory units of islets in transplantation: An index for therapeutic management of islet transplanted patients and its application to type 2 diabetes. *Diabetes Res Clin Pract*, 74(3), 222-6.

[118] Takita, M., Matsumoto, S., Qin, H., Noguchi, H., Shimoda, M., Chujo, D., et al. (2011). Secretory Unit of Islet Transplant Objects (SUITO) Index can predict severity of hypoglycemic episodes in clinical islet cell transplantation. *Cell Transplant*.

[119] Takita, M., & Matsumoto, S. (2012). SUITO Index for Evaluation of Clinical Islet Transplantation. *Cell Transplant*.

[120] Faradji, R. N., Monroy, K., Messinger, S., Pileggi, A., Froud, T., Baidal, D. A., et al. (2007). Simple measures to monitor beta-cell mass and assess islet graft dysfunction. *Am J Transplant .*, 7(2), 303-8.

[121] Ryan, E. A., Paty, B. W., Senior, P. A., Lakey, J. R., Bigam, D., & Shapiro, A. M. (2005). Beta-score: an assessment of beta-cell function after islet transplantation. *Diabetes Care*, 28(2), 343-7.

[122] Caumo, A., Maffi, P., Nano, R., Bertuzzi, F., Luzi, L., Secchi, A., et al. (2008). Transplant estimated function: a simple index to evaluate beta-cell secretion after islet transplantation. *Diabetes Care*, 31(2), 301-5.

[123] Friberg, A. S., Lundgren, T., Malm, H., Felldin, M., Nilsson, B., Jenssen, T., et al. (2012). Transplanted functional islet mass: donor, islet preparation, and recipient fac-

tors influence early graft function in islet-after-kidney patients. *Transplantation*, 93(6), 632-8.

[124] Eriksson, O., Eich, T., Sundin, A., Tibell, A., Tufveson, G., Andersson, H., et al. (2009). Positron emission tomography in clinical islet transplantation. *Am J Transplant*, 9(12), 2816-24.

[125] Eich, T., Eriksson, O., & Lundgren, T. (2007). Transplantation NNfCI. Visualization of early engraftment in clinical islet transplantation by positron-emission tomography. *N Engl J Med*, 356(26), 2754-5.

[126] Saudek, F., Jirák, D., Girman, P., Herynek, V., Dezortová, M., Kríz, J., et al. (2010). Magnetic resonance imaging of pancreatic islets transplanted into the liver in humans. *Transplantation*, 90(12), 1602-6.

[127] Medarova, Z., & Moore, A. (2009). MRI as a tool to monitor islet transplantation. *Nat Rev Endocrinol*, 5(8), 444-52.

[128] Caumo, A., Maffi, P., Nano, R., Luzi, L., Hilbrands, R., Gillard, P., et al. (2011). Comparative evaluation of simple indices of graft function after islet transplantation. *Transplantation*, 92(7), 815-21.

[129] Matsumoto, S., Takita, M., Shimoda, M., Itoh, T., Iwahashi, S., Chujo, D., et al. (2011). Usefulness of the Secretory Unit of Islet Transplant Objects (SUITO) Index for Evaluation of Clinical Autologous Islet Transplantation. *Transplant Proc*, 43(9), 3246-9.

[130] Sutherland, D. E., Gruessner, A. C., Carlson, A. M., Blondet, J. J., Balamurugan, A. N., Reigstad, K. F., et al. (2008). Islet autotransplant outcomes after total pancreatectomy: a contrast to islet allograft outcomes. *Transplantation*, 86(12), 1799-802.

Chapter 7

The Impact of Inflammation on Pancreatic β-Cell Metabolism, Function and Failure in T1DM and T2DM: Commonalities and Differences

Philip Newsholme, Kevin Keane,
Paulo I Homem de Bittencourt Jr. and
Mauricio Krause

Additional information is available at the end of the chapter

1. Introduction

Type 1 diabetes mellitus (T1DM) is a chronically progressive autoimmune disease that affects approximately 1% of the population in the developed world. This adverse immune response is induced and promoted by the interaction of both genetic and environmental factors. In contrast, in type 2 diabetes mellitus (T2DM), insulin-resistance coupled with reduced insulin output appears to be the major cause of hyperglycaemia (affecting approximately 6% of the population). Although the aetiology of diabetes may differ from T1DM to T2DM, a common feature associated with both types is the failure of pancreatic β-cells in the islets of Langerhans, thus causing a reduction in insulin secretion, cell mass and ultimately apoptotic death. However, the impact and time-course of pancreatic β-cell death, which may appear very different in T1 and T2DM, may be related through common molecular mechanisms.

Glucose-stimulated insulin secretion (GSIS) is central to the physiological control of metabolic fuel homeostasis, and its impairment is a hallmark of pancreatic β-cell failure in T2DM. β-Cells are often referred to as "fuel sensors" as they continually monitor and respond to dietary nutrients, under the modulation of additional neuro-hormonal and immunological signals, in order to secrete insulin to best meet the needs of the organism. Therefore, β-cell dysfunction and death in diabetes leads to hyperglycaemia and its complications. An intriguing characteristic of the pancreatic β-cells is their similarity to immune cells: 1) they can release cytokines; 2) they strongly respond to cytokines from other cells and tissues; 3) their function is dependent on the production of reactive oxygen (ROS) and nitrogen species (RNS); 4) they express high levels of pro-inflammatory proteins such as nuclear transcription factor κB (NFκB), inducible nitric oxide synthase (iNOS), NADPH oxidase (NOX), Toll-like receptors (TLR) and other proteins in response to immune signals, but also to metabolic challenge. However and in contrast to professional immunoinflammatory cells, such as macrophages or neutrophils, the β-cell is fragile when subjected to immune attack and is highly vulnerable to oxidative stress.

In this chapter, we intend to review the mechanisms of insulin secretion in response to a wide variety of metabolic stimuli, the 'immune-like' characteristics of the pancreatic β-cells with respect to metabolism, secretion and cell defence, the similarities between β-cell failure/death in T1DM and T2DM and finally, to suggest novel targets for the treatment of diabetes.

2. Regulation of β-cell function and insulin secretion

Control of energy metabolism is essential in maintaining cellular homeostasis in all animals across the metazoan (all animals with differentiated tissues). Insulin and glucagon are hormones produced by vertebrate organisms to regulate glycaemic homeostasis. In addition, insulin-like and glucagon-like peptide genes have been detected in invertebrate organisms including, insects, molluscs and nematodes, thus inferring a similar metabolic control that is conserved among most species [1,2]. However, in the case of vertebrates, insulin and glucagon are produced by cells located in the islets of Langerhans of the animal pancreas. Under normal physiological conditions, blood glucose concentration is maintained within narrow limits by an alternate release of these powerful proteins, regardless of nutrient intake or expenditure (*e.g.* exercise). There are four main cell types that contribute to the regulation of this pancreatic function and they include, α-cells, β-cells, δ-cells and pancreatic peptide (PP)-cells [3]. The role of α-cells is to synthesise and secrete glucagon in response to low extracellular glucose concentrations, thus replenishing the plasma carbohydrate level [3]. δ-Cells secrete somatostatin that has an inhibitory effect on insulin and glucagon release, while PP-cells secrete pancreatic peptide whose physiological function has not been fully elucidated [3]. Conversely, the function of β-cells has been extensively studied and they are responsible for the biosynthesis and release of insulin in response to elevated plasma glucose, amino acid and saturated fatty acid levels [3]. These cells represent the most abundant cell type in pancreatic islets and are the primary source of dysfunction in DM.

β-Cell responsiveness and subsequent insulin secretion is subject to a plethora of cellular regulatory mechanisms. Insulin biosynthesis and secretion is a highly controlled system that has many influencing extracellular and intracellular factors including, glucose, fatty acids, amino acids, nucleotides, calcium/potassium electrochemical gradient, metabolic coupling factors (MCFs), and level of ROS and RNS. Furthermore, the fact that cellular insulin secretion is achieved by the physical release of vesicles or granules containing the protein, suggests that the process acquires a greater degree of complexity and control, and is subject to vesicle manufacture, recruitment and finally plasma membrane docking.

Glucose-Stimulated Insulin Secretion (GSIS) is fundamental to insulin exocytosis as glucose is the most potent insulin secretagogue [4]. In an environment of excess extracellular glucose, β-cell plasma membrane transporter proteins GLUT1 and GLUT2, actively transport free glucose molecules inside the cell where glycolysis can be initiated to create the nucleotide ATP (Fig. 1). Consequently, intracellular metabolism of glucose by glycolysis, and further metabolism of pyruvate via the downstream tricarboxylic acid (TCA) cycle, leads to elevated NADH, $FADH_2$ and ultimately ATP levels [4]. The increased intracellular ATP:ADP ratio closes membrane-bound ATP-sensitive K^+ channels, resulting in plasma membrane depolarisation and a subsequent opening of membrane-bound voltage activated Ca^{2+} channels. A rapid influx of calcium ions is promoted, causing the exocytosis of insulin through fusion of the insulin containing vesicles with the plasma membrane via VAMP (vesicle-associated membrane protein) and SNARE (soluble NH2-ethylmaleimide-sensitive fusion protein attachment protein receptor) association [5]. This specific process of insulin secretion is known as K_{ATP}-dependent GSIS, and since ATP generation is critical, the metabolic control points of glycolysis, the TCA cycle and oxidative phosphorylation (i.e. activity of metabolic enzymes such as hexokinase, phosphofructokinase, pyruvate kinase, pyruvate dehydrogenase, pyruvate carboxylase, glutamate dehydrogenase and mitochondrial redox-shuttles) have a significant impact on regulation of insulin release.

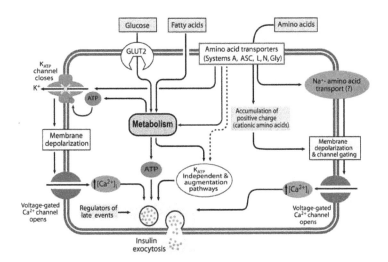

Figure 1. Mechanisms of nutrient and amino acid stimulated insulin secretion. Glucose metabolism is essential for stimulation of insulin secretion. The mechanisms by which amino acids enhance insulin secretion are understood to primarily rely on (a) direct depolarization of the plasma membrane (e.g. cationic amino acid, L-arginine); (b) metabolism (e.g. alanine, glutamine, leucine); and (c) co-transport with Na^+ and cell membrane depolarization (e.g. alanine). Notably, rapid partial oxidation may also initially increase both the cellular content of ATP (impacting on K^+ATP channel closure prompting membrane depolarization) and other stimulus secretion coupling factors. In the absence of glucose, fatty acids may be metabolised to generate ATP and maintain basal levels of insulin secretion. Adapted from [3].

However, there also remains the possibility that K_{ATP}-independent GSIS can occur in the β-cell, although the exact methodology is still not fully understood. K_{ATP}-independent GSIS has been illustrated in studies utilising diazoxide to maintain K^+ channels in the open position [6] and in mice with disrupted/deleted K$^+$ channels [7, 8]. GSIS was subsequently shown to be possible in a K$_{ATP}$-independent manner and it is believed that these two co-ordinate mechanisms of insulin secretion (*i.e.* K$_{ATP}$-dependent & K$_{ATP}$-independent GSIS), are responsible for the bi-phasic insulin response in animals. It is thought that the initial rise in insulin secretion is K$_{ATP}$-dependent, while the second phase is mediated through K$_{ATP}$-independent interactions dependent on mitochondrial activity [4,9].

Mitochondrial, lipid and amino acid metabolism plays a significant role in regulation of insulin secretion and GSIS. Lipid and amino acid metabolites can generate, or can directly become MCFs that enhance or inhibit GSIS. While individual amino acids alone at physiological concentrations do not enhance GSIS, some specific amino acids at higher concentrations, or in combination with others, can cause increments in GSIS [10]. Arginine, alanine, leucine and glutamine can increase GSIS, while homocysteine and cysteine at elevated concentration can inhibit GSIS [10]. The effect of amino acids is also dependent on whether β-cells are exposed acutely or chronically, as chronic exposure may influence the expression of genes involved in the control of insulin secretion [10,11]. In addition, another nutrient source, fatty acids, can also regulate GSIS in both a positive or negative manner depending on the level of saturation, carbon chain length, and whether exposure is under acute or chronic conditions. Saturated fatty acids like palmitic and stearic acid are known to chronically decrease GSIS *in vitro*, but palmitic acid can acutely enhance GSIS [12-14]. Conversely, chronic exposure to monounsaturated oleic acid and polyunsaturated arachidonic acid can increase insulin production in β-cells [13,15]. Fatty acids can amplify β-cell GSIS, and it is likely that they elevate insulin levels by causing changes in calcium influx and proteins associated with ion channel activity [16]. Mitochondrial metabolism of amino and fatty acid is at the hub of the reported effects on insulin secretion and GSIS, mainly because TCA-mediated metabolism of both leads to increased ATP production and protein biosynthesis, which is a prerequisite for insulin secretion (Fig. 1). The intricacies of mitochondrial-mediated metabolism of amino and fatty acids will be discussed below.

3. Pancreatic β-cell metabolism and influencing factors

Pancreatic β-cells are unique and can be distinguished from other cell types by their metabolic profile. Several key characteristics of β-cells include the ability to utilise glucose in the physiological range of 2-20mmol/L, express low levels of lactate dehydrogenase (LDH) and plasma membrane monocarboxylate pyruvate/lactate transporter, have a corresponding high activity of glycerol-3-phosphate and malate/aspartate redox shuttles, and finally possess an elevated level of pyruvate dehydrogenase (PDH) and pyruvate carboxylase (PC) activity, ensuring that both oxidative and anaplerotic metabolism of glucose and pyruvate can occur preferentially in the near absence of lactate generation (Fig. 2) (further details can be found in [4,10,11,17-21]). These adaptions are designed to specifically accelerate oxidative phosphorylation and TCA activity as a means to increase ATP output and consequently insulin exocytosis.

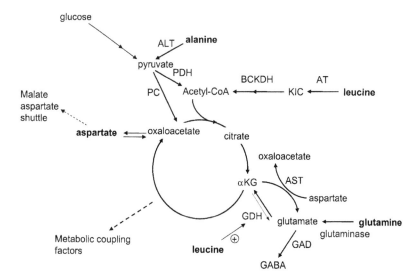

Figure 2. Schematic diagram representing the metabolism of selected amino acids, highlighting related metabolic stimulus-secretion coupling factors involved in insulin release. The pathway of glutamine metabolism via glutaminase, GDH, and entry into the TCA cycle (glutaminolysis) is shown along with key points of amino acid interaction with glutamine and glucose metabolism. KG, -ketoglutarate; ALT, alanine aminotransferase; AST, aspartate aminotransferase; AT, aminotransferase; BCKDH, branched-chain-keto-acid dehydrogenase; PC, pyruvate carboxylase; PDH, pyruvate dehydrogenase; KIC, ketoisocaproic acid. Adapted from [21].

Pancreatic β-cells regenerate NAD+ for glycolysis primarily through high expression of mitochondrial NADH shuttles like glycerol-3-phosphate and the malate/aspartate shuttle (Fig. 3), for specific details refer to [11,22]. Briefly, the glycerol-3-phosphate shuttle consists of cytosolic and mitochondrial glycerol-3-phosphate dehydrogenase that operate in unison to convert dihydroxyacetone phosphate to glycerol-3-phosphate and NAD+, with a subsequent generation of FADH$_2$ from NAD+ [4]. In contrast, the malate/aspartate shuttle is the main shuttle responsible for transferring glycolytic reducing equivalents to the mitochondria in the β-cell [11]. Here, cytosolic malate dehydrogenase reduces oxaloacetate to malate and NAD+, with a subsequent generation of NADH inside the mitochondria. Using an amino group provided by glutamate, mitochondrial oxaloacetate can be converted back to aspartate maintaining this cyclic event. The malate/aspartate shuttle is dominantly expressed in β-cells, eloquently linking glycolysis to mitochondrial & amino acid metabolism.

As alluded to previously, amino acid metabolism is essential for nutrient- and glucose-stimulated insulin secretion, and the effects of several amino acids have been reviewed extensively [3,10, 11]. To summarise these findings briefly, both arginine and alanine have been shown to promote insulin release through changes in electrogenic transport, progressing to activation of Ca^{2+} ion channels [10,23,24]. It has also been demonstrated that they enhance glutamate production and consequently may play a role in malate/aspartate shuttle-mediated generation of NADH, and/or in glutathione synthesis and antioxidant defence [25]. Therefore, both arginine and alanine may

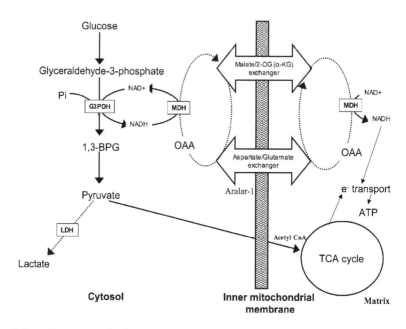

Figure 3. The malate–aspartate shuttle is the principal mechanism for the movement of reducing equivalents in the form of NADH from the cytoplasm to the mitochondrion in β-cells. Cytoplasmic malate dehydrogenase (MDH) reduces oxaloacetate (OAA) to malate while oxidizing NADH to NAD+. Malate then enters the mitochondrion where the reverse reaction is performed by mitochondrial malate dehydrogenase. Movement of mitochondrial oxaloacetate to the cytoplasm to maintain this cycle is achieved by transamination to aspartate with the amino group being donated by glutamate. The 2-oxoglutarate (α-ketoglutarate) generated leaves the mitochondrion for the cytoplasm. Adapted from [11].

protect β-cells from oxidative insult in addition to promoting insulin secretion. However, prolonged exposure of β-cells to alanine results in decreased alanine-induced insulin secretion, while reaction of arginine with inducible nitric oxide synthase (iNOS) can promote nitric oxide (NO) production [10,19]. NO is an important signalling molecule, which is essential for β-cell glucose uptake at low levels, but at high concentration may be toxic [26]. Interaction of NO with superoxide (O⁻) can also lead to the formation of peroxynitrite (ONOO⁻), a damaging free radical that can disrupt mitochondrial function [27]. In fact, ONOO⁻, which is in equilibrium with its conjugate peroxynitrous acid (ONOOH, $pK_a \approx 6.8$) [28], is a highly reactive oxidant species produced by the combination of the oxygen free radical O_2^- and NO [29] and has been demonstrated to be a more potent oxidant and cytotoxic mediator than NO or O_2^- individually, in a variety of inflammatory conditions [30]. ONOO⁻ is extremely cytotoxic to rat and human islet cells *in vitro* [31] and its *in vivo* formation has been reported in pancreatic islets where it has been associated with β-cell destruction and development of T1DM in NOD mice [32].

High levels of homocysteine and cysteine have also been shown to elicit a negative effect on β-cell function. In obese hyperinsulinaemic T2DM patients, homocysteine levels are increased, while they are increased in T1DM patients, but only following disease-related complications such as diabetic nephropathy [11,33]. It has been suggested that homocysteine can decrease GSIS in rat pancreatic β-cells [34], although the inhibitory mechanism is still not fully understood. It may decrease insulin secretion by altering enzyme and/or protein activity, or by causing oxidative stress [35,36]. In addition, homocysteine can be converted to asymmetric dimethylarginine, which is inhibitor of neuronal NOS and can also inhibit iNOS to a lesser extent and therefore may reduce NO production, which is important for β-cell insulin secretion and function [10,37]. In contrast, cysteine has been shown to increase β-cell GSIS at low concentrations [38] and is essential for antioxidant defence and glutathione synthesis, along with glycine and glutamate. Cysteine supplementation was found to protect β-cells from hydrogen peroxide (H_2O_2)-induced cell death and prevented glucotoxicity in mouse β-cells [39,40]. However, at elevated concentrations, it impaired GSIS through excessive hydrogen sulphide (H_2S) formation [41].

Glutamine is required for β-cell metabolism and function, and is consumed at rapid rates [10]. Glutamine supplementation does not induce insulin release [10], but co-treatment with leucine significantly enhances GSIS via activation of glutamate dehydrogenase (GDH), allowing entry of glutamine into the TCA cycle (Fig. 2) [42]. It has been suggested that glutamine alone does not induce insulin secretion because it is not oxidised during its metabolism. Instead, metabolism of glutamine may yield aspartate and GABA (γ-aminobutyric acid), a potent inhibitor of glucagon secretion (Fig. 2) [3]. However, using NMR studies, we found that the major products of glutamine metabolism were aspartate and glutamate. Here, glutamate entered the γ-glutamyl cycle and increased the synthesis of the antioxidant, glutathione [43]. Formation of glutamate from glutamine also has important implications in activation of the aspartate/glutamate shuttles and in ATP production from the TCA cycle, via glutamate metabolism to α-ketoglutarate. Consequently, glutamine may function to enhance ATP production and insulin release by changes in down-stream metabolism, most notably via glutamine-derived glutamate. Alternatively, glutamate can be transported externally from the cell and into the surrounding matrix, which may cause glutamate receptor activation and desensitisation if the rate of release is over extended periods [44]. Since glucagon secretion from pancreatic α-cells is sensitive to glutamate exposure, its release may represent a novel paracrine control mechanism for modulation of blood carbohydrate levels [44]. Some groups have reported that total intracellular glutamate levels increased in response to glucose, while others reported no significant change [25,45,46]. Recently, it has been suggested that glutamate is transported into insulin-containing vesicles, thereby promoting Ca^{2+}-dependent insulin secretion [47]. However, the role of glutamate in mediating insulin secretion remains hotly debated.

Taken together, this evidence suggests that a variety of amino acids may contribute significantly to regulation of pancreatic β-cell insulin secretion. However, other β-cell metabolic processes are important to insulin secretion and must be considered. These include four key metabolic shunts that divert glucose from being utilised by TCA cycle (i.e., aldose reductase, pentose-phosphate, glycogen synthesis and hexosamine pathways; please, see Fig. 4) as well as down-stream glycolytic enzymes such as PC and PDH, and also enzymes involved in fatty acid metabolism like acetyl CoA carboxylase (ACC) and fatty acid synthase.

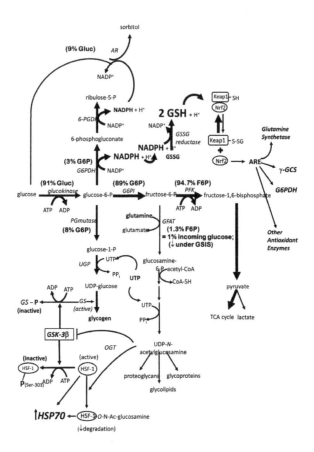

Figure 4. Flux balance analysis of glucose utilisation in β-cells. The fluxes through the biochemical pathways shown here were calculated by using Michaelis-Menten function, intracellular metabolite concentrations estimated from different works. Percentages in parentheses refer to the proportional amount of the metabolite consumed through that step. AR, aldose reductase; ARE, antioxidant response (ARE) elements in the promoter regions of target genes; F6P, fructose-6-phosphate; G6P, glucose-6-phosphate; G6PDH, glucose-6-phosphate dehydrogenase; G6PI, glucose-6-phosphate isomerase (a.k. as phosphoglucoisomerase); γ-GCS, glutamate cysteine ligase, a.k. as γ-glutamylcysteine synthetase; GFAT, glutamine:fructose-6-phosphate amidotransferase a.k. as GFPT, for glutamine-fructose-6-phosphate transaminase; Gluc, glucose; GS, glycogen synthase; GSIS, glucose-stimulated insulin secretion; GSK-3β, glycogen synthase kinase-3β; HSF-1, heat shock transcription factor-1; HSP70, the 70-kDa family of heat-shock proteins (includes both hsp72, encoded by the HSPA1A gene, and hsp73, a.k. as hsc70, encoded by the HSPA8 gene); Keap1, Kelch-like ECH-associated protein 1; Nrf2, Nuclear factor erythroid 2-related transcription factor 2; OGT, O-N-acetylglucosamine transferase, a.k. as UDP-N-acetyl-D-glucosamine:protein-O-β-N-acetyl-D-glucosaminyl transferase and uridine diphospho-N-acetylglucosamine:polypeptide β-N-acetylglucosaminyl transferase; PFK, phosphofructokinase; PGmutase, phosphoglucomutase; UGP, UDP-glucose pyrophosphorylase.

Highlighting the peculiarities of β-cell metabolism in a coordinated effort to increase the activity of a number of metabolic pathways in response to glucose, Huang & Joseph (2012) have shown, by using metabolomic analysis, during GSIS in clonal β-cells, a conspicuous accumulation of pyruvate, succinate, fumarate, malate, α-ketoglutarate, dihydroxyacetone phosphate (DHAP), (iso)citrate, palmitate, glucose-6-phosphate and 6-phosphogluconate whereas aspartate was consumed in response to glucose [48]. Here, the authors have clearly demonstrated that under glucose stimulus, β-cells strongly enhance metabolic flux towards glycolysis and TCA cycle. Indeed, there is a very delicate poise to coordinately regulate the flux of glucose towards the formation of NADPH (through the pentose-phosphate shunt) avoiding excessive formation of sorbitol (via the polyol-aldose reductase shunt) which would empty glycolytic flux (Fig. 4). It has long been recognised, for instance, that overexpression of the aldose reductase gene is able to induce apoptosis in pancreatic β-cells by causing a redox imbalance [49] while, on the contrary, pharmacological blockage of aldose reductase may impair GSIS, thus suggesting that the conversion of free intracellular glucose to sorbitol in the β-cell is an essential step in the glucose-induced release mechanism (Fig.4) [50].

Although the physiological significance is still under debate, glucose 6-phosphate may also be targeted towards glycogen synthesis in pancreatic islets, which is enhanced during GSIS and impaired in STZ-diabetic rats (Fig. 4) [51,52]. Finally, glucose may be deviated from ultimate metabolism through further glycolytic steps via the reaction of fructose-6-phosphate with glutamine through the hexosamine biochemical pathway (HBP) (Fig. 4). Increased fluxes through HBP may, on the one hand, block glycogen synthase kinase-3β (GSK-3β), thus liberating glycogen synthesis by glycogen synthase and, on the other, may reduce heat shock factor-1 (HSF-1) degradation thus allowing enhanced expression of the 70-kDa heat shock protein (HSP70), which is cytoprotective to β-cells (Fig. 4) [53,54]. Over-enhanced flux through HBP is an inducer of endoplasmic reticulum (ER) stress, while being associated with insulin-resistance [55].

PC and PDH are both highly expressed in β-cells and allow conversion of pyruvate to oxaloacetate (PC) and acetyl-CoA (PDH), with subsequent entry into the TCA cycle [4]. Interestingly, siRNA inhibition of PC reduces cell proliferation and GSIS in insulinoma cells and rat islets, while overexpression in rat islets could enhance GSIS and cell proliferation [56, 57]. The role of PDH is less understood and it is thought to support PC activity by providing acetyl-CoA for citrate production. Both enzymes are important regulators of the pyruvate/malate and pyruvate/citrate shuttles. Common to each pathway is the conversion of glycolytic-derived pyruvate to oxaloacetate by PC, as described above. In the case of the pyruvate/malate shuttle, oxaloacetate is then converted to malate and translocated to the cytosol, where malic enzyme1 (ME1) converts malate back to pyruvate along with generation of NADPH. Pyruvate can re-enter the mitochondria to repeat the cycle with further generation of NADPH [4]. However, for the pyruvate/citrate shuttle, PC-mediated oxaloacetate leads to condensation with acetyl CoA (possibly generated by PDH), and the subsequent formation of citrate. Translocation of citrate to the cytosol results in oxaloacetate and acetyl CoA regeneration from citrate by ATP-citrate lyase (ACL). Oxaloacetate re-enters the pyruvate/malate cycle with generation of NADPH as outlined previously, while acetyl CoA is carboxylated to malonyl CoA by acetyl CoA carboxylase (ACC). Malonyl CoA is then converted to long chain acyl CoA by fatty acid synthase leading to fatty acid production. Additionally, malonyl CoA can also inhibit carnitine palmitoyl transferase 1 (CPT-1), which in a low glucose state, transports fatty acids into the mitochondria to generate ATP by oxidation [4,10]. However, in high glucose situations, inhibition of CPT-1 leads to fatty acid accumulation in the cytosol and this accumulation may increase insulin exocytosis by augmenting calcium influx and ion channel proteins [10,16]. Interestingly, formation of malonyl CoA from acetyl CoA by ACC is positively regulated by the glutamine-sensitive protein phosphatase type 2A (PP2A), while it is negatively regulated by the amino acid-sensitive AMP-activated kinase (AMPK) [11,58,59]. These concepts again fully illustrate the inherent relationship between β-cell metabolism of glucose, amino acids and lipids with insulin exocytosis [11,58,59].

AMPK is crucial in lipid metabolism control and can chronically regulate β-cell function by altering the expression of vital transcription factors that govern lipogenic and glycolytic enzymes [10]. Chronic exposure of β-cells to high circulatory lipid levels, as occurs in T2DM, can inhibit glucose oxidation and result in a decreased ATP/AMP ratio along with a subsequent activation of AMPK, which inhibits fatty acid synthesis, while enhancing fatty acid oxidation, and impairing GSIS [10]. The exact metabolic mechanisms of how lipids can augment GSIS are still not fully understood but are believed to involve modulation of Ca^{2+} mobilisation via interaction with G-protein coupled receptors [60]. Recent evidence has shown that these G-protein coupled receptors are highly expressed in β-cells and correlated with insulinogenic index [10,61]. It has also been demonstrated that interaction of omega-3 fatty acids and the GPR120 receptor, plays an instrumental role in mediating insulin-sensitisation and anti-inflammatory effects in obese mice models [62].

AMPK also occupies a central position in metabolic regulation in order to avoid inflammatory dysregulation. Accordingly, in different cell types, AMPK phosphorylates and inhibit glutamine:fructose-6-phosphate amidotransferase-1 (GFAT-1), the flux-generating step of HBP (Fig. 4), thus allowing for the down-regulation of such a shunt from glycolysis under low glucose situations [63], while chronic hexosamine flux stimulates fatty acid oxidation by activating AMPK [64]. However, regulatory pathways under AMPK control are not solely intended to divert metabolic fluxes. Rather, AMPK regulation of GSK-3β allows the concomitant regulation of inflammatory cytokine production, since the inhibition of GSK-3β elicits the deinhibition of HSF-1, thus triggering the expression of HSP70, which is an intracellular anti-inflammatory protein.

It is of note that, besides the now classical molecular chaperone action, the most remarkable intracellular effect of HSP70 is the inhibition of NF- κB activation, which has profound implications for immunity, inflammation, cell survival and apoptosis. HSP70 blocks nuclear factor κB (NF—κB) activation at different levels. For instance, HSP70 inhibits the phosphorylation of inhibitor of κB (IκBs), while heat-induced HSP70 protein molecules are able to directly bind to IκB kinase gamma (IKKγ) thus inhibiting tumor necrosis factor- α (TNFα)-induced apoptosis [65]. In fact, the supposition that HSP70 might act intracellularly as a suppressor of NF- κB pathways has been raised after a number of seminal discoveries in which HSP70 was intentionally induced, such as the inhibition of TNFα-induced activation of phospholipase A_2 in murine fibrosarcoma cells [66], the suppression of astroglial iNOS expression paralleled by decreased NF—κB activation [67] and the protection of rat hepatocytes from TNFα-induced apoptosis by treating cells with the nitric oxide (NO)-donor SNAP, which reacts with intracellular glutathione molecules generating S-nitrosoglutathione (SNOG) that induces HSP70, and, consequently, HSP70 expression [68].

HSP70 confers protection against sepsis-related circulatory fatality via inhibition of iNOS (NOS-2) gene expression in the rostral ventrolateral medulla through the prevention of NF-κB activation, inhibition of IκB kinase activation and consequent inhibition of IκB degradation [69]. This is corroborated by the finding that HSP70 assembles with liver NF-κB/IκB complex in the cytosol thus impeding further transcription of NF-κB-dependent TNF-α and NOS-2 genes that worsen sepsis [70]. This may also be unequivocally demonstrated by treating cells or tissues with HSP70 antisense oligonucleotides that completely reverse the beneficial NF-κB-inhibiting effect of HSP70 and inducible HSP70 expression (see [68,69]). Hence, HSP70 is anti-inflammatory per se, when intracellularly located, which also explains why cyclopentenone prostaglandins (cp-PGs), which are the most powerful physiological inducers of HSP70 by activating HSF-1, are at the same time powerful anti-inflammatory autacoids [71-73].

Another striking effect of HSP70 is the inhibition of apoptosis. The intrinsic apoptotic pathway is characterized by the release of mitochondrial pro-apoptotic factors and activation of caspase enzymes, while stimulation of cell surface receptors triggers the extrinsic death-pathway. The inhibitory potential of HSP70 over apoptosis occurs via many intracellular downstream pathways (e.g. JNK, NF-κB and Akt), which are both directly and indirectly blocked by HSP70, or through inhibition of mitochondrial Bcl-2 release. Together, these mechanisms are responsible for HSP70's anti-apoptotic function in stressed-cells [74].

In conclusion, intracellularly activated HSPs of the 70-kDa family are cytoprotective and anti-inflammatory by avoiding protein denaturation and excessive NF-κB activation which may be damaging to the cells [75]. These observations link energy sensing (AMPK) to anti-inflammation (HSP70) and points out to the complexity of the impact of metabolic regulation for cell survival and function. In addition, expression of cytokines such as interleukin-1β (IL-1β), tumour necrosis factorα (TNFα), and interferon-γ (INF-γ) in pancreatic islets is important in inflammation and progression of both T1 and T2DM, and is associated with β-cell dysfunction and death. Therefore, agents or nutrients that promote anti-inflammatory responses may be beneficial as anti-diabetic therapies. Since interaction of the immune system with pancreatic islets is central to T1DM and is becoming increasing linked to T2DM, the precise mechanisms of pancreatic cell death in relation to immunological function will now be discussed.

4. Immune-like characteristics of β-cells and response to cytokines

The pathophysiology of pancreatic islets in T1 and T2DM is characterised by an inflammatory process that includes immune cell infiltration, presence of apoptotic cells, expression of cytokines or adipokines and even amyloid deposits [76]. Although the aetiology of T1DM differs from T2DM, a common feature of both is an immune system-mediated destruction of pancreatic β-cells, ultimately leading to pancreatic dysfunction and reduced β-cell mass. However, the immunological-mediated attack does not solely originate from invading macrophages and/or cytokines produced by T-lymphocytes, as initially occurs in early stage T1DM. In fact, it also stems from local production of pro-inflammatory cytokines by the pancreatic β-cells themselves. The similarity between pancreatic β-cells and immune cells is an intriguing characteristic. Both can release and respond to cytokines; their function is dependent on changes in concentration of ROS/RNS and they both express high levels of pro-inflammatory proteins such as NFκB, iNOS, NOX and TLR's. Pancreatic β-cells have been shown to express biologically active cytokines like the pro-inflammatory cytokine IL-1β in hyperglycaemic conditions [77,78]. Due to their potent effects, cytokine production is strin-gently regulated. Control mechanisms include down-stream activation/processing (conver-sion of pro-IL-1β to IL-1β by inflammasomes), and co-expression of binding proteins/antagonists (like the IL-1 receptor antagonist, IL-1Ra), that regulate cytokine bio-reactivity [76]. However, expression of the biologically active form of IL-1β was evident in pancreatic β-cells, indicating that similar to immune cells, these cells possess the necessary cellular machinery to allow expression of immunologically active cytokines [77]. Autocrine production of IL-1β, has been correlated with autoimmune destruction of β-cells in T1DM and is also associated with glucotoxicity in the pathogenesis of T2DM patients [76,79]. IL-1β elicits its potent cytotoxic effects through activation of NFκB, and a subsequent initiation of the extrinsic cell-death pathway [78]. Additionally, chronic exposure to IL-1β results in increased iNOS expression, and consequently excess NO production. High levels of NO inhibit mitochondrial ATP synthesis and up-regulate the expression of pro-inflammatory genes in β-cells, which may potentiate β-cell failure [78].

Similar to macrophages and dendritic cells, β-cells also express TLR's that normally function to regulate the immune system [80]. TLR's interact with a wide variety of pathogen-related molecules, including lipopolysaccharide (LPS), a component of bacterial cell walls. This allows phagocytosis of microbes before infection can be established. However, in β-cells, it is believed that TLR's play a role in insulin-resistance and inflammation in T2DM. TLR2 and TLR4 have been suggested as receptors for fatty acids, and may alter insulin signalling during dyslipidaemia. We have shown that β-cells express a range of TLR's and could indeed respond to LPS via TLR's, and this interaction decreased insulin exocytosis accordingly [80]. However, glutamine restored insulin release. Glutamine can also regu-late pro-inflammatory gene expression in mononuclear cells [11,80]. Glutamine also up-regulates nuclear factor of activated T cells (NFAT), and thus promotes β-cell growth, while suppressing β-cell death. Mutations in NFAT-dependent genes have been demonstrated to result in hereditary forms of T2DM [11]. Moreover, as discussed above, glutamine can enter HBP thus regulating GSK-3β activity and HSP70 expression which promotes anti-inflamma-tion and cytoprotection [53,54].

Pancreatic β-cells are also reported to express other cytokines, including IL-6, IL-8, granulocyte colony-stimulating factor (G-CSP) and MIP-1 (macrophage inflammatory protein-1) that not only induce apoptotic β-cell death, but also signal patrolling macrophages, enhancing islet immune cell infiltration [76]. Macrophages, monocytes, neutrophils and dendritic cells perform their function by engulfing invading foreign matter including bacteria or dead cells, and degrade them using super oxide (O_2^-) generated from plasma membrane-bound NOX [27].

β-Cells also express NOX in large quantities, and utilise controlled NOX-derived ROS to drive mitogenic signalling and proliferation [27]. However, during hyperglycaemia or dyslipidaemia as occurs in T2DM, levels of NOX-derived ROS may increase and overwhelm antioxidant defences, leading to mitochondrial dysfunction, DNA oxidation, lipid peroxidation and β-cell death.

These reports illustrate the immune-like characteristics of pancreatic β-cells and clearly demonstrate the ability of these cells to not only respond to cytokines, but to be capable of producing endogenous cytokines in an autocrine fashion. This suggests that the immune system plays an integral part in progression of DM and may offer potential therapeutic targets. However, to develop immune-related treatments, more research is required into understanding the mechanisms of islet inflammation in both T1 and T2DM.

5. Islet inflammation in T1DM and T2DM

T1DM is exclusively an autoimmune form of DM, and islet inflammation is characterised by the presence of leukocyte infiltrates that include B-cells, T-cells, macrophages and Natural Killer (NK) cells [81]. Macrophages play a critical role since they phagocytose apoptotic and necrotic β-cells, as well as produce ROS and cytokines (TNFα, INF-γ and IL-1β), that can promote β-cell death, which leads to patient insulin-dependence. However, effector CD4-helper and CD8-cytotoxic T-cells represent the predominant pancreatic infiltrate for this disease, and recent evidence has suggested that T1DM progression may be dependent on a precarious equilibrium between migration and activation of effector and regulatory T-cells (Treg) [82]. An important element in T1DM disease development is the generation of autoreactive effector T-cells that kill pancreatic β-cells through expression of Fas, lytic granules and cytokines such as INF-γ [82]. Research into formation of these autoreactive cell types is still at an early stage, and it was only definitively shown in 2012, that autoreactive effector cytotoxic-CD8 T-cells were indeed present in T1DM human pancreatic islets [81]. Furthermore, the means by which these "homicidal" immune cells are generated and go on to attack β-cells is still not fully understood. However, part of the process is believed to involve dendritic cell migration to draining lymph nodes following antigen presentation, and stimulation of autoreactive T-cell differentiation [82,83]. T-cells sub-sets such as T_h1, T_h2 and T_h17 are thus formed and they express the necessary weaponry that is responsible for β-cell death in T1DM [82], this being exacerbated by strong psychological stress [84], one of the possible triggering factors for the onset of T1DM (for review, please see [85]). Additionally, T-cell–mediated release of INF-γ and TNFα can up-regulate expression of pro-apoptotic proteins (Bim and PUMA) leading to β-cell death, along with promoting recruitment and clearance of damaged-cells by macrophages [77,86]. On the other hand, in normal individuals, activity of these autoimmune cells is normally controlled by Treg cells and it is the failure to control the action of effector T-cells that result in autoimmune disease. The mechanisms by which Treg cells prevent autoimmune attack is also not fully elucidated, but they are thought to prevent cytotoxic action of T-cells by use of contact inhibition and release of soluble signalling factors, such as IL-10 and TGFβ (transforming growth factorβ) [82]. It is also unclear whether the precise causes of inflammation in T1DM are a consequence of T-cell failure to respond to Treg, or whether defective or low Treg numbers are to blame for disease progression. Nonetheless, the interplay between these cell populations offers a potential therapeutic strategy for T1DM treatment [82].

Interestingly, an autoimmune element has also been reported in patients with T2DM, along with the accepted thesis of insulin-resistance [76,87]. Hyperglycaemia, dyslipidaemia and low-grade inflammation (consisting of circulating inflammatory cytokines or adipokines released by adipocyte expansion), are considered important factors in the progression of T2DM and are generally present in obese individuals who are at risk of T2DM development [77]. These conditions lead to β-cell stress through a variety of processes that mainly include uncontrolled generation of ROS/RNS and cytokine-dependent initiation of death signals. Both processes combine to reduce β-cell function and decrease β-cell mass by inducing apoptotic cell death, leading to further hyperglycaemic and dyslipidaemic complications, and causing amplification of ROS/RNS generation, cytokine release and cytokine-mediated recruitment of the immune system (i.e. inflammation). These inflammatory factors are all detrimental for β-cell survival. As mentioned previously, IL-1β is elevated in the hyperglycaemic state, is increased in T1DM and is also expressed by β-cells in T2DM [77-79,88]. Moreover, concomitant down-regulation of the receptor antagonist IL-1Ra was also observed in β-cells cultured in hyper-glycaemic conditions [76]. β-Cells are similar to immune cells and dysregulated expression of IL-1β in islets can cause auto-stimulation and subsequent release of IL-1β by other β-cells, via NFκB activation [76,88]. In addition, IL-1β can promote the local expression of other cytokines, for example IL-6 and IL-8. These cytokines aid in the recruitment of patrolling macrophages, which may subsequently become activated by high microenvironment levels of IL-1β and amplify IL-1β content in their own right [76]. In terms of islet inflammation, IL-1β expression and its effects on β-cell death appears to be a uniting factor, in both T1 and T2DM and is being considered a possible therapeutic target [77,89].

While inflammation is essential to maintain tissue homeostasis, it is also beneficial and allows repair of damaged organs. However, it is the presence of chronic, out of control and unchecked inflammatory factors that contribute to β-cell death and ensuing DM. Ultimately, increased local microenvironment cytokine production in islets is detrimental and understanding the mechanisms of cytokine release and regulation, and also suppression of β-cell function, will allow the development of new treatment regimens.

6. Inflammatory mediators and suppression of β-cell function

Since inflammation and β-cell death is common to both T1 and T2DM, it is reasonable to assume that shared inflammatory mediators may exist between the two conditions. It is these mediators that promote infiltration of immune cells, suppression of β-cell function, culminat-ing in reduced insulin exocytosis and increased β-cell apoptosis. These mediators can be loosely classified into four categories, cytokines, chemokines, ROS/RNS and other inflamma-tory products. However, it must be noted that the activity of these modulators can be heavily influenced by nutrient availability, such as in hyperglycaemia and dyslipidaemia conditions. Further to this, there is significant crossover between the molecules in these categories, and several can significantly impact on the others, indicating a complex role in both T1 and T2DM.

T1DM is an autoimmune disease and it comes as no surprise that cytokine expression is elevated in these patients [79]. Interestingly, it is becoming more evident that cytokines also play a critical role in T2DM progression, and increased levels have been reported in T2DM patients [76,87]. The most obvious source of cytokine production is from islet invading immune cells, although other researchers have illustrated that islet β-cells could also express cytokines [76,79]. Cytokine and adipokine release also occurs from adipose tissue since it expands rapidly in obese patients. Here, hypoxia also plays a key part in cytokine release due to an inflammatory response to lack of vasculature in rapidly growing adipose tissue [90,91]. Recent evidence has suggested that adipocyte invading macrophages are a significant supplier of TNFα to the circulation in obese T2DM patients, and this could be a contributing-factor that modulates inflammation in disease progression [92,93]. It is likely that all sources contribute in some way or another to elevate cytokine levels, and consequently compound inflammation in DM patients.

The main cytokines that are responsible for inflammation in T1 and T2DM, include IL-1β, TNFα, INF-γ, IL-6 and IL-8. Central to the inflammatory role of each is stimulation of stress-induced kinases, IKKβ (inhibitor of nuclear factor kappaB kinase subunit β) and/or c-JNK (c-Jun-N-terminal kinase) [90]. Activation of IKKβ leads to translocation and activation of the NFκB. This factor targets transcription of genes associated with inflammation, and can cause subsequent up-regulation and release of IL-1β, TNFα, IL-6 and IL-8 [94,95]. Therefore, the aforementioned cytokines can initiate an auto-stimulatory or feed-forward inflammatory effect through NFκB-signalling in β-cells, resulting in amplification of inflammation. IL-1β and TNFα initiate NFκB-signalling directly via association with their relative receptors (IL-1R and TNFR) [96] and can also activate the apoptotic JNK pathway indirectly by intracellular interaction of TNF receptor associated factor (TRAF) with the cytoplasmic portion of IL-1R or TNFR [97]. NFκB can play either a pro-survival or pro-death role given the correct circumstances [98]. Both NFκB and JNK are intrinsically connected, and NFκB can prevent JNK-mediated cell death, the regulatory interactions of which have been reviewed expertly elsewhere [99]. An important component of NFκB activation and function is the presence/absence of ROS/RNS. Therefore, ROS/RNS can influence NFκB-dependent cytokine expression and consequently immune response [98].

ROS/RNS can activate nuclear translocation of NFκB which promotes gene expression. However, ROS/RNS can also have an inhibitory effect when NFκB has already translocated to the nucleus [98]. The process by which ROS/RNS affects NFκB function is not entirely known but is believed to involve alteration of the NFκB catalytic site through interaction with cysteine residues, or by inhibiting specific kinase enzymes such as IκBα, that results in phosphorylation of NFκB [98]. Cellular ROS can be generated from Electron Transport Chain (ETC) respiratory complexes or from specific enzymes (e.g. NOX-mediated production for phagocytosis) [27,98]. Most notably, in hyperglycaemic/glucotoxic conditions (in T1 or T2DM), mitochondria are the major source of ROS/RNS primarily because of high oxidative phosphorylation and ATP production [100]. As a result of unavoidable oxidative chemistry and prolonged ETC activity, superoxide (O_2^-) anions can be formed and may "leak" from the mitochondria and elicit cellular damage [100]. Additionally, excess glucose can cause increased intracellular calcium, which may enhance mitochondrial O_2^- output, but also activate NOX-derived ROS via protein kinase C (PKC) [100]. High glucose can also induce NOX activity through NADPH production from the conversion of glucose-6-phosphate to pentose leading to increased O_2^- [100]. Superoxide is a precursor reactive species and can be converted to other forms of strong oxidants including H_2O_2, and free radicals such as hydroxyl radicals and also peroxynitrite following reaction with NO [27,100]. These reactive species can cause DNA, lipid and protein damage and can also activate/regulate NFκB, who in turn can promote cytokine release and increased NO/O_2^- production by activation of iNOS and NOX expression [100,101]. Thus, ROS/RNS can exacerbate the immunological response and lead to cell death in a cyclic fashion (Fig. 5).

Lipid- and adipose-derived factors are considered other inflammatory mediators. In T2DM patients, dyslipidaemia occurs along with hyperglycaemia and consequently vascular circulation and intracellular accumulation of lipids can have a profound effect on the inflammatory response. Excess fatty acids can induced ROS generation through increased TCA metabolite production, increased NADH/NAD+ ratio and elevated intracellular Ca^{2+} [100]. They can also increase O_2^- and NO production via activation of NOX and iNOS, respectively, all potentially activating the NFκB pathway [97,100,102]. Formation of ceramide from long chain fatty acids also contributes to precipitation of lipotoxicity in β-cells and results in ROS generation and apoptotic death [97,100]. Ceramide, synthesised by serine palmitoyltransferase from long chain fatty acids like palmitic acid [100], is capable of inhibiting the pro-survival PI3K pathway, activating caspase-9 [100]. Like other fatty acids, ceramide can associate with and activate TLR's, which may elicit an immune response [90].

Since adipose tissue expands in obese patients, increased adipose-derived factors have been detected in patient serum, including leptin, TNFα and IL-6. Leptin and adiponectin can play a role in the immune reaction in DM patients. Leptin, an appetite control endocrine factor, inhibits feeding by interaction with receptors in the hypothalamus and a subsequent stimulation of neurotransmitter release, for example norepinephrine [103]. It is considered a cytokine due to its homology in structure with IL-6, and its receptor-mediated effects [77,103,104]. It has been shown to induce β-cell death by up-regulating IL-1β, and has also been implicated in exacerbation of T1DM in animal models [77,105]. Conversely, adiponectin is considered an anti-inflammatory protein, and enhances IL-1Ra and IL-10 expression [90,106], leading to reduced IL-1β and enhanced suppression of T-cell mediated inflammation.

Chemokines can also be secreted from adipose tissue and are elevated in the adipose tissue of obese mice and humans [90,107]. CC-chemokine ligand-2 (CCL-2) functions to recruit monocytes to adipose tissue resulting in differentiation into activated macrophages [108]. Others such as CCL-3, CCL-6, CCL-7, CCL-8 and CCL-9, have also been reported to be elevated in high-fat fed mice, suggesting they may play a role in immune cell recruitment and inflammation [90].

Several mechanisms and modulators may contribute to the inflammatory response observed in T1 and T2DM. Cytokines, ROS and NFκB-signalling appear to be critical in mediating immune cell infiltration and further cytokine production. The balance between β-cell survival

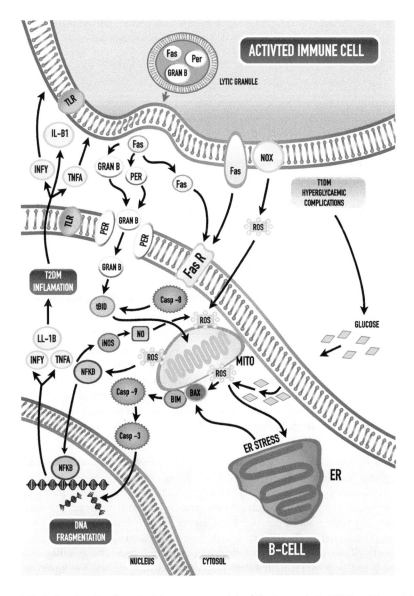

Figure 5. Illustration depicting the potential convergence points of the immunological NFκB and the metabolic ROS/ER stress pathways in pancreatic β-cells. Islet inflammation is characterised by the presence of leukocyte infiltrates that mediate the destruction of β-cells by release of cytokines, generation of ROS (NO, cytokine-NFκB-dependent]) and by activating the granzyme b- and death-receptor-mediated death pathways. Also shown is the effect of excess glucose on ROS production and ER stress that ultimately activates caspase enzymes via mitochondrial- and ER-mediated death pathways. ROS/RNS can also activate and regulate the NFκB stress pathway, which may lead to expression of cytokines that promotes immune cell infiltration exacerbating β-cell death.

and death is dependent on the interactions of these mediators, but also on the glycaemic and lipidaemic environment. We will now discuss the precise mechanisms of β-cell death in T1 and T2DM, and examine the commonalities between both.

7. Pancreatic β-cell failure and death in T1DM

Pancreatic β-cell failure can be defined as a reduction in insulin secretion or a failure to respond to plasma glucose (i.e. insulin-resistance). β-cell dysfunction in T1DM is characterised by an autoimmune-mediated destruction of β-cells leading to a decrease in pancreatic β-cell mass and reduced insulin secretion [109]. On the other hand, progression of T2DM is more variable and β-cell death occurs against the backdrop of insulin-resistance [109]. Here, the pathogenesis of T2DM usually involves a response to increased metabolic load by increased β-cell mass and enhanced insulin secretion [110]. A period of normoglycaemia ensues before a reduction in insulin secretion and β-cell function is observed. Finally, this phase is followed by a decrease in β-cell mass due to apoptotic cell death and is referred to as overt diabetes [110,111]. The shared feature associated with both T1 and T2DM is the failure of pancreatic β-cells resulting in reduced cell mass, dysfunction and ultimately apoptotic death. While there are commonalities associated with both types, the main mechanism of cell death associated with T1DM is immune-related.

At the time of diagnosis, T1DM patients present with a 70-80% reduction β-cell mass [109]. Insulitis and infiltration of leukocytes into islets is common in these patients. Several types of leukocytes are present including B-cells, macrophages and Natural Killer (NK) cells, but the principal invading cell type is the cytotoxic T-cell (CD4 and CD8) [81,82]. Immune cells promote β-cell death via several mechanisms, and these can be simplified to include phagocytosis, production of cytokines and T-cell-induced initiation of death-receptor-mediated apoptosis. The intracellular generation of ROS/RNS and activation of caspase enzymes occurs inside target cells and ultimately seals the fate of these cells.

Generation of autoreactive effector T-cells is extremely important in the pathogenesis of T1DM, but the precise biochemical mechanisms behind release of self-antigen and development of autoreactive T-cells remains unknown. However, work in this field has identified a potential role for decreased expression of peripheral tissue antigens (PTA) in pancreatic draining lymph nodes, which possibly allows unchallenged escape of differentiated autoreactive T-cells [82,83,112]. These T-cells kill pancreatic β-cells through expression of Fas ligand and expression of extracellular cytotoxic factors including cytokines, and lytic granules containing granzyme B and perforin [113]. In death-receptor-mediated apoptosis, Fas ligand or TNFα initiates death signals through association with FasR (Fas receptor) or TNFR (tumour necrosis factor receptor). An intracellular conformational change occurs that results in activation of caspase-8 [114,115]. This in turn serves to activate caspase-3 downstream promoting the apoptotic cascade [116].

T-cell-mediated release of granzyme B and perforin also leads to caspase activation in target cells. Here, perforin creates pores in the plasma membrane of the target cell, while granzyme

B is released into the cytosol and activates caspase-3 [113,117]. Interestingly, in order to yield activation of caspase-3, both caspase-8 from the death-receptor pathway outlined above, and granzyme B converge and initiate the mitochondrial-mediated death pathway via cleavage of BID [a member of the B-cell lymphoma-2 (Bcl-2) family of proteins], to truncated BID (tBID). In this process, cytosolic tBID translocates to the mitochondrial membrane and activates other Bcl-2-related proteins, such as BAX. Release of cytochrome c is then stimulated, which acts as the trigger for mitochondrial-mediated activation of caspase -9 and -3 [118,119,120]. Therefore, both the death-receptor and granzyme B-mediated death pathways activate the mitochondrial-mediated death pathway.

Conversely, macrophages induce β-cell death through production of ROS, cytokines and eventually phagocytosis. Macrophages express high levels of NOX, and use O_2^- to kill invading organisms or possibly damaged β-cells. Expression of high amounts of ROS/RNS or reduced antioxidant defences, results in mitochondrial dysfunction, which can culminate in mitochondrial-mediated apoptosis. Briefly, this involves major structural changes caused by ROS/RNS-mediated lipid/protein oxidation on both the inner and outer mitochondrial membranes, thus increasing the membrane permeability to proteins [121]. This is regulated by the interaction of pro- and anti-apoptotic Bcl-2 family proteins (Bcl-2, Bcl-X_L, BAX, BAK, BIM, BID and BAD) [122]. The release of cytochrome c to the cytosol and its association with apoptosis protease activation factor-1 (Apaf-1) and pro-caspase-9, forms a heptameric wheel-like caspase-activating complex, known as the apoptosome, which subsequently leads to activation of caspase-9 and effector caspase-3, further down-stream [123]. Caspase activation promotes cell death by degradation of DNA and cytoskeletal proteins [124].

In addition, immune cells release cytokines (e.g. TNFα, INF-γ and IL-1β) that also promote up-regulation of ROS/RNS via activation of NFκB (e.g. NO), who in turn can be regulated by ROS [100,101]. Induction of NO expression can cause activation of tumour suppressor protein (p53) leading to inhibition of cell cycle and death [109]. Cytokines can also inflict cell death via stimulation of the JNK pathway [97]. Here, IL-1β and TNFα activate mitochondrial translocation of JNK, who is a regulator of Bcl-2 proteins. JNK phosphorylates BIM, which results in the release of BAX-dependent cytochrome c and initiation of mitochondrial-mediated apoptosis [125,126]. Additionally, release of INF-γ by T-cells, can also phosphorylate BIM in β-cells, promoting cell death in a similar manner [77,86].

A variety of biochemical signalling pathways are available by which autoimmune cells utilise to initiate β-cell destruction. Consequently, due to a complete lack of insulin secretion and subsequent diminished glucose-uptake by muscle and adipose tissue, hyperglycaemia ensues in T1DM patients. High levels of blood glucose leads to further complications including, glucotoxicity, lipotoxicity and glucolipotoxicity and these are key players in exacerbation of the disease, and can lead to the clinical complications of T2DM [108]. Therefore, the precise way in which these factors affect β-cell turnover and survival will be discussed in the next section. Nonetheless, β-cell death in T1DM is based on classical immune-related death processes, but also relies on involvement of ROS and mitochondrial mediated which may occur in a sub-population of beta cells in T2DM.

8. Pancreatic β-cell failure and death in T2DM

Failure of pancreatic β-cells is essential in the progression of both T1 and T2DM. The development of T2DM is more gradual than T1, and appears to occur in specific stages. It is dependent on the establishment of insulin-resistance and displays increased degrees of variability in comparison with T1DM. Therefore, determination of the precise mechanisms of T2DM-related cell death remains difficult and, these are still not fully understood.

T2DM patients have a 30-50% reduction in β-cell mass on average post-mortem and the primary candidate pathways leading to β-cell apoptosis are oxidative stress, ER stress, amyloid accumulation, ectopic lipid deposition, lipotoxicity and glucotoxicity [127]. These stresses can all be caused by over-nutrition and neatly connects T2DM to obesity [90]. Glucose, the most important insulin secretatogue, is also the most important regulator of β-cell mass and function [128]. Impaired glucose-tolerance and hyperglycaemia are hallmarks of T2DM and prolonged glucose exposure can promote glucose-desensitisation, decreased insulin secretion and generation of oxidative stress in β-cells [128]. Consequently, glucotoxicity plays a significant part in pancreatic β-cell death in T2DM.

Understandably, excess glucose increases β-cell glucose metabolism and oxidative phosphorylation. Elevated ETC activity promotes increased superoxide (O_2^-) anion leakage from the mitochondria and may cause oxidative cellular damage [100]. Furthermore, high glucose levels induces NOX activity via NADPH production from metabolism of glucose to pentose, and through the TCA cycle, both leading to increased O_2^- output [100]. O_2^- can be converted to the less reactive H_2O_2 via superoxide dismutase, to the highly reactive hydroxyl anion by the iron-catalysed Fenton reaction, or to peroxynitrite ($ONOO^-$) via reaction with iNOS-derived NO [27,129]. β-cells are considered vulnerable to ROS/RNS generation because they express relatively low levels of antioxidant enzymes, like glutathione and catalase [27,128,129]. These enzymes immediately convert H_2O_2 to molecular oxygen and water. However, the detrimental combination of reduced activity of antioxidant enzymes, along with ROS/RNS generation can result in oxidative damage to DNA, lipids and proteins, thereby promoting mitochondrial-mediated apoptosis. In addition, ROS/RNS can also activate and regulate biochemical stress pathways, such as the NFκB, leading to further negative effects in β-cells [100,101].

Excess glucose can cause increased intracellular calcium, as outlined previously, which may enhance mitochondrial O_2^- production, but also deplete ER Ca^{2+}, promoting activation of the ER-stress-mediated death pathway [111,128] alongside unfolded protein response (UPR) (for review, please see [130]). In normal conditions, proteins are synthesised in the ER and are subsequently secreted or routed into a variety of sub-cellular compartments. However, accumulation of native or unfolded proteins within the lumen of the ER can activate caspase enzymes and ultimately promote cell death [131,132]. Reaction of ROS with the ER leads to protein accumulation via dysregulation of the ER oxidative folding pathway [111]. It also results in oxidative activation of Ca^{2+} release channels in the ER membrane, thereby depleting the ER of Ca^{2+} [111]. This ER stress activates pro-caspase-12, located on the cytoplasmic side of the ER, in a manner similar to caspase-9 [133,134]. Caspase-12 apoptosomes also causes translocation of JNK to the mitochondrial membrane inducing BIM phosphorylation, ultimately leading to cytochrome c release and initiation of mitochondrial-dependent apoptosis [111,135,136].

Lipid accumulation (lipotoxicity) in the ER may also play a significant function in mediating ER stress in β-cells. Obesity is a primary risk factor associated with T2DM, and is accompanied with increased plasma glucose and lipid levels due to high carbohydrate- and fat-based diets [137]. The process by which free fatty acids modulate ER stress is not entirely known [111] but, it has been shown that palmitic acid could deplete ER Ca^{2+} levels and augment ER morphology and integrity, which may cause activation of ER stress by the mechanisms mentioned above [137,138]. Furthermore, excess fatty acid esterification in the ER, may divert ER machinery and delay the processing and export of proteins in the ER [137]. Since there is a large demand for protein/insulin production in pancreatic islets, β-cells have a highly active and well developed ER. This suggests that β-cells may be more susceptible to ER stress during protein synthesis [109,137]. Given the effects of elevated plasma glucose and lipids in T2DM patients, ER stress could be a vital mechanism facilitating glucotoxicity-, lipotoxicity- or glucolipotoxicity-mediated β-cell failure and death [137].

Moreover, accumulation of islet amyloid polypeptide (IAPP) may also contribute to β-cell dysfunction and death in a manner similar to that described above [110,111,139]. IAPP precipitates into lethal oligomers inside the ER and like unfolded proteins, activates the ER stress-mediated death pathway [139]. IAPP deposits are present in over 90% of T2DM islets, post-mortem, indicating a substantial participation in T2DM progression [109,111].

In summary, several biochemical mechanisms have been suggested to be responsible for pancreatic β-cell failure and death in T2DM. However, there appears to be significant interplay between the purported pathways and conditions of glucotoxicity-, lipotoxicity- and glucolipotoxicity, which are common in the aetiology of T2DM and require further investigation. Interestingly, from this review there are noteworthy commonalities associated with T1 and T2DM mechanisms of β-cell failure and death. In the following section we will attempt to summarise these, with a view to identifying the potential therapeutic targets that are of interest to the research community.

9. Similarities between β-cell failure and death in T1DM and T2DM

T1DM is considered a chronic autoimmune disease and the major mechanisms responsible β-cell death and dysfunction are immune-related. In contrast, the main mechanisms responsible β-cell death and dysfunction in T2DM are related to metabolism. Thus, the convergence points of these two aetiologically-different disorders appear to be the immunological NFκB pathway and, the metabolic ROS/ER stress pathways (Fig. 5).

Islet inflammation in T1DM is characterised by the presence of leukocyte infiltrates [81]. In particular, macrophages and T-cells mediate the destruction of β-cells by phagocytosis, release of cytokines, generating ROS (NO, cytokine-NFκB-dependent [82]) and by activating the granzyme b- and death-receptor-mediated death pathways (Fig. 5). At the biochemical level, production of cytokines such as INF-γ, TNFα and IL-1β act in synergy to promote expression of iNOS and consequently NO, via stimulation of NFκB in mouse islet β-cells [82]. If not regulated, this generation of ROS may impact on ER stress and possibly promote cell death, which has been shown to be an import cell death process in T2DM (Fig. 5). Furthermore, cytokine–mediated activation of β-cell NFκB may result in an autocrine production of similar cytokines by β-cells, amplifying these death signals [76,79]. Another complication that arises with T1DM and immune-mediated reduction of β-cell mass is impaired insulin secretion, which may possibly promote additional hyperglycaemia and dyslipidaemia in these patients. Therefore, and as explained earlier, glucolipotoxicity may follow, along with further cell death that is achieved through mitochondrial- and/or ER-mediated death processes (Fig. 5).

In T2DM, hyperglycaemia and dyslipidaemia are critical factors and are generally present in obese individuals with the disease [77]. Consequently, excess glucose and circulating free fatty acids may promote increased ROS production and ER stress by enhancing oxidative phosphorylation and causing a build-up of unfolded proteins in the ER. Elevated ROS and ER stress will activate caspase enzymes via mitochondrial- and ER-mediated death pathways, respectively (Fig. 5). Interestingly, ROS/RNS can also activate and regulate the NFκB stress pathway, which may possibly lead to transcription of genes coding either cytokines or immune cell chemo-attractants (Fig. 5) [98]. Given the spontaneous reactivity of ROS, it is not clear yet exactly how it influences NFκB activation. However, it has been shown to react in a variety of ways promoting stimulation or inhibition of NFκB, with effects dependent on context [98]. For example, if ROS does promote expression of NFκB-derived cytokines or immune cell chemo-attractants, these signals may alert nearby macrophages and T-cells to the elevated level of β-cell ROS, and initiate the removal of these damaged cells. Consequently, this could result in immune cell infiltration into pancreatic islets of T2DM patients and possibly β-cell death (Fig. 5).

Interestingly, an autoimmune element has been reported in obese patients with T2DM, who have presented with elevated circulatory cytokine and acute-phase protein levels [77,87]. A common denominator that may link both T1 and T2DM is IL-1β. Autocrine production of IL-1β by β-cells has been observed in T1DM and in T2DM patients [76,79]. Furthermore, *in vitro* culture of islets from non-diabetic doners in high glucose, caused increased production and secretion of IL-1β, along with subsequent NFκB activation, Fas up-regulation, reduced insulin secretion and β-cell DNA fragmentation [77,78]. Chronic exposure to IL-1β also increases expression of iNOS, and consequently may up-regulate ROS generation and the expression of other pro-inflammatory cytokines like IL-6 and IL-8, which may further potentiate β-cell failure [78]. These reports clearly demonstrate the inherent link between glucotoxicity and the inflammatory processes [77]. In addition, investigators took a step further and showed that exogenous addition of IL-1Ra, the IL-1 receptor antagonist (Anakinra), protected the islets from IL-1β, but also reduced glycated haemoglobin in a small clinical trial of T2DM patients [77,140]. Clinical trials utilising IL-1Ra, still continue [90].

In conclusion, T1 and T2DM are different diseases, but do appear to share some common biochemical ground in terms of disease development. Although T1DM is mostly an autoimmune-related syndrome, elements of metabolic dysregulation are evident. Likewise, even though T2DM is very much a metabolic disease, there are also immunological-related factors that may exacerbate disease progression. NFκB, IL-1β, ER-stress and generation of ROS/RNS are instrumental players in both diseases, and may warrant further investigation with regard to development of novel therapies.

10. β-cell therapies and possible targets for prevention of β-cell failure

The traditionalistic concept of separate T1 and T2DM syndromes has become clouded with knowledge of the involvement of inflammation in T2DM and the metabolic syndrome in T1DM [108]. It is now apparent that treatment modalities that were specifically designed for one form of diabetes may have application in the other. Exercise, weight loss and diet are the most effective strategies to delay T2DM disease development, but similar strategies have shown significant efficacy in T1DM [108,128].

Researchers have targeted TNFα in children with newly diagnosed T1DM and showed that a recombinant TNFR fusion protein preserved c-peptide function, along with enhancing insulin production [82,141]. However, to date, anti-TNFα treatment has failed to improve blood glucose in T2DM patients [90]. Infiltration of cytotoxic T-cells in T1DM has been well characterised [82]. Therefore, some developing treatment strategies for this precise component of T1DM disease is the generation of T-cell targeted therapy to prevent the destruction of transplanted islets, some of which include introduction of anti-inflammatory Tregs that regulate T-cell activation [89]. Since inflammation has been detected in T2DM, these approaches may have similar applications. Directing treatment towards the immunological pathways is quite attractive and recent evidence has suggested that the most promising results involve blockade of IL-1β or NFκB activation [90]. Again, it is noteworthy to highlight that enhanced HSP70 expression has been convincingly demonstrated to protect against obesity-induced insulin-resistance [142], while low HSP70 contents in skeletal muscle of T2DM patients are associated with insulin-resistance [143,144]. Hence, pharmacological (e.g. the hydroxylamine derivative BGP-15, now under clinical trial) as well as physiological (hyperthermic, hot tube) treatments have started to be cogitated as promising therapeutic approaches in T2DM [142,145]. Moreover, physical exercise, which is a powerful antidiabetic intervention, is one of the strongest ways to increase intracellular HSP70 expression in many tissues (for reviews, please see [75,146]), including in pancreatic β-cells (A. Bittencourt et al., manuscript in preparation).

Elevated IL-1β and reduced IL-1Ra is known to correlate with T1DM, but the recent identification of inflammation in T2DM has meant that the IL-1 receptor antagonist (Anakinra), has been trialed in both T2DM and T1DM patients with successful results [77,140,147]. Here, the agent lowered blood glucose, reduced inflammation, improved insulin-sensitivity and secretion. These reports again illustrate the pivotal role played by IL-1β in mediating DM development, and thus clinical trials continue [90].

Salicylate-derivatives, such as salsalate, are also being used in an anti-inflammatory capacity to inhibit the activation of NFκB, although the precise mechanisms of action are not fully understood. These agents have the clear advantages of being orally available and well tolerated. Salsalate has been shown to improve insulin sensitivity and production, increase secretion of the anti-inflammatory cytokine adiponectin, reduce blood glucose and C-reactive protein (CRP) and decrease fatty acid and triglyceride levels [90].

From our own studies we have shown how different amino and fatty acid combinations may affect β-cell metabolism. This proposes the concept of diet manipulation as an additional treatment for hyperglycaemia and lipidaemia in T2 and even T1DM patients. We demonstrated the antioxidant activities of arachidonic acid, arginine and glutamine, and this data may suggests that dietary supplementation, high in specific amino or fatty acids, may have favourable effects in DM patients. Given the role of ROS and ER stress in β-cell death, dietary or pharmacological agents that target these pathways may also represent novel treatments for the delay or prevention of DM.

11. Conclusions and perspectives

Over-nutrition and diminished physical activity in the modern lifestyle has led to a staggering increase in T2DM onset in Western cultures [108]. However, the epidemic is also progressing into the developing world, indicating that T2DM has become a major global health issue [108]. Since the 1990's, T1DM has more than doubled in number and is expected to double again before 2020 [108,148]. The traditional classification of distinct criteria for T1 and T2DM syndromes has become blurred due to the global increase in obese individuals and the incidence of obesity-related insulin-resistance [108]. Currently the paradigm of T1 and T2DM treatment appears to be changing in line with the clarification of dysfunctional pathways that are common to both disease types. Although diet-and-exercise still remains the most effective (and cheapest) treatment, new therapies will be required going into the future. Consequently, an increased understanding of the molecular and biochemical mechanisms that lead to disease onset and progression are mandatory.

In this manuscript, we have examined some of the key pathways that are essential in the pathogenesis of both T1 and T2DM, and we have reviewed some of the novel treatments that are currently being developed to counteract these dysfunctional processes. It is clear that inflammation, generation of ROS/RNS and ER stress leads to significant damage to pancreatic β-cells, culminating in cell dysfunction, and ultimately cell death. It is hoped that further study of the NFκB and the ER stress-mediated pathways, will reveal novel therapeutic targets that can be developed into a new generation of anti-diabetic treatments, that will improve β-cell function, survival and regeneration in T1 and T2DM.

Acknowledgements

The authors would like to thank Mr. Peter McEvoy for assistance with design and illustration of Figure 5.

Abbreviations

ACC - Acetyl coA carboxylase

ACL - ATP-citrate lyase

AMPK - AMP-activated kinase

Apaf-1 - Apoptosis protease activation factor-1

Bcl-2 - B-cell lymphoma-2

Cp-PGs - Cyclopentenone prostaglandins

CPT-1 - Carnitine palmitoyl transferase 1

DHAP - Dihydroxyacetone phosphate

ER - Endoplasmic reticulum

ETC - Electron transport chain

FasR - Fas receptor

GABA - γ-aminobutyric acid

G-CSP - Granulocyte colony-stimulating factor

GDH - Glutamate dehydrogenase

GFAT-1 - Glutamine:fructose-6-phosphate amidotransferase-1

GSIS - Glucose-stimulated insulin secretion

GSK3β - Glycogen synthase kinase-3β

HBP - Hexosamine biochemical pathway

HSF-1 - Heat shock factor-1

HSP70 - Heat shock protein-70

iNOS - Inducible nitric oxide synthase

JNK - c-Jun-N-terminal kinase

LDH - Lactate dehydrogenase

MCFs - Metabolic coupling factors

ME1 - Malic enzyme1

MIP-1 - Macrophage inflammatory protein-1

NFAT - Nuclear factor of activated T cells

NFκB - Nuclear factor κB

NOD - Non-obese diabetic

NOX - NADPH oxidase

PC - Pyruvate carboxylase

PDH - Pyruvate dehydrogenase

PP2A - Protein phosphatase type 2A

PTA - Peripheral tissue antigens

RNS - Reactive nitrogen species

ROS - Reactive oxygen species

SNARE -Soluble NH2-ethylmaleimide-sensitive fusion protein attachment protein receptor

SNOG - S-nitrosoglutathione

T1DM - Type 1 diabetes mellitus

T2DM - Type 2 diabetes mellitus

TCA - Tricarboxylic acid

TGFβ – Transforming growth factorβ

TLR - Toll-like receptors

TNFR - TNFα receptor

TRAF - TNF receptor associated factor

Tregs - Regulatory T-cells

VAMP - Vesicle-associated membrane protein

Author details

Philip Newsholme[1], Kevin Keane[1], Paulo I Homem de Bittencourt Jr.[2,3] and
Mauricio Krause[4,5]

1 School of Biomedical Sciences, Curtin University, Western Australia

2 Department of Physiology, Institute of Basic Health Sciences, Federal University of Rio
Grande do Sul, Porto Alegre, Brazil

3 National Institute of Hormones and Women's Health, Brazil

4 Institute of Technology Tallaght and Institute for Sport and Health UCD Dublin, Ireland

5 School of Public Health and Physiotherapy, UCD Dublin, Ireland

References

[1] Chan, S. J, & Steiner, D. F. Insulin Through the Ages: Phylogeny of a growth promoting and metabolic regulatory hormone. American Zoologist (2000). , 40, 213-22.

[2] Irwin, D. M, Humer, O, & Youson, J. H. Lamprey Proglucagon and the origin of glucagon-like peptides. Molecular Biology and Evolution (1999). , 16(11), 1548-57.

[3] Newsholme, P, Abdulkader, F, Rebelato, E, Romanatto, T, Pinheiro, C. H, Vitzel, K.
F, Silva, E. P, Bazotte, R. B, Procopio, J, Curi, R, Gorjao, R, & Pithon-curi, T. C. Amino
acids and diabetes: implications for endocrine, metabolic and immune functions.
Frontiers in Bioscience (2011). , 16, 315-39.

[4] Jitrapakdee, S, Wutthisathapornchai, A, Wallace, J. C, & MacDonald, M.J. Regulation
of insulin secretion: role of mitochondrial signalling. Diabetologia (2010). , 53(6),
1019-32.

[5] Rutter, G. A, & Hill, E. V. Insulin vesicle release: walk, kiss, pause…then run. Physiology (Bethesda, Md.) (2006). , 21, 189-96.

[6] Gembal, M, Gilon, P, & Henquin, J. C. Evidence that glucose can control insulin release independently from its action on ATP-sensitive K+ channels in mouse B cells.
Journal of Clinical Investigations (1992). , 89(4), 1288-95.

[7] Remedi, M. S, Rocheleau, J. V, Tong, A, Patton, B. L, Mcdaniel, M. L, Piston, D. W,
Koster, J. C, & Nichols, C. G. Hyperinsulinism in mice with heterozygous loss of
K(ATP) channels. Diabetologia (2006). , 49(10), 2368-78.

[8] Miki, T, Nagashima, K, Tashiro, F, Kotake, K, Yoshitomi, H, Tammamoto, A, Gonoi,
T, Iwanaga, T, Miyazaki, J. I, & Seino, S. Defective insulin secretion and enhanced insulin action in KATP channel-deficient mice. Proceedings of the National Academy
of Sciences (1998). , 95, 10402-06.

[9] Straub, S. G, & Sharp, G. W. G. Glucose-stimulated signalling pathways in biphasic
insulin secretion. Diabetes and Metabolism Research and Reviews (2002). , 18(6),
451-63.

[10] Newsholme, P, & Krause, M. Nutritional Regulation of Insulin Secretion: Implications for Diabetes. The Clinical Biochemist Reviews (2012). , 33(2), 35-47.

[11] Newsholme, P, Bender, K, Kiely, A, & Brennan, L. Amino acid metabolism, insulin
secretion and diabetes. The Biochemical Society Transactions (2007). Pt 5): 1180-6.

[12] Opara, E. C, Garfinkel, M, Hubbard, V. S, Burch, W. M, & Akwari, O. E. Effect of fatty acids on insulin release; role of chain length and degree of unsaturation. The
American Journal of Physiology (1994). Pt 1): E, 635-9.

[13] Keane, D. C, Takahashi, H. K, Dhayal, S, Morgan, N. G, Curi, R, & Newsholme, P.
Arachidonic acid actions on functional integrity and attenuation of the negative ef-

fects of palmitic acid in a clonal pancreatic β-cell line. Clinical Science (London) (2011). , 120(5), 195-206.

[14] Hosokawa, H, Corkey, B. E, & Leahy, J. L. Beta-cell hypersensitivity to glucose following 24-h exposure of rat islets to fatty acids. Diabetologia (1997). , 40(4), 392-7.

[15] Vassiliou, E. K, Gonzalez, A, Garcia, C, Tadros, J. H, Chakraborty, G, & Toney, J. H. Oleic acid and peanut oil high in oleic acid reverse the inhibitory effect of insulin production of the inflammatory cytokine TNF-α both *in vitro* and *in vivo* systems. Lipids in Health and Disease (2009).

[16] Keane, D, & Newsholme, P. Saturate and unsaturated (including arachidonic acid) non-esterified fatty acid modulation of insulin secretion from pancreatic β-cells. The Biochemical Society Transactions (2008). Pt 5): 955-8.

[17] Jensen, M. V, Joseph, J. W, Ronnebaum, S. M, Burgess, S. C, Sherry, A. D, & Newgard, C. B. Metabolic cycling in control of glucose-stimulated insulin secretion. The American Journal of Physiology Endocrinology and Metabolism (2008). E, 1287-97.

[18] Newsholme, P, Keane, D, Welters, H. J, & Morgan, N. G. Life and death decisions of the pancreatic beta-cell: the role of fatty acids. Clinical Science (London) (2007). , 112(1), 27-42.

[19] Mcclenaghan, N. H, Scullion, S. M, Mion, B, Hewage, C, Malthouse, J. P, Flatt, P. R, Newsholme, P, & Brennan, L. Prolonged L-alanine exposure induces changes in metabolism, Ca2+ handling and desensitisation of insulin secretion clonal pancreatic beta-cells. Clinical Science (London) (2009). , 116(4), 341-51.

[20] Bender, K, Maechler, P, Mcclenaghan, N. H, Flatt, P. R, & Newsholme, P. Overexpression of malate-aspartate NADH shuttle member Aralar1 in the clonal beta-cell line BRIN-BD11 enhances amino-acid-stimulated insulin secretion and cell metabolism. Clinical Science (London) (2009). , 117(9), 321-30.

[21] Newsholme, P, Brennan, L, & Bender, K. Amino acid metabolism, β-cell function and diabetes. Diabetes (2006). S, 39-47.

[22] Maassen, J. A, Hart, t, Janssen, L. M, Reiling, G. M, Romijn, EJ. A, & Lemkes, . Mitochondrial diabetes and its lesson for common type 2 diabetes. The Biochemical Society Transactions (2006). Pt 5): 819-23.

[23] Sener, A, Best, L. C, Yates, A. P, Kadiata, M. M, Oliveares, E, Louchami, K, Jijakli, H, Ladriere, L, & Malaisse, W. J. Stimulus-secretion coupling of arginine-induced insulin-release: comparison between the cationic amino acid and its methyl ester. Endocrine (2000). , 13(3), 329-40.

[24] Mcclenaghan, N. H, Barnett, C. R, & Flatt, P. R. Na+ cotransport by metabolizable and nonmetabolizable amino acids stimulates a glucose-regulated insulin-secretory response. Biochemical and Biophysical Research Communications (1998). , 249(2), 299-303.

[25] Broca, C, Brennan, L, Petit, P, Newsholme, P, & Maechler, P. Mitochondria-derived glutamate at the interplay between branched-chain amino acid and glucose-induced insulin secretion. FEBS Letters (2003).

[26] Krause, M, Rodrigues-krause, J, Hagan, O, De Vito, C, Boreham, G, Susta, C, Newsholme, D, & Murphy, P. C. Differential nitric oxide levels in the blood and skeletal muscle of type 2 diabetic subjects may be a consequence of adiposity: a preliminary study. Metabolism: Clinical and Experimental (2012). , 61(11), 1528-37.

[27] Newsholme, P, Rebelato, E, Abdulkader, F, Krause, M, Carpinelli, A, & Curi, R. Reactive oxygen and nitrogen species generation, antioxidant defences and β-cell function: a critical role for amino acids. The Journal of Endocrinology (2012). , 214(1), 11-20.

[28] Pryor, W. A, & Squadrito, G. L. The chemistry of peroxynitrite: a product from the reaction of nitric oxide with superoxide. American Journal of Physiology (1995). Pt 1): L, 699-722.

[29] Beckman, J. S, Beckman, T. W, Chen, J, Marshall, P. A, & Freeman, B. A. Apparent hydroxyl radical production by peroxynitrite: implications for endothelial injury from nitric oxide and superoxide. Proceedings of the National Academy of Sciences (1990). , 87(4), 1620-24.

[30] Crow, J. P, & Beckman, J. S. The role of peroxynitrite in nitric oxide-mediated toxicity. Current Topics in Microbiology and Immunology (1995). , 196(1), 57-73.

[31] Delaney, C. A, Tyrberg, B, Bouwens, L, Vaghef, H, Hellman, B, & Eizirik, D. L. Sensitivity of human pancreatic islets to peroxynitrite-induced cell dysfunction and death. FEBS Letters (1996). , 394(3), 300-6.

[32] Rabinovitch, A, & Suarez-pinzon, W. L. Role of cytokines in the pathogenesis of autoimmune diabetes mellitus. Reviews in Endocrine and Metabolic Disorders (2003). , 4(3), 291-9.

[33] Sancez-margalet, V, Valle, M, Ruz, F. J, Gascon, F, Mateo, J, & Goberna, R. Elevated plasma total homocysteine levels in hyperinsulinaemic obese subjects. The Journal of Nutritional Biochemistry (2002). , 13(2), 75-79.

[34] Patterson, S, Flatt, P. R, & Mcclenaghan, N. H. Homocysteine and other structurally-diverse amino thiols can alter pancreatic beta cell function without evoking cellular damage. (2006). Biochemica et Biophysica Acta 2006; , 1760(7), 1109-14.

[35] Medina, M, Urdiales, J. L, & Amores-sanchez, M. I. Roles of homocysteine in cell metabolism: old and new functions. The European Journal of Biochemistry (2001). , 268(14), 3871-82.

[36] Patterson, S, Flatt, P. R, & Mcclenaghan, N. H. Homocysteine-induced impairment of insulin secretion from clonal pancreatic BRIN-BD11 beta-cells is not prevented by catalase. Pancreas (2007). , 34(1), 144-51.

[37] Baylis, C. Nitric oxide deficiency in chronic kidney disease. The American Journal of Physiology: Renal Physiology (2008). F, 1-9.

[38] Ammon, H. P, Hehl, G, Enz, G, Setaidi-ranti, A, & Verspohl, J. Cysteine analogues potentiate glucose-induced insulin release in vitro. Diabetes (1986). , 35(12), 1390-6.

[39] Rasilainen, S, Nieminen, J. M, Levonen, A. L, Otonkoski, T, & Lapatto, R. Dose-dependent cysteine-mediated protection of insulin-producing cells from damage by hydrogen peroxide. Biochemical Pharmacology (2002). , 63(7), 1297-304.

[40] Kaneko, Y, Kimura, T, Taniquchi, S, Souma, M, Kojima, Y, Kimura, Y, Kimura, H, & Niki, I. Glucose-induced production of hydrogen sulphide may protect the pancreatic beta-cells from apoptotic cell death by high glucose. FEBS Letters (2009). , 538(2), 377-82.

[41] Kaneko, Y, Kimura, T, & Kimura, H. and Niki I. L-cysteine inhibits insulin release from pancreatic beta-cells: possible involvement of metabolic production of hydrogen sulphide, a novel gasotransmitter. Diabetes (2006). , 55(5), 1391-7.

[42] Sener, A, & Malaisse, W. J. L-l. e. u. c. i. n. e. and a nonmetabolized analogue activate pancreatic islet glutamate dehydrogenase. Nature (1980). , 288(5787), 187-9.

[43] Brennan, L, Corless, M, Hewage, C, Malthouse, J. P, Mcclenaghan, N. H, Flatt, P. R, & Newsholme, P. C NMR analysis reveals a link between L-glutamine metabolism, D-glucose metabolism and gamma-glutamyl cycle activity in a clonal pancreatic beta-cell line. Diabetologia (2007). , 46(11), 1512-21.

[44] Corless, M, Kiely, A, Mcclenaghan, N. H, Flatt, P. R, & Newsholme, P. Glutamine regulates expression of key transcription factor, signal transduction, metabolic gene, and protein expression in a clonal pancreatic beta-cell line. The Journal of Endocrinology (2006). , 190(3), 719-27.

[45] Brennan, L, Shine, A, Hewage, C, Malthouse, J. P, Brindle, K. M, Mcclenaghan, N. H, Flatt, P. R, & Newsholme, P. A nuclear magnetic resonance-based demonstration of substantial oxidative L-alanine metabolism and L-alanine-enhanced glucose metabolism in a clonal pancreatic beta-cell line: metabolism of L-alanine is important to the regulation of insulin secretion. Diabetes (2002). , 51(6), 1714-21.

[46] MacDonald MJ. and Fahien L.A. Glutamate is not a messenger in insulin secretion. The Journal of Biological Chemistry (2000). , 275(44), 34025-7.

[47] Gammelsaeter, R, Coppola, T, Marcaggi, P, Storm-mathisen, J, Chaudry, F. A, Attwell, D, Regazzi, R, & Gundersen, V. A role for glutamate transporters in the regulation of insulin secretion. PLoS One (2011). e22960.

[48] Huang, M, & Joseph, J. W. Metabolomic analysis of pancreatic β-cell insulin release in response to glucose. Islets (2012). , 4(3), 210-22.

[49] Hamaoka, R, Fujii, J, Miyagawa, J, Takahashi, M, Kishimoto, M, Moriwaki, M, Yamamoto, K, Kajimoto, Y, Yamasaki, Y, Hanafusa, T, Matsuzawa, Y, & Taniguchi, N.

Overexpression of the aldose reductase gene induces apoptosis in pancreatic beta-cells by causing a redox imbalance. The Journal of Biochemistry. (1999). , 126(1), 41-7.

[50] Gabbay, K. H, & Tze, W. J. Inhibition of glucose-induced release of insulin by aldose reductase inhibitors. Proceedings of the National Academy of Sciences (1972). , 69(6), 1435-9.

[51] Ladrière, L, Louchami, K, Laghmich, A, Malaisse-lagae, F, & Malaisse, W. J. Labeling of pancreatic glycogen by D-[U-14c]glucose in hyperglycemic rats. Endocrine (2001). , 14(3), 383-97.

[52] Doherty, M, & Malaisse, W. J. Glycogen accumulation in rat pancreatic islets: in vitro experiments. Endocrine (2001). , 14(3), 303-9.

[53] He, B, Meng, Y. H, & Mivechi, N. F. Glycogen synthase kinase 3beta and extracellular signal-regulated kinase inactivate heat shock transcription factor 1 by facilitating the disappearance of transcriptionally active granules after heat shock. Molecular and Cellular Biology (1998). , 18(11), 6624-33.

[54] Kazemi, Z, Chang, H, Haserodt, S, & Mcken, C. and Zachara NE. O-linked beta-N-acetylglucosamine (O-GlcNAc) regulates stress-induced heat shock protein expression in a GSK-3beta-dependent manner. The Journal of Biological Chemistry (2010). , 285(50), 39096-107.

[55] Srinivasan, V, Tatu, U, Mohan, V, & Balasubramanyam, M. Molecular convergence of hexosamine biosynthetic pathway and ER stress leading to insulin-resistance in L6 skeletal muscle cells. Molecular and Cellular Biochemistry (2009).

[56] Hasan, N. M, Longacre, M. J, Stoker, S. W, Boonsaen, T, Jitrapakdee, S, Kendrick, M. A, & Wallace, J. C. and MacDonald M.J. Impaired anaplerosis and insulin secretion in insulinoma cells caused by small interfering RNA-mediated suppression of pyruvate carboxylase. The Journal of Biological Chemistry (2008). , 283(42), 28048-59.

[57] Xu, J, Han, J, Long, Y. S, Epstein, P. N, & Liu, Y. Q. The role of pyruvate carboxylase in insulin secretion and proliferation in rat pancreatic beta-cells. Diabetologia (2008). , 51(11), 2022-30.

[58] Gaussin, V, Hue, L, Stalmans, W, & Bollen, M. Activation of hepatic acetyl-CoA carboxylase by glutamate and Mg^{2+} is mediated by protein phosphatase-2A. The Biochemical Journal (1996). Pt 1): 217-24.

[59] Xiang, X, Saha, A. K, Wen, R, Ruderman, N. B, & Luo, Z. AMP-activated protein kinase activators can inhibit the growth of prostate cancer cells by multiple mechanisms. Biochemical and Biophysical Research Communications (2004). , 321(1), 161-7.

[60] Shapiro, H, Shachar, S, Sekler, I, Hershfinkel, M, & Walker, M. D. Role of GPR40 in fatty acid action on the beta-cell line INS-1E. Biochemical and Biophysical Research Communications (2005). , 335(1), 97-104.

[61] Tomita, T, Masuzaki, H, Iwakura, H, Fujikura, J, Noguchi, M, Tanaka, T, Ebihara, K, Kawamura, J, Komoto, I, Kawaquchi, Y, Fujimoto, K, Doi, R, Shimada, Y, Hosoda, K, Imamura, M, & Nakao, K. Expression of the gene for a membrane-bound fatty acid receptor in the pancreas and islet cell tumours in humans: evidence for GPR40 expression in pancreatic beta-cells and implications for insulin secretion. Diabetologia (2006). , 49(5), 962-8.

[62] Krause, M. S, Mcclenaghan, N. H, & Flatt, P. R. Homem de Bittencourt P.I., Murphy C. and Newsholme P. L-arginine is essential for pancreatic b-cell functional integrity, metabolism and defence from inflammatory challenge. The Journal of Endocrinology (2011). , 211(1), 87-97.

[63] Eguchi, S, Oshiro, N, Miyamoto, T, Yoshino, K, Okamoto, S, Ono, T, Kikkawa, U, & Yonezawa, K. AMP-activated protein kinase phosphorylates glutamine : fructose-6-phosphate amidotransferase 1 at Ser243 to modulate its enzymatic activity. Genes to Cells (2009). , 14(2), 179-89.

[64] Luo, B, Parker, G. J, Cooksey, R. C, Soesanto, Y, Evans, M, Jones, D, & Mcclain, D. A. Chronic hexosamine flux stimulates fatty acid oxidation by activating AMP-activated protein kinase in adipocytes. The Journal of Biological Chemistry (2007). , 282(10), 7172-80.

[65] Ran, R, Lu, A, Zhang, L, Tang, Y, Zhu, H, Xu, H, Feng, Y, Han, C, Zhou, G, Rigby, A. C, & Sharp, F. R. Hsp70 promotes TNF-mediated apoptosis by binding IKK gamma and impairing NF-kappa B survival signaling. Genes and Development (2004). , 18(12), 1466-81.

[66] Jaattela, M. Overexpression of major heat shock protein hsp70 inhibits tumor necrosis factor-induced activation of phospholipase A2. The Journal of Immunology (1993). , 151(8), 4286-94.

[67] Feinstein, D. L, Galea, E, Aquino, D. A, Li, G. C, Xu, H, & Reis, D. J. Heat shock protein 70 suppresses astroglial-inducible nitric-oxide synthase expression by decreasing NFkappaB activation. The Journal of Biological Chemistry (1996). , 271(30), 17724-32.

[68] Kim, Y. M, De Vera, M. E, Watkins, S. C, & Billiar, T. R. Nitric oxide protects cultured rat hepatocytes from tumor necrosis factor-alpha-induced apoptosis by inducing heat shock protein 70 expression. The Journal of Biological Chemistry (1997). , 272(2), 1402-11.

[69] Chan, J. Y, Ou, C. C, Wang, L. L, & Chan, S. H. Heat shock protein 70 confers cardiovascular protection during endotoxemia via inhibition of nuclear factor-kappaB activation and inducible nitric oxide synthase expression in the rostral ventrolateral medulla. Circulation (2004). , 110(23), 3560-66.

[70] Chen, H. W, Kuo, H. T, Wang, S. J, Lu, T. S, & Yang, R. C. In vivo heat shock protein assembles with septic liver NF-kappaB/I-kappaB complex regulating NF-kappaB activity. Shock (2005). , 24(3), 232-8.

[71] Rossi, A, Kapahi, P, Natoli, G, Takahashi, T, Chen, Y, Karin, M, & Santoro, M. G. An-
      ti-inflammatory cyclopentenone prostaglandins are direct inhibitors of IkappaB kin-
      ase. Nature (2000). , 403(6765), 103-18.

[72] Homem de Bittencourt P.I. Jr. and Curi R. Antiproliferative prostaglandins and the
      MRP/GS-X pump role in cancer immunosuppression and insight into new strategies
      in cancer gene therapy. Biochemical Pharmacology (2001). , 62(7), 811-19.

[73] Gutierrez, L. L, Maslinkiewicz, A, & Curi, R. and Homem de Bittencourt P.I. Jr. Athe-
      rosclerosis: a redox-sensitive lipid imbalance suppressible by cyclopentenone prosta-
      glandins. Biochemical Pharmacology (2008). , 75(12), 2245-62.

[74] Beere, H. M. The stress of dying": the role of heat shock proteins in the regulation of
      apoptosis. The Journal of Cell Science (2004). Pt 13): 2641-51.

[75] Heck, T. G, & Schöler, C. M. and Homem de Bittencourt P.I. HSP70 expression: does
      it a novel fatigue signalling factor from immune system to the brain? Cell Biochemis-
      try and Function (2011). , 29(3), 215-26.

[76] Ehses, J. A, Boni-schnetzler, M, Faulenbach, M, & Donath, M. Y. Macrophages, cyto-
      kines and b-cell death in type 2 diabetes. The Biochemical Society Transactions
      (2008). Pt 3): 340-2.

[77] Donath, M. Y, Schumann, D. M, Faulenbach, M, Ellingsgaard, H, Perren, A, & Ehses,
      J. A. Islet inflammation in type 2 diabetes. Diabetes Care (2008). Suppl 2): S, 161-4.

[78] Wang, C, Guan, Y, & Yang, J. Cytokines in the progression of pancreatic β-cell dys-
      function. The International Journal of Endocrinology (2010). , 1, 1-10.

[79] Mandrup-poulsen, T. The role of interleukin-1 in the pathogenesis of IDDM. Diabeto-
      logia (1996). , 39(9), 1005-29.

[80] Kiely, A, Robinson, A, Mcclenaghan, N. H, Flatt, P. R, & Newsholme, P. Toll-like re-
      ceptor agonist induced changes in clonal rat BRIN-BD11 β-cell insulin secretion and
      signal transduction. The Journal of Endocrinology (2009). , 202(3), 365-73.

[81] Coppieters, K. T, Dotta, F, Amirian, N, Campbell, P. D, Kay, T. W, Atkinson, M. A,
      Roep, B. O, & Von Herrath, M. G. Demonstration of islet-autoreactive CD8 T cells in
      insulitic lesions from recent onset and long-term type 1 diabetes patients. The Journal
      of Experimental Medicine (2012). , 209(1), 51-60.

[82] Bending, D, Zaccone, P, & Cooke, A. Inflammation and type one diabetes. Interna-
      tional Immunology (2012). , 24(6), 339-46.

[83] Turley, S, Poirot, L, Hattori, M, Benoist, C, & Mathis, D. Physiological beta-cell death
      triggers priming of self-reactive T cells by dendritic cells in type-2 diabetes model.
      The Journal of Experimental Medicine (2003). , 198(10), 1527-37.

[84] Elenkov, I. J, & Chrousos, G. P. Stress Hormones, Th1/Th2 patterns, Pro/Anti-inflam-matory Cytokines and Susceptibility to Disease. Trends in Endocrinology and Metab-olism (1999). , 10(9), 359-68.

[85] Homem de Bittencourt Jr, P.I. and Newsholme P. A novel L-arginine/L-glutamine coupling hypothesis: implications for type 1 diabetes, Type 1 Diabetes- Complica-tions, Pathogenesis, and Alternative Treatments, Chih-Pin Liu (Ed.), 978-9-53307-756-7InTech (2011). Available from: http://www.intechopen.com/books/type-1 diabetes-complications-pathogenesis-and-alternative-treatments/a-novel-l-ar-ginine-l-glutamine-coupling-hypothesis-implications-for-type-1-diabetes

[86] Barthson, J, Germano, C. M, Moore, F, Maida, A, Drucker, D. J, Marchetti, P, Gyse-mans, C, Mathieu, C, Nunez, G, Juriscova, A, Eizirik, D. L, & Gurzov, E. N. Cyto-kines tumour necrosis factor-(alpha) and interferon-(gamma) induce pancreatic (beta)-cell apoptosis through STAT1-mediated Bim activation. The Journal of Biologi-cal Chemistry (2011). , 286(45), 39632-43.

[87] Ehses, J. A, Perren, A, Eppler, E, Ribaux, P, Pospisilik, J. A, Maor-cahn, R, Gueripel, X, Ellingsgaard, H, Schneider, M. K, Biollaz, G, Fontana, A, Reinecke, M, Homo-de-larche, F, & Donath, M. Y. Increased cell number of islet associated macrophages in type 2 diabetes. Diabetes (2007). , 56(9), 2356-70.

[88] Boni-schnetzler, M. M. L, Ehses, J. A, Weir, G. C, & Donath, M. Y. (2007). IL-1beta expression is induced by glucose and IL-1beta auto-stimulation, and increased in be-ta cells of type 2 diabetics. Diabetes 2007; 56(Suppl 1): A413.

[89] Ryan, A, Murphy, M, Godson, C, & Hickey, F. B. Diabetes mellitus and apoptosis: in-flammatory cells. Diabetes and Apoptosis (2009). , 14(12), 1435-50.

[90] Donath, M. Y, & Shoelson, S. E. Type 2 diabetes as an inflammatory disease. Nature Reviews Immunology (2011). , 11(2), 98-107.

[91] Pasarica, M, Rood, J, Ravussin, E, Schwarz, J. M, Smith, S. R, & Redman, L. M. Re-duced oxygenation in human obese adipose tissue is associated with impaired insu-lin suppression of lipolysis. The Journal of Clinical Endocrinology and Metabolism (2010). , 95(8), 4052-5.

[92] Weisberg, S. P, Mccann, D, Desai, M, Rosenbaum, M, Leibel, R. L, & Ferrante Jr., A. W. Obesity is associated with macrophage accumulation in adipose tissue. The Jour-nal of Clinical Investigations (2003). , 112(12), 1796-808.

[93] Xu, H, Barnes, G. T, Yang, Q, Tan, G, Yang, D, Chou, C. J, Sole, J, Nichols, A, Ross, J. S, Tartaglia, L. A, & Chen, H. Chronic inflammation in fat plays a crucial role in the development of obesity-related insulin-resistance. The Journal of Clinical Investiga-tions (2003). , 112(12), 1821-30.

[94]   Arkan, M. C, Hevener, A. L, Greten, F. R, Maeda, S, Li, Z. W, Long, J. M, Wynshaw-boris, A, Poli, G, Olefsky, J, & Karin, M. IKK-β links inflammation to obesity-induced insulin-resistance. Nature Medicine (2005). , 11(2), 191-8.

[95]   Bowie, A, & O Neill, L.A.J. The interleukin-1 receptor/toll-like receptor superfamily: signal generators for pro-inflammatory interleukins and microbial products. Journal of Leukocyte Biology (2000).

[96]   Nishikori, M. Classical and alternative NFκB activation pathways and their role in lymphoid malignancies. The Journal of Clinical and Experimental Hematopathology (2005). , 45(1), 15-24.

[97]   Donath, M. Y, Storling, J, Maedler, K, & Mandrup-poulsen, T. Inflammatory media-tors and islet β-cell failure: a link between type 1 and type 2 diabetes. The Journal of Molecular Medicine (Berlin) (2003). , 81(8), 455-70.

[98]   Morgan, M. J, & Liu, Z. G. Crosstalk of reactive oxygen species and NFκB signalling. Cell Research (2011). , 21(1), 103-15.

[99]   Wullaert, A, Heyninck, K, & Bayaert, R. Mechanisms of crosstalk between TNF-in-duced NFκB and JNK activation in hepatocytes. Biochemical Pharmacology (2006). , 72(9), 1090-101.

[100] Newsholme, P, Haber, E. P, Hirabara, S. M, Rebelato, E. L. O, Procopio, J, Morgan, D, Oliveira-emilio, H. C, Carpinelli, A. R, & Curi, R. Diabetes associated cell stress and dysfunction: role of mitochondria and non-mitochondrial ROS production and activ-ity. The Journal of Physiology (2007). Pt 1): 9-24.

[101] Schoonbroodt, S, & Piette, J. Oxidative stress interference with nuclear factor-κ B acti-vation pathways. Biochemical Pharmacology (2000). , 60(8), 1075-83.

[102] Shimabukuro, M, Zhou, Y. T, Levi, M, & Unger, R. H. Fatty acid-induced beta-cell apoptosis: a link between obesity and diabetes. Proceedings of the National Acade-my of Sciences (1998). , 95(5), 2498-502.

[103] Otero, M, Lago, R, Lago, F, Casanueva, F. F, Dieguez, C, Gomez-reino, J. J, & Gualil-lo, O. Leptin, from fat to inflammation: old questions and new insights. FEBS Letters (2005). , 579(2), 295-301.

[104] Zhang, F, Basinski, M. B, Beals, J. M, Briggs, S. L, Churgay, J. M, & Clawson, D. K. DiMarchi R.D., Furman T.C., Hale J.E., Hsiung H.M., Schoner B.E., Smith D.P., Zhang X.Y., Wery J.P. and Schevitz R.W. Crystal structure of the obese protein leptin-E100. Nature (1997). , 387(6629), 206-9.

[105] Matarese, G, Sanna, V, Lechler, R. I, Sarvet-nick, N, Fontana, S, & Zappacosta, S. and La Cava A. Leptin accelerates autoimmune diabetes in female NOD mice. Diabetes (2002). , 51(5), 1356-61.

[106] Wolf, A. M, Wolf, D, Rumpold, H, Enrich, B, & Tilg, H. Adiponectin induces the anti-inflammatory cytokines IL-10 and IL-1RA in human leukocytes. Biochemical and Biophysical Research Communications (2004). , 323(2), 630-5.

[107] Harman-boehm, I, Bluher, M, Redel, H, Sion-vardy, N, Ovadia, S, Avinoach, E, Shai, I, Kloting, N, Stumvoll, M, Bashan, N, & Rudich, A. Macrophage infiltration into omental versus subcutaneous fat across different populations: effects of regional adiposity and the comorbidities of obesity. The Journal of Clinical Endocrinology and Metabolism (2007). , 92(6), 2240-7.

[108] Odegaard, J. I, & Chawla, A. Connecting type 1 and type 2 diabetes through innate immunity. Cold Spring Harbour Perspectives in Medicine (2012). a007724.

[109] Cnop, M, Welsh, N, Jonas, J. C, Jorns, A, Lenzen, S, & Eizirik, D. L. Mechanisms of pancreatic β-cell death in type 1 and type 2 diabetes: Many differences, few similarities. Diabetes (2005). Suppl 2): S, 97-107.

[110] Lee, S. C, & Pervaiz, S. Apoptosis in the pathophysiology of diabetes mellitus. The International Journal of Biochemistry and Cell Biology (2007). , 39(3), 497-504.

[111] Back, S. H, Kang, S. W, Han, J, & Chung, H. T. Endoplasmic reticulum stress in the β-cell pathogenesis of type 2 diabetes. Experimental Diabetes Research (2012).

[112] Yip, L, Su, L, & Sheng, D. Deaf1 isoforms control the expression of genes encoding peripheral tissue antigens in the pancreatic lymph nodes during type 1 diabetes. Nature Immunology (2009). , 10(9), 1026-33.

[113] Clark, R, & Griffiths, G. M. Lytic granules, secretory lysosome and disease. Current Opinion in Immunology (2003). , 15(5), 516-21.

[114] Ashkenazi, A, & Dixit, V. M. Death receptors: signalling and modulation. Science (1998). , 281(5381), 1305-8.

[115] Sakamoto, S, & Kyprianou, N. Targeting anoikis-resistance in prostate cancer metastasis. Molecular Aspects of Medicine (2010). , 31(2), 205-14.

[116] Chang, H. Y, & Yang, X. Proteases for cell suicide: functions and regulation of caspases. Microbiology & Molecular Biology Reviews (2007). , 64(4), 821-46.

[117] Batinac, T, Zamolo, G, Coklo, M, & Hadzisejdic, I. Possible key role of granzyme B in keratoacanthoma regression. Medical Hypotheses (2006). , 66(6), 1129-32.

[118] Sutton, V. R, Wowk, M. E, Cancilla, M, & Trapani, J. Caspase activation by granzyme B is indirect, and caspase autoprocessing requires the release of pro-apoptotic mitochondrial factors. Immunity (2003). , 18(3), 319-29.

[119] Li, H, Zhu, H, Xu, C. J, & Yuan, J. Cleavage of Bid by caspase-8 mediates the mitochondrial damage in the Fas pathway of apoptosis. Cell (1998). , 94(4), 494-501.

[120] Yang, S. H, Chein, C. M, Lu, M. C, Hu, X. W, & Lin, S. R. Up-regulation of Bax and endonuclease G, and down-modulation of Bcl-XL involved in cardiotoxin III-induced apoptosis in K562 cells. Experimental and Molecular Medicine (2006). , 38(4), 435-44.

[121] Green, D. R, & Reed, J. C. Mitochondria and apoptosis. Science (1998). , 281(5381), 1309-12.

[122] Breckenridge, D. G, & Xue, D. Regulation of mitochondrial membrane permeabiliza-tion by BCL-2 family proteins and caspases. Current Opinion in Cell Biology (2004). , 16(6), 647-52.

[123] Wang, Z. B, Liu, Y. Q, & Cui, Y. F. Pathways to caspase activation. Cell Biology Inter-national (2005). , 29(7), 489-96.

[124] Portt, L, Norman, G, Clapp, C, Greenwood, M, & Greenwood, M. T. Anti-apoptosis and cell survival: A review. Biochimica et Biophysica Acta (2011). , 1813(1), 238-59.

[125] Ferri, K. F, & Kroemer, G. Organelle-specific initiation of cell death pathways. Nature Cell Biology (2001). E, 255-63.

[126] Brandt, B, Abou-eladab, E. F, Tiedge, M, & Walzel, H. Role of the JNK/c-Jun/AP-1 signalling pathway in galectin-induced T-cell death. Cell Death and Disease (2010). e23., 1.

[127] Rahier, J, Guiot, Y, Goebbels, R. M, Sempoux, C, & Henquin, J. C. Pancreatic beta-cell mass in European subjects with type 2 diabetes. Diabetes, Obesity and Metabolism (2008). Suppl 4): 32-42.

[128] Chang-chen, K. J, Mullur, R, & Bernal-mizrachi, E. cell failure as a complication of diabetes. Reviews in Endocrine Metabolic Disorders (2008). , 9(4), 329-43.

[129] Gehrmann, W, Elsner, M, & Lenzen, S. Role of metabolically generated reactive oxy-gen species for lipotoxicity in pancreatic β-cells. Diabetes, Obesity and Metabolism (2010). Suppl 2): 149-58.

[130] Chakrabarti, A, Chen, A. W, & Varner, J. D. A review of the mammalian unfolded protein response. Biotechnology and Bioengineering (2011). , 108(12), 2777-93.

[131] Kaufman, R. J Stress signalling from the lumen of the endoplasmic reticulum: coordi-nation of gene transcriptional and translational controls. Genes & Development (1999). , 13(10), 1211-33.

[132] Szegezedi, E, Logue, S. E, Gorman, A. M, & Samali, A. Mediators of endoplasmic re-ticulum stress-induced apoptosis. EMBO Reports (2006). , 7(9), 880-5.

[133] Nakagawa, T, & Yuan, J. Cross-talk between two cysteine protease families. Activa-tion of caspase-12 by calpain in apoptosis. Journal of Cell Biology (2000). , 150(4), 887-94.

[134] Rao, R. V, Peel, A, & Loqvinova, A. del Rio G., Hermel E., Yokota T., Goldsmith P.C., Ellerby L.M., Ellerby H.M. and Bredesen D.E. Coupling endoplasmic reticulum stress to the cell death program: role of the ER chaperone GRP78. FEBS Letters (2002).

[135] Putcha, G. V, Le, S, Frank, S, Besirli, C. G, Clark, K, Chu, B, Alix, S, & Youle, R. J. LaMarche A., Maroney A.C. and Johnson E.M. Jr. JNK-mediated BIM phosphorylation potentiates BAX-dependent apoptosis. Neuron (2003). , 38(6), 899-914.

[136] Donath, M. Y, Ehses, J. A, Maedler, K, Schumann, D. M, Ellingsgaard, H, Eppler, E, & Reinecke, M. Mechanisms of β-cell death in type 2 diabetes. Diabetes (2005). Suppl 2): S, 108-13.

[137] Cunha, D. A, Hekerman, P, Ladriere, L, Bazarra-castro, A, Ortis, F, Wakeham, M. C, Moore, F, Rasschaert, J, Cardozo, A. K, Bellomo, E, Overbergh, L, Mathieu, C, Lupi, R, Hai, T, Herchuelz, A, Marchetti, P, Rutter, G. A, Eizirik, D. L, & Cnop, M. Initiation and execution of lipotoxic ER stress in pancreatic β-cells. The Journal of Cell Science (2008). Pt 14): 2308-18.

[138] Cnop, M. Fatty acids and glucolipotoxicity in the pathogenesis of type 2 diabetes. The Biochemical Society Transactions (2008). Pt 3): 1180-6.

[139] Haataja, L, Gurlo, T, Huang, C. J, & Butler, P. C. Islet amyloid in type 2 diabetes, and the toxic oligomer hypothesis. Endocrine Reviews (2008). , 29(3), 303-16.

[140] Larsen, C. M, Faulenbach, M, Vaag, A, Volund, A, Ehses, J. A, Seifert, B, Mandrup-poulsen, T, & Donath, M. Y. Interleukin-1-receptor antagonist in type 2 diabetes mellitus. New England Journal of Medicine (2007). , 356(15), 1517-26.

[141] Mastrandrea, L, Yu, J, Behrens, T, Buchlis, J, Albini, C, Fourtner, S, & Quattrin, T. Etanercept treatment in children with new-onset type 1 diabetes: pilot randomised, placebo-controlled, double blind study. Diabetes Care (2009). , 32(7), 1244-9.

[142] Chung, J, Nguyen, A. K, Henstridge, D. C, Holmes, A. G, Chan, M. H, Mesa, J. L, Lancaster, G. I, Southgate, R. J, Bruce, C. R, Duffy, S. J, Horvath, I, Mestril, R, Watt, M. J, Hooper, P. L, Kingwell, B. A, Vigh, L, Hevener, A, & Febbraio, M. A. HSP72 protects against obesity-induced insulin-resistance. Proceedings of the National Academy of Sciences (2008). , 105(5), 1739-44.

[143] Kurucz, I, Morva, A, Vaag, A, Eriksson, K. F, Huang, X, Groop, L, & Koranyi, L. Decreased expression of heat shock protein 72 in skeletal muscle of patients with type 2 diabetes correlates with insulin-resistance. Diabetes (2002). , 51(4), 1102-9.

[144] Rodrigues-krause, J, Krause, M, Hagan, O, De Vito, C, Boreham, G, Murphy, C, Newsholme, C, & Colleran, P. G. Divergence of intracellular and extracellular HSP72 in type 2 diabetes: does fat matter? Cell Stress Chaperones. (2012). , 17(3), 293-302.

[145] Gupte, A. A, Bomhoff, G. L, Swerdlow, R. H, & Geiger, P. C. Heat treatment improves glucose tolerance and prevents skeletal muscle insulin-resistance in rats fed a high-fat diet. Diabetes (2009). , 58(3), 567-78.

[146] Krause, M. S. and Homem de Bittencourt P.I. Jr. Type 1 diabetes: can exercise impair the autoimmune event? The L-arginine/glutamine coupling hypothesis. Cell Bio-chemistry and Function (2008). , 26(4), 406-33.

[147] Mandrup-poulsen, T, Pickersgill, L, & Donath, M. Y. (2010). Blockade of interleukin-1 in type 1 diabetes. Nature Reviews Endocrinology 2010; , 6(3), 158-66.

[148] Patterson, C. C, Dahlquist, G. G, Gyurus, E, Green, A, & Soltesz, G. and EURODIAB Study Group. Incidence t rends for childhood type 1 diabetes in Europe during 1989-2003 and predicted new cases 2005-20: a multicentre prospective registration study. Lancet (2009). , 373(9680), 2027-33.

Chapter 8

Biochemical Evaluation of Oxidative Stress in Type 1 Diabetes

Donovan A. McGrowder,

Lennox Anderson-Jackson and

Tazhmoye V. Crawford

Additional information is available at the end of the chapter

1. Introduction

1.1. Type 1 diabetes mellitus

Diabetes mellitus is considered to be one of the most common chronic diseases worldwide, and recognized as one of the leading causes of morbidity and mortality (American Diabetes Association, 2010). It has been reported that the prevalence of diabetes mellitus will increase from 6% to over 10% in the next decade (Rosen et al., 2001). According to the World Health Organization in 2000, a total of 171 million people in all age groups worldwide (2.8% of the global population) have been affected by diabetes mellitus, and the number of persons is expected to increase to 366 million (4.4% of the global population) by 2030 (Wild et al., 2004).

Type 1 diabetes mellitus accounts for 5-10% of all diagnosed cases of diabetes mellitus, and exhibits hyperglycemia as its hallmark. It is caused by pancreatic β-islet cell failure with resulting insulin deficiency mortality and risk factors may be autoimmune, genetic, or environmental (American Diabetes Association, 2004). Type 1 diabetes mellitus is an autoimmune disorder involving immune-mediated recognition of islet β-cells by auto-reactive T cells. This subsequently leads to the liberation of pro-inflammatory cytokines and reactive oxygen species. There is destruction of pancreatic β-cells in the islets of Langerhans and loss of insulin secretion (Delmastro & Piganelli, 2011). The Jun kinase pathway is also activated by the pro-inflammatory cytokines, and there is evidence that oxidative stress is involved in β-cell destruction (Kaneto et al., 2007). The loss of β-cell mass consequential to the activation of pro-apoptotic signaling events is increasingly recognized as a causal and committed stage in the development of type 1 diabetes mellitus (Watson & Loweth, 2009).

Moreover, pancreatic β-cells are sensitive to cytotoxic damage caused by reactive oxygen species as gene expression and activity of antioxidant enzymes such as glutathione peroxidase activity is decreased in these cells (Lenzen et al., 1996).

Increasing evidence in both experimental and clinical studies suggests that oxidative stress plays a central role in the onset of diabetes mellitus as well as in the development of vascular and neurologic complications of the disease (Niedowicz & Daleke, 2005). Studies advancing the role of oxidative stress in vascular endothelial cells proposed that oxidative stress mediate the diversion of glycolytic intermediates into pathological pathways (Rolo & Palmeira, 2006; Turk, 2010). Oxidative stress is increased in diabetes mellitus owing to an increase in the production of oxygen free radicals and a deficiency in antioxidant defense mechanisms. Free radicals are formed disproportionately in diabetes by glucose oxidation, non-enzymatic glycation of proteins, and the subsequent oxidative degradation of glycated proteins (Rodiño-Janeiro et al., 2010). Abnormally high levels of free radicals and the simultaneous decline of antioxidant defense mechanisms can lead to damage of cellular organelles and enzymes, increased lipid peroxidation, and development of insulin resistance (Ceriello, 2006).

This review will explore recent evidence in the literature of the use of biomarkers to assess oxidative stress which is recognized as a significant mediator in the development of macrovascular or cardiovascular complication in type 1 diabetes mellitus, as well as the potential for prevention of complications through the use of antioxidants. There is also a search for other biomarker of oxidative stress which might be clinically useful in patients with diabetes mellitus. Such a biomarker could potentially indicate the severity of disease, identify those at increased risk of complications and monitor response to treatment.

2. Oxidative stress and beta-cell destruction

Impairment in the oxidant/antioxidant equilibrium creates a condition known as oxidative stress. There is a complex interaction between antioxidants and oxidants such as reactive oxygen species, which modulates the generation of oxidative stress. Oxidative stress takes place in a cellular system when the generation of reactive oxygen species increases and overwhelms the body's antioxidant capacity and defenses (Baynes, 1991). If the free radicals are not removed by the cellular antioxidants, they may attack and damage lipids, carbohydrates, proteins and nucleic acids (Baynes & Thorpe, 1999).

Oxidative stress is known to be a component of molecular and cellular tissue damage mechanisms in a wide spectrum of human diseases (Maritim et al., 2003; Isabella et al., 2006). There is growing evidence that have connected oxidative stress to a variety of pathological conditions, including cancer, cardiovascular diseases, chronic inflammatory disease, post-ischaemic organ injury, diabetes mellitus, xenobiotic/drug toxicity, and rheumatoid arthritis (El Faramawy & Rizk, 2011; Samanthi et al., 2011). In recent years, much attention has been focused on the role of oxidative stress. It has been reported that oxidative stress participates in the progression and pathogenesis of secondary diabetic complications. This includes impairment of insulin action and elevation of the complication incidence (Ceriello, 2006). Furthermore, there is evidence for the role of reactive oxygen species and oxidative stress in the development of type 1 diabetic complications including retinopathy, nephropathy, neuropathy, and accelerated coronary artery disease (Phillips et al., 2004; Niedowicz & Daleke, 2005).

It has also been reported that oxidative stress induced by reactive oxygen and nitrogen species is critically involved in the impairment of β-cell function, and thus play a role in the pathology of type 1 diabetes mellitus (West, 2000). Islet β-cells are highly susceptible to oxidative stress because of their reduced levels of endogenous antioxidants (*Azevedo-Martins et al., 2003; Kajikawa et al., 2002*). With decreased antioxidant capacity, β-cells are extremely sensitive towards oxidative stress. Cell metabolism and potassium (adenosine-5'-triphosphate) channels in β-cells are important targets for reactive oxygen species and other oxidants. The alterations of potassium (adenosine-5'-triphosphate) channel activity by the oxidants, is crucial for oxidant-induced dysfunction as genetic ablation of potassium (adenosine-5'-triphosphate) channels attenuates the effects of oxidative stress on β-cell function (Drews, 2010).

Oxidative stress may reduce insulin sensitivity and damage the β-cells within the pancreas. The reactive oxygen species produced by oxidative stress can penetrate through cell membranes and cause damage to the β-cells of pancreas (Chen et al., 2005; Lepore et al., 2004). Reactive oxygen species produced from free fatty acids can cause mitochondrial deoxyribonucleic acid damage and impaired pancreatic β-cell function (Rachek et al., 2006). Mitochondrial and nitrogen oxides (NO_x)-derived reactive oxygen species have been implicated in β-cell destruction and subsequently type 1 diabetes mellitus. Furthermore, increased glucose can cause rapid induction of the Krebs cycle within the β-cell mitochondria, leading to augmented reactive oxygen species production (Newsholme et al., 2007). The superoxide leaked from the mitochondria can contribute to the formation of hydrogen peroxide which may play a role in uncoupling glucose metabolism from insulin secretion (Maechler et al., 1999).

3. Oxidative stress induced by hyperglycaemia in type 1diabetes

3.1. Pathways involved in the production of oxidants

There are multiple sources of reactive oxygen species production in diabetes including those of non-mitochondrial and mitochondrial origins. Reactive oxygen species accelerates four important molecular mechanisms that are involved in oxidative tissue damage induced by hyperglycemia. These four pathways are increased advanced glycation end product, increased hexosamine pathway flux, activation of protein kinase C, and increased polyol pathway flux (also known as the sorbitol-aldose reductase pathway) (Rolo & Palmeira, 2006).

In the polyol pathway, the two enzymes aldose reductase and sorbitol dehydrogenase cause reactive oxygen species production. Glucose is reduced to sorbitol through the use of reduced nicotinamide adenine dinucleotide phosphate, a reaction catalyzed by aldose reductase. This pathway metabolizes 30 - 35% of the glucose present during hyperglycemia. The available reduced nicotinamide adenine dinucleotide phosphate is depleted resulting in the reduction of glutathione regeneration and nitric oxide synthase activity (Ramana et al., 2003). The oxidation of sorbitol to fructose with the concomitant production of reduced nicotinamide adenine dinucleotide is catalyzed by sorbitol dehydrogenase. The reduced nicotinamide adenine dinucleotide phosphate may be used by nicotinamide adenine dinucleotide phosphate oxidases to generate superoxide anion (Moore & Roberts, 1998). Vitamin C supplementation has been found to be effective in reducing sorbitol accumulation in the red blood cells of diabetic patients. In a study conducted by Cunningham et al. (1994) who investigated the effect of two different doses of vitamin C supplements (100 and 600 mg) during a 58 day trial on young adults with type 1 diabetes mellitus, vitamin C supplementation at either dose within 30 days normalized sorbitol levels.

Glucose at high concentrations undergoes non-enzymatic reactions with primary amino groups of proteins to form glycated residues called Amadori products. These early glycation products undergo further complex reactions, such as rearrangement, dehydration, and condensation, to become irreversibly cross-linked, heterogeneous fluorescent derivatives called advanced glycation end products (Thornalley, 2002). The advanced glycation end products binds to a cell surface receptor known as receptor for advanced glycation end product. As a result of interaction of advanced glycation end products, with receptor for advanced end product, there is the induction of the synthesis of reactive oxygen species via a mechanism which involves localization of pro-oxidant molecules at the cell surface (Yan et al., 1994) and the participation of activated nicotinamide adenine dinucleotide phosphate oxidase (Wautier et a., 2001). The reactive aldehydes methylglyoxal and glyoxal are produced from enzymatic and non-enzymatic degradation of glucose, lipid and protein catabolism, and lipid peroxidation. These aldehydes form advanced glycation end products with proteins that are implicated in diabetic complications. Han et al. (2007) assessed plasma methylglyoxal and glyoxal using a novel liquid chromatography-mass spectrophotometry method in 56 young patients (6 - 22 years) with type 1 diabetes mellitus without complications. They found that mean plasma methylglyoxal and glyoxal levels were higher in the diabetic patients compared with their non-diabetic counterparts. They suggest that increased plasma methylglyoxal and glyoxal levels give an indication of future diabetic complications and emphasized the need for aggressive management (Han et al., 2007).

It has been shown that through receptor for advanced glycation end products mediated effects, advanced glycation end product induces reactive oxygen species production possibly through an nicotinamide adenine dinucleotide phosphate oxidase, and the subsequent expression of inflammatory mediators and activation of redox-sensitive transcription factors (Wautier et al., 2001; Schmidt et al., 1996). Furthermore, advanced glycation end products, binding to receptor for advanced glycation end product activate protein kinase C-α-mediated activation of nuclear factor-κB (NFκβ) and nicotinamide adenine dinucleotide phosphate oxidase. This may cause the generation of mitochondrial reactive oxygen species and induce the production of various inflammatory cytokines further aggravating oxidative stress (Simm et al., 1997).

Advanced glycation end product in high concentration in body is toxic and can modify the structure of intracellular proteins especially those involved in gene transcription, and can cause damage to biological membranes and the endothelium. It may diffuse to the extracellular space and directly modify extracellular proteins such as laminin and fibronectin to disturb signaling between the matrix and cells that act via receptor for advanced glycation end products, which is present on many vascular cells (Bierhaus et al. 1998). In addition, advanced glycation end products can modify blood proteins such as albumin, causing them to bind to advanced glycation end product receptors on macrophages/mesangial cells and increase the production of growth factors and proinflammatory cytokines (Brownlee, 2005). Kostolanská et al. (2009) observed significantly higher glycated hemoglobin, serum advanced glycation end products and advanced oxidation protein products concentrations in 81 patients with type 1 diabetes mellitus compared with controls. They suggest that the measurement of glycated hemoglobin, serum advanced glycation end products and advanced oxidation protein products may be useful to predict the risk of development of diabetic complications (Kostolanská et al., 2009).

Antioxidants or antibodies against receptor for advanced glycation end product prevent both oxidative stress and the downstream signaling pathways that can be activated by ligation of receptor for advanced glycation end product. Advanced glycation end product-mediated reaction oxygen species production is implicated in diabetic vascular complications and in blood vessel endothelial activation (Cameron & Cotter, 1999; Mullarkey et al., 1990). The formation and accumulation of advanced glycation end products have been involved in the development and progression of diabetic micro- and macroangiopathy. The advanced glycation end product-receptor for advanced glycation end product interaction produces oxidative stress and subsequently evokes thrombosis and vascular inflammation, thereby playing an important role in diabetic vascular complications (Yamagishi, 2009; Niiya et al., 2006). In a recent study, median levels of malondialdehyde and increased plasma levels of soluble receptor for advanced glycation end product were found in 42 type 1 diabetic patients during the early years after diagnosis (0-10 years). These findings suggest that increased plasma levels of soluble receptor for advanced glycation end product in type 1diabetes may provide protection against cell damage and may be sufficient to eliminate excessive circulating malondialdehyde during early years after disease onset (Reis et al., 2012).

4. Free radicals formed during oxidative stress

4.1. Reactive oxygen species in type 1 diabetes

Reactive oxygen species consist of oxygen free radicals such as superoxide anion ($O_2^{\bullet-}$), hydrogen peroxide (H_2O_2), hydroxyl radical ($^{\bullet}OH$), singlet oxygen, nitric oxide, and peroxynitrite (Chong et al., 2005). Most of these free radicals are produced at low concentrations during normal physiological conditions in the body and are scavenged by endogenous enzymatic and non-enzymatic antioxidant systems that include superoxide dismutase, glutathione peroxidase, catalase, and small molecule substances such as vitamins C and E.

Reactive oxygen species induced tissue injury as well as they are involved in signaling pathways and gene expression (Ha & Lee, 2000). Excess generation of reactive oxygen species such as superoxide anion, hydrogen peroxide, hydroxyl radical and reactive nitrogen species such as nitric oxide oxidize target cellular proteins, nucleic acids, or membrane lipids and damage their cellular structure and function (Brownlee, 2001). There is also evidence that reactive oxygen species also regulate the expression of genes encoding for proteins involved in immune response, inflammation and cell death (Ho & Bray, 1999).

Hydroxyl radicals, hydrogen peroxide, and superoxide anion are byproducts of xanthine oxidase. Xanthine oxidase and xanthine dehydrogenase catalyze the conversion of hypoxanthine to xanthine and then to uric acid, with the former reducing oxygen as an electron acceptor while the latter can reduce either oxygen or nicotinamide adenine dinucleotide (NAD^+) (Fatehi-Hassanabad et al., 2010). Superoxide anion is also produced by nicotinamide adenine dinucleotide phosphate oxidases and cytochrome P450, and is the most commonly occurring oxygen free radical that produces hydrogen peroxide by dismutation. This is achieved via the Haber-Weiss reaction in the presence of ferrous iron by copper (Cu)-superoxide dismutase or manganese (Mn)-superoxide dismutase. Mitochondrial superoxide anion is produced from excess reduced nicotinamide adenine dinucleotide produced in the Krebs cycle (Fubini & Hubbard, 2003). Elevated free or non-esterified fatty acids in type 1 diabetic patients enter the Krebs cycle causing the production of acetyl-CoA to subsequently excess reduced nicotinamide adenine dinucleotide (Steinberg & Baron, 2002). The superoxide anion undergo dismutation to hydrogen peroxide, which if not degraded by catalase or glutathione peroxidase, and in the presence of transition metals, can lead to production of hydroxyl radical, the most active oxygen free radical. Hydroxyl radical alternatively may be formed through an interaction between superoxide anion and nitric oxide (Fubini & Hubbard, 2003; Wolff, 1993).

Superoxide anion can also react with nitric oxide to form the reactive peroxynitrite radicals (Hogg & Kalyanaraman, 1998). Excess production of superoxide anion by the mitochondrial electron transport chain, induced by hyperglycaemia has been reported to have a role in triggering protein kinase C, hexosamine and polyol pathway fluxes, and advanced glycation end product formation pathways which are involved in the pathogenesis of diabetic complications (Nishikawa et al., 2000; Brownlee, 2001). In a study conducted by Hsu et al. (2006), plasma superoxide anion (determined by a chemiluminescent assay) gave photoemission which was considerably higher in 47 type 1 diabetic children than those in controls. The findings confirm the presence of oxidative stress in children with type 1 diabetes mellitus (Hsu et al., 2006).

4.2. Reactive nitrogen species in type 1 diabetes

Nitric oxide is an important regulator of endothelial function and the impairment of its activity is determinant of the endothelial dysfunction (Ignarro, 2002). It is an important vascular target for ROS and is produced by constitutive and inducible nitric oxide synthases. These enzymes oxidize L-arginine to citrulline in the presence of biopterin, reduced nicotinamide adenine dinucleotide phosphate, and oxygen (Alp & Channon, 2004). Constitutive endothelial nitric oxide synthase contains reductase and oxygenase domains that are con-nected by a calmodulin-binding region and requires cofactor groups such as heme, flavin mononucleotide, flavin adenine dinucleotide, tetrahydrobiopterin, and Ca^{2+}-calmodulin for activation (Gorren & Mayer, 2002; Andrew & Mayer, 1999). If there is none or insufficient L-arginine, the endothelial nitric oxide synthase produce superoxide instead of nitric oxide and this is referred to as the uncoupled state of nitric oxide synthase (Channon, 2004).

Oxidative stress decreases the bioavailability of endothelium-derived nitric oxide in diabetic patients. In a 3-year longitudinal study involving 37 patients with recent-onset (less than 2 years) type 1 diabetes, oxidative stress was evident by elevated malondialdehyde excretion and serum NO_x (nitrate and nitrite) (Hoeldtke et al., 2011). In a latter study, NO_x was also higher in 99 female subjects with uncomplicated type 1 diabetes (duration disease <10 years) compared with 44 sex-matched controls (Pitocco et al., 2009). Mylona Karayanni et al. (2006) examined possible correlation between oxidative stress parameters and adhesion molecules derived from endothelial/platelet activation, P-selectin and tetranectin in a group of juve-niles with type 1 diabetes mellitus. Significantly elevated NO_x and lipid hydroperoxide lev-els, elevated tetranectin and P-selectin plasma levels, and lower glutathione peroxidase activity were found in the diabetic children compared with healthy controls. Based on these findings the authors suggested that decreased anti-oxidative protection from overproduc-tion of lipid hydroperoxide and NO_x overproduction is present in juveniles with type 1 dia-betes mellitus. There is also a parallel endothelial/platelet activation which contributes to the vascular complications of type 1 diabetes mellitus (Mylona-Karayanni et al., 2006).

Nitric oxide can react with superoxide to form peroxynitrite which in turn oxidizes tetrahy-drobiopterin and causes further uncoupling of nitric oxide formation (Yung et al., 2003). In diabetes mellitus, elevated glucose may cause an increase in the expression of both reduced nicotinamide adenine dinucleotide phosphate and of inducible nitric oxide synthase via the activation of NF-κB, (Spitaler & Graier, 2002). The upregulated inducible nitric oxide syn-thase will synthesize the superoxide anion instead of nitric oxide, leading to oxidative and nitrosative stress (Llorens & Nava, 2003). The stable protein adduct, nitrotyrosine, is a mark-er of peroxynitrite (Ischiropoulos, 1998) and nitrogen dioxide (Prutz et al., 1985). Moreover, increased oxidative and nitrosative stress activates poly(ADP-ribose) polymerase-1, which substrate, nicotinamide adenine dinucleotide (NAD^+) as well as slows the rate of glycolysis, electron transport, and adenosine triphosphate formation (Pacher & Szabó, 2006).

The formation of peroxynitrite can further lead to the generation of peroxynitrous acid. The spontaneous decomposition of peroxynitrous acid results in the formation of hydroxyl radi-cals that can cause endothelial damage (Elliott et al., 1993; Beckman & Koppenol, 1996) thereby reduces the efficacy the endothelium-derived vasodilator system that participates in the general homeostasis of the vasculature (Benz et al., 2002). Overproduction of both nitric oxide and superoxide anion has been reported in response to hyperglycemia (Cosentino et al., 1997; Ceriello et al., 2002), and nitric oxide may work through peroxynitrite to directly alter cellular structure and function (Pfeiffer et al., 2001). Increased nitric oxide levels have been reported in both saliva and plasma of diabetic patients in comparison to healthy sub-jects (Astaneie et al., 2005).

5. Enzymatics and non-enzymatic antioxidants

5.1. Intracellular enzymes activity in type 1 diabetes

A number of natural antioxidants are present in the body to scavenge oxygen free radicals and prevent oxidative damage to biological membranes. Antioxidant defense mechanisms involve both non-enzymatic and enzymatic strategies. One group of these antioxidants is intracellular enzymes such as manganese superoxide dismutase, catalase, glutathione peroxidase, and glutathione-S-transferases. These enzymes represent a protective mechanism against the damage caused by the oxidative stress and most of these enzymes are polymorphic (Fang et al., 2002; Mates et al., 1999).

Superoxide dismutase is considered a primary enzyme since it is involved in the direct elimination of reactive oxygen synthase (Halliwell, 1994). Isoforms of superoxide dismutase are Cu/Zn-superoxide dismutase which is found in both the cytoplasm and the nucleus, and Mn-superoxide dismutase that is present in the mitochondria. The latter can be released into extracellular space (Reiter et al., 2000). Cu/Zn-superoxide dismutase over-expression inhibits oxidized low density lipoprotein which is can elevate deoxyribonucleic acid binding activity of activator protein-1 and NF-κB (Yung et al., 2006). Superoxide dismutase catalyzes the conversion of superoxide anion radicals produced in the body to hydrogen peroxide. This decreases the possibility of superoxide anion interacting with nitric oxide to form reactive peroxynitrite (Reiter et al., 2000). Low Cu/Zn-superoxide dismutase is a potential early marker of susceptibility to diabetic vascular disease. Suys et al. (2007) found that erythrocyte superoxide dismutase activity and Cu/Zn-superoxide dismutase were higher in type 1 diabetic subjects and was positively associated with flow-mediated dilatation. Based on these findings the authors suggest that higher circulating Cu/Zn-superoxide dismutase could protect type 1 diabetic children and adolescents against endothelial dysfunction (Suys et al., 2007). Furthermore, Reznick and colleagues analyzed both serum and salivary superoxide dismutase activity in 20 patients with type 1 diabetes mellitus. A significant association was found between the level of glycemic control as indicated by the glycated hemoglobin values and an increase in both salivary and serum superoxide dismutase activity (Reznick et al., 2006). On the contrary, in a study which assessed correlations between increase of oxidative stress and the development of microalbuminuria in 87 type 1 diabetic patients (44 with normal urinary protein excretion, and 43 with microalbuminuria), there was a decreased in activity of superoxide dismutase. This was associated with an increased microalbuminuria in type 1 diabetic patients (Artenie et al., 2005).

Selenium-dependent glutathione peroxidase works in conjunction with superoxide dismutase in protecting cell proteins and membranes against oxidative damage. In the literature, glutathione peroxidase response to diabetes has been conflicting. Diabetics have been reported to be associated with increased glutathione peroxidase activity in 90 pregnant women with type 1 diabetes mellitus (Djordjevic et al., 2004) and in young diabetic patients (Ndahimana et al., 1996). On the other hand, decreased glutathione peroxidase activity was reported in the early stages of type 1 diabetes in children and adolescents (Dominguez et al., 1998) or unchanged in type 1 diabetic patients with early retina degenerative lesions (Faure et al., 1995). The low glutathione peroxidase activity could be directly explained by either low glutathione content or enzyme inactivation under sever oxidative stress (Faure et al., 1995). However, some authors found no differences between glutathione peroxidase activity of type 1 diabetic patients and control subjects (Jain et al., 1994; Murakami et al., 1993; Majchrzak et al., 2001).

Catalase, located in peroxisomes, decomposes hydrogen peroxide to water and oxygen (Winterbourn & Metodiewa, 1994). In addition, glutathione peroxidase in the mitochondria and the lysosomes also catalyses the conversion of hydrogen peroxide to water and oxygen (Yung et al., 2006). A significant increase in the catalase activity in lymphocytes was found in 40 children with type 1 diabetes during all phases (at the beginning of diabetes, in remission period and in the later chronic course) compared with the control group. The highest catalase activity occurs in the early course of disease followed by a linear decrease and the lowest activity in chronic course (Zivić, 2008). Conversely Dave and colleagues (2007) reported significant decreased glutathione peroxidase, catalase and glutathione, and significant increase in thiobarbituric acid reactive substances concentration in type 1 diabetic patients with and without nephropathy compared with normal healthy individuals (Dave et al., 2007).

5.2. Non-enzymatic antioxidant levels in type 1 diabetes

In addition to enzymatic antioxidants, the major natural antioxidants, most of which are derived from dietary sources are vitamin A, vitamin C or ascorbic acid, vitamin E and carotenoids. Water-soluble vitamin C and fat-soluble vitamin E together make up the antioxidant system for mammalian cells (Engler et al., 2003). Vitamins A, C, and E are obtained from the diet and function to directly detoxify free radicals. Vitamin C forms the first line of defense against plasma lipid peroxidation is considered the most important antioxidant in plasma (Frei et al., 1990). Vitamin C under certain conditions may foster toxicity by generating pro-oxidants, and is also engaged in the recycling processes which involved the generation of reduced forms of the vitamins. In the processes of regeneration, α-tocopherol is reconstituted when ascorbic acid recycles the tocopherol radical; dihydroascorbic acid, which is formed, is recycled by glutathione (Weber, 1997).

Vitamin E involves all tocopherol and tocotrienol derivatives that comprise the major lipophilic exogenous antioxidant in tissues (Di Mambro et al., 2003). Vitamin E, a component of the total peroxyl radical-trapping antioxidant system reacts directly with superoxide and peroxyl radicals, and singlet oxygen and in so doing protects membranes from lipid peroxidation (Weber & Bendich, 1997). In a study by Gupta et al. 2011 that evaluated the oxidative stress in 20 type 1 diabetic children, reduced glutathione and vitamin E levels were decreased and malondialdehyde levels were elevated compared with controls. After supplementation with vitamin E (600 mg/daily for three months) there was a significant decrease in malondialdehyde levels and significant increase in glutathione and vitamin E. The findings indicate that vitamin E ameliorates oxidative stress in type 1 diabetes mellitus patients and improves antioxidant defense system. In a latter study high-dose vitamin E supplementation (1200 mg/day) reduces markers of oxidative stress and improves antioxidant defense in young patients with type 1 diabetes mellitus. However vitamin E supplementation did not decreased albumin excretion rate in these patients (Giannini et al., 2007).

α-Tocopherol is very effective in lipid peroxidation inhibition and is the primary *in vivo* chain-breaking, lipid-soluble antioxidant in human serum. A reduction in serum α-tocopherol could be attributed to its consumption while scavenging free radicals in lipoproteins or biomembranes (Frei, 1994). In the Pittsburgh Epidemiology of Diabetes Complications Study cohort, a 10-year prospective study of childhood-onset type 1 diabetes, α-tocopherol or γ-tocopherol did not showed protection against incident coronary artery disease overall. However, high α-tocopherol levels among patients with renal disease and in those using vitamin supplements were associated with lower coronary artery disease risk in type 1 diabetes (Costacou et al., 2006). All the antioxidants work in a synergistic manner with each other and against different types of free radicals. This is shown in the way in which vitamin E suppresses the propagation of lipid peroxidation, and vitamin C working with vitamin E inhibits hydroperoxide formation (Laight et al., 2000).

Glutathione functions as a direct free-radical scavenger, and as a co-substrate for glutathione peroxidase activity (Meister & Anderson, 1983). Glutathione, a tri-peptide present in millimolar concentrations is the most prevalent low-molecular weight peptide antioxidant in cells. Reduced glutathione normally plays the role of a direct intracellular free-radical scavenger through interaction with free radicals and is the substrate of many xenobiotic elimination reactions (Gregus et al., 1996). It is also involved in other cellular functions such as the elimination of hydrogen peroxide, detoxification processes such as protection of the sulfhydryl group of cysteine in proteins, and regeneration of oxidized vitamin E (Lu, 1999). In 30 children with type 1 diabetes at onset, there was a significant reduction in all glutathione forms (total, reduced, oxidized, and protein-bound glutathione). This indicates that there is glutathione depletion upon early onset of type 1 diabetes mellitus (Pastore et al., 2012). In another study, Likidlilid et al. (2007) compared the glutathione level, and glutathione peroxidase activity in 20 type 1 diabetic patients (with fasting glucose > 140 mg/dL) and a normal healthy group. They found that the level of red cell reduced glutathione was significantly lower in type 1 diabetic patients but red cell glutathione peroxidase activity was significantly increased. The decrease of red cell glutathione may be due to its higher rate of consumption, increasing glutathione peroxidase activity or a reduction of pentose phosphate pathway, stimulated by insulin, resulting in lowered glutathione recycle (Likidlilid et al., 2007). In a recent study, reduced glutathione and vitamin E levels were decreased and malondialdehyde levels were higher in 20 type 1 diabetic children compared with healthy controls. After supplementation with vitamin E (600 mg/daily for three months), there was a significant decrease in malondialdehyde levels and significant increase in glutathione and vitamin E levels. This shows that vitamin E ameliorates oxidative stress in type 1 diabetic patients and improves antioxidant defense system (Gupta et al., 2011).

Other nonenzymatic antioxidants include α-lipoic acid, mixed carotenoids, coenzyme Q_{10}, several bioflavonoids, antioxidant minerals (copper, zinc, manganese and selenium), and the cofactors (folic acid, vitamins B_1, B_2, B_6, B_{12}). β-carotene is a lipid soluble and chain-breaking antioxidant that effectively quenches singlet oxygen and inhibits lipid peroxidation. At low physiological oxygen pressures, it exhibits effective radical-trapping antioxidant behaviour (Frei, 1994). Coenzyme Q_{10} has been found to have a very important role in mitochondrial bioenergetics. It is an electron carrier-proton translocator in the respiratory chain and potent antioxidant which works by directly scavenging radicals or indirectly by regenerating vitamin E. In a study by Menke and colleagues (2008), plasma concentrations of coenzyme Q_{10} in 39 children with type 1 diabetes mellitus were higher than in healthy children. The findings suggest that elevated plasma concentration and the intracellular redox capacity of coenzyme Q_{10} in diabetic children may contribute to the body's self-protection during a state of enhanced oxidative stress (Menke et al., 2008). In another study, Salardi and colleagues (2004) determine whether serum hydroperoxides as oxidative markers and vitamin E and coenzyme Q_{10} as indexes of antioxidant capacity could be related to metabolic control in 75 unselected children, adolescents, and young adults with type 1 diabetes. Vitamin E and coenzyme Q_{10} were not significantly different from age-matched control subjects. However, there were significant positive correlations between coenzyme Q_{10} and glycated hemoglobin, and vitamin E and glycated hemoglobin. It was also observed that diabetic patients with poor metabolic control and complications had elevated vitamin E levels and coenzyme Q_{10} levels (Salardi et al., 2004).

Small molecules that have antioxidant capacity such as glutathione and uric acid are synthesized or produced within the body (Engler et al., 2003). A study by Maxwell et al. (1997) found significantly reduced total serum antioxidant status in 28 patients with type 1 diabetes mellitus as attributed by lower uric acid and vitamin C levels. Furthermore, multiple regression analysis showed that uric acid, vitamin E and vitamin C were the main contributors to serum total antioxidant activity.

6. Markers of oxidative stress in type 1 diabetes

6.1. Biomarkers of lipid peroxidation in type 1 diabetes

Oxidative stress and its contribution to low-density lipoprotein oxidation have been implicated in the pathogenesis of vascular diabetic complications. Diabetes produces disturbances of lipid profiles, especially an increased susceptibility to lipid peroxidation, which is responsible for increased incidence of atherosclerosis, a major complication of diabetes mellitus (Siu & To, 2002). Polyunsaturated fatty acids with multiple bonds and lipoproteins in the plasma membrane are very susceptible to attack by reactive oxygen species (Esterbauer & Schaur, 1991). The hydroxyl radicals extract a hydrogen atom from one of the carbon atoms in the polyunsaturated fatty acid and lipoproteins, initiating a free radical chain reaction which leads to lipid peroxidation. This characterized by membrane protein damage through subsequent free radical attacks (Halliwell, 1995). Lipid peroxidation can produce advanced products of oxidation, such as aldehydes, alkanes and isoprostanes (Moore & Roberts, 1998). Elevation of lipid peroxidation negatively affects membrane function causing reduced membrane fluidity and changing the activity of membrane bound enzymes and receptors (Acworth et al., 1997).

In diabetes mellitus, persistence of hyperglycemia was reported to cause increased production of oxidative parameters of lipid peroxidation including malondialdehyde. In a study by Firoozrai and colleagues (2007), malondialdehyde levels were significantly elevated in diabetic patients. The level of malondialdehyde was positively correlated with duration of diabetes and glycated hemoglobin and negatively with ferric reducing ability of plasma (Firoozrai et al., 2007). In a latter study that investigated the effect of glycemic control on oxidative stress and the lipid profile of pediatric type 1 diabetes mellitus patients, total cholesterol, low density lipoprotein-cholesterol, apolipoprotein A, apolipoprotein B, and malondialdehyde levels were significantly elevated compared with controls. In addition, serum malondialdehyde levels and malondialdehyde/low density lipoprotein-cholesterol index were significantly elevated in metabolically poorly controlled in relation to metabolically well-controlled diabetic patients. Based on these findings the authors suggested that type 1 diabetic children, especially those who are metabolically poorly controlled are at high risk of atherosclerosis and vascular complications of diabetes mellitus, and that there is a significant relationship between the lipid profile and oxidative stress (Erciyas et al., 2004).

Isoprostanes are prostaglandin-like compounds formed through peroxidation of arachidonic acid, and have been used extensively as biomarkers of lipid peroxidation as a risk factor for atherosclerosis and other diseases (Roberts & Marrow, 2000). Oxidative stress parameters such as advanced oxidation protein products, total peroxyl radical-trapping antioxidant parameter, and F2-isoprostanes (8-epi-prostaglandin-F2: 8-isoPGF2alpha) were not significantly different in 27 pre-pubertal patients with type 1 diabetes mellitus (with less than 5 years of disease) compared with controls (Gleisner et al., 2006). In another study, Flores and colleagues (2004) evaluated the effect of the normalization of blood glucose levels on urinary F2-isoprostanes at the onset of type 1 diabetes in 14 patients. There was a statistically significant reduction in F2-isoprostanes after insulin therapy (after 16 weeks) which was accompanied by a significant reduction in glycated hemoglobin (Flores et al., 2004).

Lipid hydroperoxides are potentially atherogenic and are degraded by enzymes such as paraoxonase-1 and lipoprotein-associated phospholipase A_2 (Van Lenten et al., 2001; Macphee et al., 2005). Paraoxonase-1 is an enzyme associated with high density lipoprotein surface and the antioxidant effect of the latter is partially related to paraoxonase. This enzyme is able to hydrolyze lipid hydroperoxides and to delay or inhibit the initiation of oxidation of lipoproteins induced by metal ions (Watson et al., 1995). It has been suggested that individuals with low paraoxonase-1 activity may have a greater risk of developing diseases such as diabetes mellitus in which oxidative damage and lipid peroxidation are involved, compared with those with high paraoxonase-1 activity (Durrington et al., 2001; Nourooz-Zadehet al., 1995).

Wegner et al. (2011) reported that 80 type 1 diabetic patients had lower paraoxonase-1 arylesterase activity and higher lipid hydroperoxide levels, and that there was a negative correlation between paraoxonase-1arylesterase activity and lipid hydroperoxide levels. In a latter study, paraoxonase-1 activity was reduced in patients with type 1 diabetes mellitus with retinopathy, confirming that oxidative stress could play a role in pathogenesis of diabetic retinopathy (Nowak et al., 2010). A similar finding of lower high density lipoprotein-paraoxonase-1 activity in 31 type 1 diabetic patients compared with the same number of sex-

and age-matched healthy subjects was reported by Ferretti et al. (2004). These findings confirm a linkage between paraoxonase-1 activity and lipid peroxidation of lipoproteins and suggest that the ability of high density lipoprotein to protect erythrocyte membranes might be related to the paraoxonase-1 activity (Ferretti et al., 2004). The low paraoxonase-1 aryles-terase activity suggests insufficient high density lipoprotein capacity to protect against lipid oxidation in patients with type 1 diabetes (Wegner et al., 2011). It is also hypothesized that the lower high density lipoprotein protective action against membrane peroxidation and de-crease paraoxonase-1 activity in diabetic patients could contribute to acceleration of arterio-sclerosis in patients with type 1 diabetes mellitus (Ferretti et al., 2004). Furthermore, there are several studies linking diabetes and even postprandial hyperglycemia with increased low density lipoprotein oxidative susceptibility (Ceriello, 2000). Decreased insulin in diabe-tes mellitus increases the activity of fatty acyl coenzyme A oxidase, which intiates β-oxida-tion of fatty acids, resulting in lipid peroxidation (Horie et al., 2006).

6.2. Biomarkers of protein peroxidation and oxidative damage to DNA in type 1 diabetes

High plasma glucose concentrations can increase the levels of glycation and oxidative dam-age to cellular and plasma proteins in diabetes mellitus. Glycation of proteins is a complex series of reactions where early-stage reactions leads to the formation of the early glycation adduct, fructosyl-lysine and NH_2-terminal fructosyl-amino acids, and later-stage reactions form advanced glycation end products (Thornalley, 2002). The oxidation of proteins produ-ces nitrotyrosine and protein carbonyl derivatives and nitrotyrosine (Adams et al., 2001). The oxidized or nitrosylated products of free radical attack have reduced biological activity, leading to loss of cell signaling, energy metabolism, transport, and other major cellular func-tions. These altered oxidized products also are targeted for proteosome degradation, further reducing cellular function. There is also cell death through necrotic or apoptotic mecha-nisms as a result of the accumulation of cellular injury (Rosen et al., 2001).

Carbonyl group formation is considered an early and stable marker for protein oxidation in the body. Diabetes mellitus is associated with carbonyl stress where there is an increase of reactive carbonyl compounds caused by their enhanced formation and/or decreased degra-dation or excretion (Miyata et al., 1999.) This leads to the formation of advanced glycation end products such as pentosidin and carboxymethyllysine and advanced oxidation protein products, and damage to a number of biologically important compounds (Miayta et al. 1999; Witko-Sarsat et al., 1996). Telci et al. (2000) examined the influence of oxidative stress on oxi-dative protein damage in 51 young type 1 diabetic patients clinically free of complications and 48 healthy normolipidaemic age-matched controls. The levels of plasma carbonyl and plasma lipid hydroperoxide were increased in adolescent and young adult type 1 diabetic patients compared with controls.

Modifications in endothelial cell function are proposed to play an important role in athero-genesis. These perturbations include increased permeability to circulating lipoproteins par-ticularly low density lipoprotein, increased retention of these lipoproteins, the loss of endothelial cell-directed vasodilatation, and the increased expression of intercellular cell ad-hesion molecule-1 and vascular cell adhesion molecule-1 (Ross, 1999). Koitka et al. (2004) reported evidence of endothelial dysfunction in patients with type 1 diabetes. In another study of 45 type 1 diabetic children, there was significantly lower peak brachial artery flow-mediated dilation response and increased carotid artery intima-media thickness. This suggests that altered endothelium function in children with type 1 diabetes may predispose them to the development of early atherosclerosis (Jarvisalo et al., 2004). Furthermore, in a double-blind, placebo-controlled, randomized study of 41 young subjects with type I diabetes mellitus, vitamin E supplementation (1,000 IU for three months) had a positive effect on the endothelial function as evident by improved endothelial vasodilator function in both the conduit and resistance vessels (Skyrme-Jones, 2000).

In addition to lipids and proteins, reactive oxygen species reacts with deoxyribonucleic acid resulting in various products, such as 8-hydroxydeoxyguanosine, that is excrete in urine owing to deoxyribonucleic acid repair processes. Urinary 8-hydroxydeoxyguanosine has been proposed as an indicator of oxidative damage to deoxyribonucleic acid. Goodarzi and colleagues (2010) evaluated the relationship between oxidative damage to deoxyribonucleic acid and protein glycation in 32 patients with type 1 diabetes. There were elevated levels of urinary 8-hydroxydeoxyguanosine, glycated hemoglobin, plasma malondialdehyde, and glycated serum protein in 32 patients with type 1 diabetes. There was a significant correlation between urinary 8-hydroxydeoxyguanosine and glycated hemoglobin. The findings indicate that that deoxyribonucleic acid is associated to glycemic control level (Goodarzi et al., 2010). In a study which investigated whether advanced glycation end product production and oxidative stress are augmented in young patients with type 1 diabetes at early clinical stages of the disease, advanced glycation end products, pentosidine, and 8-hydroxydeoxyguanosine and acrolein-lysine were significantly higher in the patients with type 1 diabetes compared with healthy control subjects (Tsukahara et al., 2003).

6.3. Biomarkers of oxidative stress present in breath

Oxidative stress has been implicated in the major complications of diabetes mellitus, including retinopathy, nephropathy, neuropathy and accelerated coronary artery disease (Ceriello & Morocutti, 2000; Androne et al., 2000; Mackness et al., 2002). There is a clinical need for markers of oxidative stress which could potentially identify diabetic patients at increased risk for these complications. The introduction of breath microassays has enhanced the detection of oxidative stress because reactive oxygen species oxidize polyunsaturated fatty acids in membranes to alkanes such as ethane and pentane. These are excreted in the breath as volatile organic compounds (Kneepkens & Lepage, 1994). Another marker of oxidative stress is the breath methylated alkane contour, comprising a three-dimensional display of C4 to C20 alkanes and monomethylated alkanes in the breath (Phillips et al., 2004). Phillips et al. (2004) reported significantly increased volatile organic compounds and breath methylated alkane contour in the breath of type 1 diabetic patients which was independent of glycemic as they did with blood glucose concentration or with glycation hemoglobin levels.

7. Conclusion

This review presented convincing experimental and clinical evidence that the aetiology of oxidative stress in diabetes mellitus arises from a number of mechanisms that includes excessive reactive oxygen species production from the peroxidation of lipids, auto-oxidation of glucose, glycation of proteins, and glycation of antioxidative enzymes, which limit their capacity to detoxify oxygen radicals. There is also evidence that supports the role of hyperglycemia in producing oxidative stress and, eventually, severe endothelial dysfunction in blood vessels of individuals with type 1 diabetes mellitus. The induction of oxidative stress is a key process in the onset and development of diabetic complications, but the precise mechanisms has not been fully elucidated. A number of biomarkers of oxidative stress have been studied in type 1 diabetic patients such as malondialdehyde, F2-isoprostanes, advanced glycation end product and nitrotyrosine. The introduction of breath microassays has enhanced the detection of oxidative stress.

Type 1 diabetic patients have been found to have decreased amounts and efficiency of antioxidant defenses (both enzymatic and non-enzymatic) due to increased consumption of distinct antioxidant components (e.g. intracellular glutathione) or to primarily low levels of antioxidant substances (flavonoids, carotenoids, vitamin E and C). This review also presents small clinical studies that have demonstrated improvements in a variety of oxidative stress biomarkers in type 1 diabetic patients who have received vitamin A, C or E supplements. However, the findings of key prospective randomized controlled antioxidant clinical trials have failed to demonstrate a significant benefit, in the prevention of cardiovascular events. There is a need for continued investigation of the association between reactive oxygen species, type 1 diabetes mellitus and its complications in order to clarify the molecular mechanisms by which increased oxidative stress accelerates the development of diabetic complications. This will have implication for the prevention and development of therapeutic choices for type 1 diabetic patients.

Author details

Donovan A. McGrowder[1], Lennox Anderson-Jackson[2] and Tazhmoye V. Crawford[3]

1 Department of Pathology, Faculty of Medical Sciences, The University of the West Indies, Mona, Kingston, Jamaica

2 Radiology West, Montego Bay, Jamaica

3 Health Policy Department, Independent Health Policy Consultant, Christiana, Manchester, Jamaica

References

[1] Acworth, I.N., Mccabe, D.R. & Maher, T. (1997). The analysis of free radicals, their reaction products, and antioxidants, in: S.I. Baskin, H. Salem (Eds.), Oxidants, Antioxidants and Free Radicals, Taylor and Francis, Washington, DC, Chapter 2.

[2] Adams, S., Green, P., Claxton, R., Simcox, S., Williams, M.V., Walsh, K. & Leeuwenburgh, C. (2001). Reactive carbonyl formation by oxidative and non-oxidative pathways. Front Biosci Vol. 6, pp. A17-A24.

[3] Alp, N.J. & Channon, K.M. (2004). Regulation of endothelial nitric oxide synthase by tetrahydrobiopterin in vascular disease. Arterioscler Thromb Vasc Biol Vol. 24, pp. 413-420.

[4] American Diabetes Association (2010). Diagnosis and classification of diabetes mellitus. J Diabetes Care Vol 33, pp. S62-S69.

[5] American Diabetes Association (2004). Diagnosis and classification of diabetes mellitus. J Diabetes Care Vol. 27, pp. S5-S10.

[6] Andrew, P.J. & Mayer, B. (1999). Enzymatic function of nitric oxide synthases. Cardiovasc Res Vol. 43, pp. 521-531.

[7] Artenie, A., Artenie, R., Ungureanu, D. & Covic, A. (2004). Correlation between increase of oxidative stress and microalbuminuria in type 1 diabetic patients. Rev Med Chir Soc Med Nat Iasi Vol. 108, pp. 777-781.

[8] Astaneie, F., Afshari, M., Mojtahedi, A., Mostafalou, S., Zamani, M.J., Larijani, B. & Abdollahi, M. (2005).Total antioxidant capacity and levels of epidermal growth factor and nitric oxide in blood and saliva of insulin-dependent diabetic patients. Arch Med Res Vol. 36, pp. 376-381.

[9] Azevedo-Martins, A.K., Lortz, S., Lenzen, S., Curi, R., Eizirik, D.L. & Tiedge, M. Improvement of the mitochondrial antioxidant defense status prevents cytokine-induced nuclear factor-kappaB activation in insulin-producing cells. Diabetes Vol. 52, pp. 93-101.

[10] Baynes, J. & Thorpe, S. (1999). Role of oxidative stress in diabetic complications: a new perspective on an old paradigm. Diabetes Vol. 48, pp. 1-9.

[11] Baynes, J.W. (1991). Role of oxidative stress in development of complications in diabetes. Diabetes Vol. 40, pp. 405-412.

[12] Beckman, J.S. & Koppenol, W.H. (1996). Nitric oxide, superoxide, and peroxynitrite: the good, the bad, and ugly. Am J Physiol Vol. 271, pp. C1424-C1437.

[13] Benz, D., Cadet, P., Mantione, K., Zhu, W. & Stefano, G.B. (2002). Total nitric oxide and health - a free radical and scavenger of free radicals. Med Sci Monit Vol. 8, pp. RA1-RA4.

[14] Bierhaus, A., Hofmann, MA, Ziegler, R. & Nawrothn, P.P. (1998). AGEs and their interaction with AGE-receptors in vascular disease and diabetes mellitus 1. The AGE concept. Cardiovasc Res Vol. 37, pp. 586-600.

[15] Brownlee, M. (2001). Biochemistry and molecular cell biology of diabetic complications. Nature Vol. 414, pp. 813-820.

[16] Brownlee, M. (2005). The pathobiology of diabetic complications: a unifying mechanism. Diabetes. Vol. 54, pp. 1615-1625.

[17] Cameron, N.E. & Cotter, M.A. (1999). Effects of antioxidants on nerve and vascular dysfunction in experimental diabetes. Diabetes Res Clin Pract Vol. 45, pp. 137-146.

[18] Ceriello, A. (2006). Oxidative stress and diabetes-associated complications. Endocr Pract Vol. 12(Suppl 1), pp. 60-62.

[19] Ceriello, A. (2000). The post-prandial state and cardiovascular disease: relevance to diabetes mellitus. Diabetes Metab Res Rev Vol. 16, pp. 125-132.

[20] Ceriello, A., Morocutti, A., Mercuri, F., Quagliaro, L., Moro, M., Damante, G. & Viberti GC. (2000). Defective intracellular antioxidant enzyme production in type 1 diabetic patients with nephropathy. Diabetes Vol. 49, pp. 2170-2177.

[21] Ceriello, A., Quagliaro, L., Catone, B., Pascon, R., Piazzola, M., Bais, B., Marra, G., Tonutti, L., Taboga, C. & Motz, E. (2002). Role of hyperglycemia in nitrotyrosine postprandial generation. Diabetes Care Vol. 25, pp. 1439-1443.

[22] Channon, K.M. (2004). Tetrahydrobiopterin: regulator of endothelial nitric oxide synthase in vascular disease. Trends Cardiovasc Med Vol. 14, pp. 323-327.

[23] Chen, H., Li, X. & Epstein, P.N. (2005). MnSOD and catalase transgenes demonstrate that protection of islets from oxidative stress does not alter cytokine toxicity. Diabetes Vol. 54, pp. 1437-1446.

[24] Chong, Z.Z., Li, F. & Maiese, K. (2005). Oxidative stress in the brain: Novel cellular targets that govern survival during neurodegenerative disease. Prog Neurobiol Vol. 75, pp. 207-246.

[25] Cosentino, F., Hishikawa, K., Katusic, Z.S. & Lüscher, T.F. (1997). High glucose increases nitric oxide synthase expression and superoxide anion generation in human aortic endothelial cells. Circulation Vol. 96, pp. 25-28.

[26] Costacou, T., Zgibor, J.C., Evans, R.W., Tyurina, Y.Y., Kagan, V.E. & Orchard, T.J. (2006). Antioxidants and coronary artery disease among individuals with type 1 diabetes: Findings from the Pittsburgh Epidemiology of Diabetes Complications Study. J Diabetes Complications Vol. 20, pp. 387-394.

[27] Dalle-Donne, I., Ranieri, R., Roberto, C., Daniela, G. & Aldo, M. (2006). Biomarkers of oxidative damage in human disease. Clinical Chemistry Vol. 52, pp. 601-623.

[28] Dave, G.S. & Kalia, K. (2007). Hyperglycemia induced oxidative stress in type-1 and type-2 diabetic patients with and without nephropathy. Cell Mol Biol (Noisy-le-grand). Vol. 53, pp. 68-78.

[29] Delmastro, M.M. & Piganelli J. D. (2011). Oxidative stress and redox modulation potential in type 1 diabetes. Clin Dev Immunol Vol. 1.

[30] Di Mambro, V.M., Azzolini, A.E., Valim, Y.M. & Fonseca, M.J. (2003). Comparison of antioxidant activities of tocopherols alone and in pharmaceutical formulations. Int J Pharm Vol. 262, pp. 93-99.

[31] Djordjevic, A., Spasic, S., Jovanovic-Galovic, A., Djordjevic, R. & Grubor- Lajsic, G. (2004). Oxidative stress in diabetic pregnancy: SOD, CAT and GSH-Px activity and lipid peroxidation products. J Matern Fetal Neonatal Med Vol. 16, pp. 367-372.

[32] Dominguez, C., Ruiz, E., Gussinye, M. & Carrascisa, A. (1998). Oxidative stress at onset and in early stages of type I diabetes in children and adolescents. Diabetes Care Vol. 21, pp. 1736-1742.

[33] Drews, G., Krippeit-Drews, P. & Düfer M. (2010). Oxidative stress and beta-cell dysfunction. Pflugers Arch Vol. 460, pp. 703-718.

[34] Durrington, P.N., Mackness, B. & Mackness, M.I. (2001). Paraoxonase and atherosclerosis. Arterioscler Thromb Vasc Biol Vol. 21, pp.473-480.

[35] El Faramawy, S.M. & Rizk, R.A. (2011). Spectrophotometric studies on antioxidants-doped liposomes. J Am Sci Vol. 7, pp. 363-369.

[36] Elliott, T.G., Cockcroft, J.R., Groop, P.H., Viberti, G.C. & Ritter, J.M. (1993). Inhibition of nitric oxide synthesis in forearm vasculature of insulin- dependent diabetic patients: blunted vasoconstriction in patients with microalbuminuria. Clin Sci Vol. 85, pp. 687-693.

[37] Engler, M.M., Engler, M.B., Malloy, M.J., Chiu, E.Y., Schloetter, M.C., Paul, S.M., Stuehlinger, M., Lin, K.Y., Cooke, J.P., Morrow, J.D., Ridker, P.M., Rifai, N., Miller, E., Witztum, J.L. & Mietus-Snyder, M. (2003). Antioxidant vitamins C and E improve endothelial function in children with hyperlipidemia: Endothelial Assessment of Risk from Lipids in Youth (EARLY) Trial. Circulation Vol. 108, pp. 1059-1010.

[38] Erciyas, F., Taneli, F., Arslan, B. & Uslu, Y. (2004). Glycemic control, oxidative stress, and lipid profile in children with type 1 diabetes mellitus. Arch Med Res Vol. 35, pp. 134-40.

[39] Fang, Y-Z., Yang, S. & Wu, G. (2002). Free radicals, antioxidants and nutrition. Nutrition Vol. 18, pp. 872-879.

[40] Fatehi-Hassanabad, Z., Chan, C.B. & Furman, B.L. (2010). Reactive oxygen species and endothelial function in diabetes. European Journal of Pharmacology Vol. 636, pp. 8-17.

[41] Faure, P., Benhamou, P.Y., Perard, A., Halimi, S. & Roussel, A.M. (1995). Lipid perox-idationin insulin dependent diabetic patients with early retina degenerative lesions: Effects of an oral zinc supplementation. Eur J Clin Nutr Vol. 49, pp. 282-288.

[42] Ferretti, G., Bacchetti, T., Busni, D., Rabini, R.A. & Curatola G. (2004). Protective ef-fect of paraoxonase activity in high-density lipoproteins against erythrocyte mem-branes peroxidation: a comparison between healthy subjects and type 1 diabetic patients. Clin Endocrinol Metab. Vol. 89, pp. 2957-2962.

[43] Firoozrai, M., Nourbakhsh, M., Razzaghy-Azar, M. (2007). Erythrocyte susceptibility to oxidative stress and antioxidant status in patients with type 1 diabetes. Diabetes Res Clin Pract Vol. 77, pp. 427-432.

[44] Flores, L., Rodela, S., Abian, J., Clària, J. & Esmatjes, E. (2004). F2 isoprostane is al-ready increased at the onset of type 1 diabetes mellitus: effect of glycemic control. Metabolism Vol. 53, pp. 1118-1120.

[45] Frei, B. (1994). Reactive oxygen species and antioxidant vitamins: mechanisms of ac-tion. Am Med Vol. 97, pp. 5S-13S.

[46] Frei, B., Stocker, R., England, L. & Ames, B.N. (1990). Ascorbate: the most effective antioxidant in human blood plasma. Adv Exp Med Biol Vol. 264, pp. 155-163.

[47] Fubini, B. & Hubbard, A. (2003). Reactive oxygen species (ROS) and reactive nitrogen species (RNS) generation by silica in inflammation and fibrosis. Free Radic Biol Med. Vol. 34, pp. 1507-1516.

[48] Giannini, C., Lombardo, F., Currò, F., Pomilio, M., Bucciarelli, T., Chiarelli, F. & Mohn, A. (2007). Effects of high-dose vitamin E supplementation on oxidative stress and microalbuminuria in young adult patients with childhood onset type 1 diabetes mellitus. Diabetes Metab Res Rev Vol. 23, pp. 539-546.

[49] Gleisner, A., Martinez, L., Pino, R., Rojas, I.G., Martinez, A., Asenjo, S. & Rudolph, M.I. (2006). Oxidative stress markers in plasma and urine of prepubertal patients with type 1 diabetes mellitus. J Pediatr Endocrinol Metab Vol. 19, pp. 995-1000.

[50] Goodarzi, M.T., Navidi, A.A., Rezaei, M. & Babahmadi-Rezaei, H. (2010). Oxidative damage to DNA and lipids: correlation with protein glycation in patients with type 1 diabetes. J Clin Lab Anal. Vol. 24, pp. 72-76.

[51] Gorren, A.C. & Mayer, B. (2002). Tetrahydrobiopterin in nitric oxide synthesis: a nov-el biological role for pteridines. Curr Drug Metab Vol. 3, pp. 133-157.

[52] Gregus, Z., Fekete, T., Halaszi, E. & Klaassen, C.D. (1996). Lipoic acid impairs glycine conjugation of benzoic acid and renal excretion of benzoylglycine, Drug Metab Dis-pos Vol. 24, pp. 682-688.

[53] Gupta, S., Sharma, T.K., Kaushik, G.G. & Shekhawat, V.P. (2011). Vitamin E supple-mentation may ameliorate oxidative stress in type 1 diabetes mellitus patients. Clin Lab Vol. 57, pp. 379-386.

[54] Ha, H. & Lee, H.B. (2000). Reactive oxygen species as glucose signaling molecules in mesangial cells cultured under high glucose. Kidney Int Vol. Suppl 77, pp. S19-S25.

[55] Halliwell, B. (1994). Free radicals, antioxidants, and human disease: cause or consequence? Lancet Vol. 344, pp. 721-724.

[56] Halliwell, B. (1995). Oxidation of low-density lipoproteins: questions of initiation, propagation, and the effect of antioxidants. J Clin Nutr Vol. 61, pp. 670-677S.

[57] Han, Y., Randell, E., Vasdev, S., Gill, V., Gadag, V., Newhook, L.A., Grant, M. & Hagerty D. (2007). Plasma methylglyoxal and glyoxal are elevated and related to early membrane alteration in young, complication-free patients with Type 1 diabetes. Mol Cell Biochem Vol. 305, pp. 123-131.

[58] Ho, E. & Bray, T.M. (1999). Antioxidants, NFkappaB activation, and diabetogenesis. Proc Soc Exp Biol Med Vol. 222, pp. 205-213.

[59] Hoeldtke, R.D., Bryner, K.D. & VanDyke, K. (2011). Oxidative stress and autonomic nerve function in early type 1 diabetes. Clin Auton Res Vol. 21, pp. 19-28.

[60] Hogg, N. & Kalyanaraman, B. (1998). The use of NO gas in biological systems. Methods Mol Biol Vol. 100, pp. 231-234.

[61] Horie, S., Ishii, H. & Suga, T. (1981). Changes in peroxisomal fatty acid oxidation in diabetic rat

[62] liver. J Biochem (Tokyo) Vol. 90, pp. 1691-1696.

[63] Hsu, W.T., Tsai, L.Y., Lin, S.K., Hsiao, J.K. & Chen, B.H. (2006). Effects of diabetes duration and glycemic control on free radicals in children with type 1 diabetes mellitus. Ann Clin Lab Sci Vol. 36, pp. 174-178.

[64] Ignarro, L.J. (2002). Nitric oxide as a unique signaling molecule in the vascular system: a historical overview. J Physiol Pharmacol Vol. 53, pp. 503-514.

[65] Ischiropoulos, H. (1998). Biological tyrosine nitration: a pathophysiological function of nitric oxide and reactive oxygen species. Arch Biochem Biophys Vol. 356, pp. 1-11.

[66] Jain, S.K. & McVie, R. (1994). Effect of glycemic control race (white vs. black), and duration of diabetes on reduced glutathione content in erythrocytes of diabetic patients. Metabolism Vol. 43, pp. 306-309.

[67] Järvisalo, M.J., Raitakari, M., Toikka, J.O., Putto-Laurila, A., Rontu, R., Laine, S., Lehtimäki, T., Rönnemaa, T., Viikari, J. & Raitakari OT. Endothelial dysfunction and increased arterial intima-media thickness in children with type 1 diabetes. Circulation Vol. 109, pp. 1750-1755.

[68] Kaneto, H., Katakami, N., Kawamori, D., Miyatsuka, T., Sakamoto, K., Matsuoka, T.A., Matsuhisa, M. & Yamasaki, Y. (2007). Involvement of oxidative stress in the pathogenesis of diabetes. Antioxid Redox Signal Vol. 9, pp. 355-366.

[69] Kajikawa, M., Fujimoto, S., Tsuura, Y., Mukai, E., Takeda, T., Hamamoto, Y., Take-hiro, M., Fujita. J., Yamada, Y. & Seino Y. (2002). Ouabain suppresses glucose-in-duced mitochondrial ATP production and insulin release by generating reactive oxygen species in pancreatic islets. Diabetes Vol. 51, pp. 2522-2529.

[70] Kostolanská, J., Jakus, V. & Barák, L. (2009). HbA1c and serum levels of advanced glycation and oxidation protein products in poorly and well controlled children and adolescents with type 1 diabetes mellitus. J Pediatr Endocrinol Metab Vol. 22, pp. 433-442.

[71] Laight, D.W., Carrier, M.J. & Anggard, E.E. (2000). Antioxidants, diabetes and endo-thelial dysfunction. Cardiovasc Res Vol. 47, pp. 457-464.

[72] Lenzen, S., Drinkgern, J. &Tiedge, M. (1996). Low antioxidant enzyme gene expres-sion in pancreatic islets compared with various other mouse tissues. Free Radio Biol Med Vol. 20, pp. 463-466.

[73] Lepore, D.A., Shinkel, T.A., Fisicaro, N., Mysore, T.B., Johnson, L.E., d'Apice, A.J. & Cowan P.J. (2004). Enhanced expression of glutathione peroxidase protects islet beta cells from hypoxia-reoxygenation. Xenotransplantation Vol. 11, pp. 53-59.

[74] Li, F., Chong, Z.Z. & Maiese, K. (2006). Cell life versus cell longevity: the mysteries surrounding the NAD(+) precursor nicotinamide. Curr Med Chem Vol. 13, pp. 883-895.

[75] Likidlilid, A., Patchanans, N., Poldee, S. & Peerapatdit, T. (2007). Glutathione and glutathione peroxidase in type 1 diabetic patients. J Med Assoc Thai Vol. 90, pp. 1759-1767.

[76] Llorens, S. & Nava, E. (2003). Cardiovascular diseases and the nitric oxide pathway. Curr Vasc Pharmacol Vol. 1, pp. 335-346.

[77] Lu, S.C. (1999). Regulation of hepatic glutathione synthesis: current concepts and controversies, FASEB J Vol. 13, pp. 1169-1183.

[78] Mackness, B., Durrington, P.N., Boulton, A.J., Hine, D. & Mackness, M.I. (2002). Se-rum paraoxonase activity in patients with type 1 diabetes compared to healthy con-trols. Eur J Clin Invest Vol. 32, pp. 259-264.

[79] Macphee, C.H., Nelson, J.J. & Zalewski, A. (2005). Lipoprotein-associated phospholi-pase A2 as a target of therapy. Curr. Opin. Lipidol Vol. 16, pp. 442-446.

[80] Maechler, P., Jornot, L. & Wollheim, C.B. (1999). Hydrogen peroxide alters mitochon-drial activation and insulin secretion in pancreatic beta cells. Journal of Biological Chemistry, Vol. 274, pp. 27905-27913.

[81] Majchrzak, A., Zozulińska, D. & Wierusz-Wysocka, B. (2001). Evaluation of selected components in antioxidant systems of blood in patients with diabetes. Pol Merkur Lekarski Vol. 10, pp. 150-152.

[82] Maritim, A.C., Sanders, R.A. & Watkins, J.B. 3rd. (2003). Diabetes, oxidative stress, and antioxidants: a review. J Biochem Mol Toxicol Vol. 17, pp. 24-38.

[83] Mates, J.M., Perez-Gomez, C. & Castro, I.N. (1999). Antioxidant enzymes and human diseases. Clinical Biochemistry Vol. 32, pp. 595-603.

[84] Maxwell, S.R., Thomason, H., Sandler, D., Leguen, C., Baxter, M.A., Thorpe, G.H., Jones, A.F. & Barnett, A.H. (1997). Antioxidant status in patients with uncomplicated insulin-dependent and non-insulin-dependent diabetes mellitus. Eur J Clin Invest Vol. 27, pp. 484-490.

[85] Meister, A. Anderson, M.E. (1983). Glutathionne. Annu Rev Biochem Vol. 52, pp. 711-760.

[86] Menke, T., Niklowitz, P., Wiesel, T. & Andler, W. (2008). Antioxidant level and redox status of coenzyme Q10 in the plasma and blood cells of children with diabetes mellitus type 1. Pediatr Diabetes. Vol. 9, pp. 540-545.

[87] Miyata, T., Van Ypersele S.C., Kurokawa, K. & Baynes, J.W. (1999). Alterations in nonenzymatic biochemistry in uremia: origin and significance of .carbonyl stress. in long-term uremic complications. Kidney Int Vol. 55, pp. 389-399.

[88] Moore, K. & Roberts, L.J. 2nd. (1998). Measurement of lipid peroxidation. Free Radic Res Vol. 28, pp. 659-671.

[89] Mullarkey, C.J., Edelstein, D. & Brownlee, M. (1990). Free radical generation by early glycation products: a mechanism for accelerated atherogenesis in diabetes. Biochem Biophys Res Commun Vol. 173, pp. 932-939.

[90] Murakami, K., Kondo, T., Ohtsuka, Y., Fujiwara, Y., Shimada, M. & Kawakami, Y. (1989). Impairment of glutathione metabolism in erythrocytes from patients with diabetes mellitus. Metabolism Vol. 38, pp. 753-758.

[91] Mylona-Karayanni, C., Gourgiotis, D., Bossios, A. & Kamper, E.F. (2006). Oxidative stress and adhesion molecules in children with type 1 diabetes mellitus: a possible link. Pediatr Diabetes Vol. 7, pp. 51-59.

[92] Ndahimana, J., Dorchy, H. & Vertongen, E.C. (1996). Erythrocyte and plasma antioxidant activity in type I diabetes mellitus. Press Med Vol. 25, pp. 188-192.

[93] Newsholme, P., Haber, E. P., Hirabara, M., Rebelato, E. L., Procopio, J., Morgan, D., Oliveira-Emilio, H.C., Carpinelli, A. & Curi, R. (2007). Diabetes associated cell stress and dysfunction: role of mitochondrial and non-mitochondrial ROS production and activity. Journal of Physiology, Vol. 583, pp. 9-24.

[94] Niedowicz, D. & Daleke, D. (2005). The role of oxidative stress in diabetic complications. Cell Biochem Biophys Vol. 43, pp. 289-330.

[95] Niiya, Y., Abumiya, T., Shichinohe, H., Kuroda, S., Kikuchi, S., Ieko, M., Yamagishi, S.I., Takeuchi, M., Sato, T. & Iwasaki, Y. (2006). Susceptibility of brain microvascular

endothelial cells to advanced glycation end products-induced tissue factor upregulation is associated with intracellular reactive oxygen species. Brain Res Vol. 1108, pp. 179-187.

[96] Nishikawa, T., Edelstein, D., Du, X., Yamagishi, S., Matsumura, T., Kaneda, Y., Yorek, M., Beebe, D., Oates, P., Hammes, H., Giardino, I. & Brownlee, M. (2000). Normalizing mitochondrial superoxide production blocks three pathways of hyperglycemic damage. Nature Vol. 404, pp. 787-790.

[97] Nourooz-Zadeh, J., Tajaddini-Sarmadi, J., McCarthy, S., Betteridge, D.J. & Wolff, S.P. (1995). Elevated levels of authentic plasma hydroperoxides in NIDDM. Diabetes Vol. 44, pp. 1054-1058.

[98] Nowak, M., Wielkoszyński, T., Marek, B., Kos-Kudła, B., Swietochowska, E., Siemińska, L., Karpe, J., Kajdaniuk, D., Głogowska-Szelag, J. & Nowak, K. (2010). Antioxidant potential, paraoxonase 1, ceruloplasmin activity and C-reactive protein concentration in diabetic retinopathy. Clin Exp Med Vol. 10, pp. 185-192.

[99] Pacher, P. & Szabo, C. (2006). Role of peroxynitrite in the pathogenesis of cardiovascular complications of diabetes. Curr Opin Pharmacol Vol. 6, pp. 136-141.

[100] Pastore, A., Ciampalini, P., Tozzi, G., Pecorelli, L., Passarelli, C., Bertini, E. & Piemonte, F. (2012). All glutathione forms are depleted in blood of obese and type 1 diabetic children Diabetes Care Vol. 23, pp. 1182-1186.

[101] Pfeiffer, S., Lass, A., Schmidt, K. & Mayer, B. (2010). Protein tyrosine nitration in mouse peritoneal macrophages activated in vitro and in vivo: evidence against an essential role of peroxynitrite. FASEB J Vol. 15, pp. 2355-2364.

[102] Phillips, M., Cataneo, R.N., Cheema, T. & Greenberg, J. (2004). Increased breath biomarkers of oxidative stress in diabetes mellitus. Clin Chim Acta Vol. 344, pp. 189-194.

[103] Pitocco, D., Zaccardi, F., Di Stasio, E., Romitelli, F., Martini, F., Scaglione, G.L., Speranza, D., Santini, S., Zuppi, C. & Ghirlanda, G. (2009). Role of asymmetric-dimethyl-L-arginine (ADMA) and nitrite/nitrate (NOx) in the pathogenesis of oxidative stress in female subjects with uncomplicated type 1 diabetes mellitus. Diabetes Res Clin Pract Vol. 86, pp. 173-176.

[104] Prutz, W.A., Monig, H., Butler, J. & Land, E.J. (1985). Reactions of nitrogen dioxide in aqueous model systems: oxidation of tyrosine units in peptides and proteins. Arch Biochem Biophys Vol. 243, pp. 125-134.

[105] Rachek, L.I., Thornley, N.P., Grishko, V.I., LeDoux, S.P. & Wilson, G.L. (2006). Protection of INS-1 cells from free fatty acid-induced apoptosis by targeting hOGG1 to mitochondria. Diabetes Vol. 55, pp. 1022-1028.

[106] Ramana, K.V., Chandra, D., Srivastava, S., Bhatnagar, A. & Srivastava, S.K. (2003). Nitric oxide regulates the polyol pathway of glucose metabolism in vascular smooth muscle cells. The FASEB Journal Vol. 17, pp. 417-425.

[107] Reis, J.S., Veloso, C.A., Volpe, C.M., Fernandes, J.S., Borges, E.A., Isoni, C.A., Dos Anjos, P.M. & Nogueira-Machado, J.A. (2012). Soluble RAGE and malondialdehyde in type 1 diabetes patients without chronic complications during the course of the disease. Diab Vasc Dis Res Vol.

[108] Feb 15. [Epub ahead of print].

[109] Reiter, R.J., Tan, D.X., Osuna, C. & Gitto, E. (2000). Actions of melatonin in the reduction of oxidative stress. A review. J Biomed Sci Vol. 7, pp. 444-458.

[110] Reznick, A.Z., Shehadeh, N., Shafir, Y. & Nagler, R.M. (2006). Free radicals related effects and antioxidants in saliva and serum of adolescents with Type 1 diabetes mellitus. Arch Oral Biol Vol. 51, pp. 640-648.

[111] Roberts, L.J. & Morrow, J.D. (2000). Measurement of F_2-isoprostanes an index of oxidative stress in vivo. Free Radic Biol Med Vol. 28, pp. 505-513.

[112] Rodiño-Janeiro, B.K., González-Peteiro, M., Ucieda-Somoza, R., González-Juanatey, J.R. Alvarez, E. (2010). Glycated albumin, a precursor of advanced glycation end-products, up-regulates NADPH oxidase and enhances oxidative stress in human endothelial cells: molecular correlate of diabetic vasculopathy. Diabetes Metab Res Rev Vol. 26, pp. 550-558.

[113] Rolo, A.P. & Palmeira, C.M. (2006). Diabetes and mitochondrial function: role of hyperglycemia and oxidative stress. Toxicol Appl Pharmacol Vol. 212, pp. 167-178.

[114] Rosen, P., Nawroth, P.P., King, G., Moller, W., Tritschler, H.J. & Packer, L. (2001). The role of oxidative stress in the onset and progression of diabetes and its complications: A summary of a Congress Series sponsored by UNESCO MCBN, the American Diabetes Association and the German Diabetes Society. Diabetes Metab Res Rev Vol. 17, pp. 189-912.

[115] Ross, R. (1999). Atherosclerosis-an inflammatory disease. N Engl J Med Vol. 340, pp. 115-126.

[116] Salardi, S., Zucchini, S., Elleri, D., Grossi, G., Bargossi, A.M., Gualandi, S., Santoni, R., Cicognani, A. & Cacciari, E. (2004). High glucose levels induce an increase in membrane antioxidants, in terms of vitamin E and coenzyme Q10, in children and adolescents with type 1 diabetes. Diabetes Care Vol. 27, pp. 630-631.

[117] Samanthi, R.P.M., Rolf, E.A., Jelena, A.J., Maria, A. & Paresh, C.D. (2011). Novel conjugates of 1,3-diacylglycerol and lipoic acid: synthesis, DPPH assay, and RP-LC-MS-APCI analysis. J Lipids Vol. 10, pp. 1-10.

[118] Schmidt, A.M., Hori, O., Cao, R., Yan, S.D., Brett, J., Wautier, J.L., Ogawa, S., Kuwabara, K., Matsumoto, M. & Stern, D. (1996). RAGE: a novel cellular receptor for advanced glycation end products. Diabetes Vol. 45(Suppl 3), pp. S77-S80.

[119] Simm, A., Münch, G., Seif, F., Schenk, O., Heidland, A., Richter, H., Vamvakas, S. & Schinzel R. (1997). Advanced glycation endproducts stimulate the MAP-kinase pathway in tubuluscell line LLC-PK1. FEBS Lett Vol. 410. pp. 481-484.

[120] Siu, A.W. & To, C.H. (2002). Nitric oxide and hydroxyl radical-induced retinal lipid peroxidation in vitro. Clin Exp Optom. Vol. 85, pp. 378-382.

[121] Skyrme-Jones, R.A., O'Brien, R.C., Berry, K.L. & Meredith, I.T. (2000). Vitamin E supplementation improves endothelial function in type I diabetes mellitus: a randomized, placebo-controlled study. J Am Coll Cardiol Vol. 36, pp. 94-102.

[122] Spitaler, M.M. 7 Graier, W.F. (2002). Vascular targets of redox signalling in diabetes mellitus. Diabetologia Vol. 45, pp. 476-494.

[123] Steinberg, H.O. & Baron, A.D. (2002). Vascular function, insulin resistance and fatty acids. Diabetologia Vol. 45, pp. 623-634.

[124] Suys, B., de Beeck, L.O., Rooman, R., Kransfeld, S., Heuten, H., Goovaerts, I., Vrints, C., de Wolf, D., Matthys, D. & Manuel-y-Keenoy, B. (2007). Impact of oxidative stress on the endothelial dysfunction of children and adolescents with type 1 diabetes mellitus: protection by superoxide dismutase? Pediatr Res Vol. 62, pp. 456-461.

[125] Telci, A., Cakatay, U., Salman, S., Satman, I. & Sivas, A. (2000). Oxidative protein damage in early stage Type 1 diabetic patients. Diabetes Res Clin Pract Vol. 50, pp. 213-223.

[126] Thornalley, P.J. (2002). Glycation in diabetic neuropathy: characteristics, consequences, causes, and therapeutic options. Int Rev Neurobiol Vol. 50, pp. 37-57.

[127] Tsukahara, H., Sekine, K., Uchiyama, M., Kawakami, H., Hata, I., Todoroki, Y., Hiraoka, M., Kaji, M., Yorifuji, T, Momoi, T., Yoshihara, K., Beppu, M. & Mayumi, M. (2003). Formation of advanced glycosylation end products and oxidative stress in young patients with type 1 diabetes. Pediatr Res Vol. 54, pp. 419-424.

[128] Turk, Z. (2010). Glycotoxines, carbonyl stress and relevance to diabetes and its complications. Physiol Res Vol. 59, pp. 147-156.

[129] Van Lenten, B. J., Navab, M., Shih, D., Fogelman, A. M. & Lusis, A. J. (2001). The role of high-density lipoproteins in oxidation and inflammation. Trends Cardiovasc Med Vol. 11, pp. 155-161.

[130] Watson, A.D., Berliner, J.A., Hama, S.Y., La Du, B.N., Faull, K.F., Fogelman, A.M. & Navab, M. (1995). Protective effect of high density lipoprotein associated paraoxonase. Inhibition of the biological activity of minimally oxidized low density lipoprotein. J Clin Invest Vol. 6, pp. 2882-2891.

[131] Watson, D. & Loweth, A.C. (2009). Oxidative and nitrosative stress in beta-cell apoptosis: their contribution to beta-cell loss in type 1 diabetes mellitus. Br J Biomed Sci Vol. 66, pp. 208-215.

[132] Wautier, M.P., Chappey, O., Corda, S., Stern, D.M., Schmidt, A.M & Wautier, J.L. (2001). Activation of NADPH oxidase by AGE links oxidant stress to altered gene expression via RAGE. Am J Physiol Vol. 280, pp. E685-E694.

[133] Weber, P., Bendich, A. & Machlin, L.J. (1997). Vitamin E and human health: rationale for determining recommended intake levels. Nutrition Vol. 13, pp. 450-460.

[134] Wegner, M., Pioruńska-Stolzmann, M., Araszkiewicz, A., Zozulińska-Ziołkiewicz, D. & Wierusz-Wysocka, B. (2011). Evaluation of paraoxonase 1 arylesterase activity and lipid peroxide levels in patients with type 1 diabetes. Pol Arch Med Wewn Vol. 121, pp. 448-455.

[135] West, I.C. (2000). Radicals and oxidative stress in diabetes. Diabetic Med Vol. 17, pp. 171-180.

[136] Wild, S., Roglic, G., Green, A., Sicree, R. & King, H. (2004). Global prevalence of diabetes: estimates for the year 2000 and projections for 2030. Diabetes Care Vol. 27, pp. 1047-1053.

[137] Winterbourn, C.C. & Metodiewa, D. (1994). The reaction of superoxide with reduced glutathione. Arch Biochem Biophys Vol. 314, pp. 284-290.

[138] Witko-Sarsat, V., Friedlander, M., Capeillère-Blandin, C., Nguyen-Khoa, T., Nguyen, A.T., Zingraff, J., Jungers, P., Descamps-Latscha, B. (1996). Advanced oxidation protein products as a novel marker of oxidative stress in uraemia. Kidney Int Vol. 49, pp. 1304-1313.

[139] Yamagishi, S. (2009). Advanced glycation end products and receptor-oxidative stress system in diabetic vascular complications. Ther Apher Dial Vol. 13, p. 534-539.

[140] Yan, S.D., Schmidt, A.M., Anderson, G.M., Zhang, J., Brett, J., Zou, Y.S., Pinsky, D. & Stern, D. (1994). Enhanced cellular oxidant stress by the interaction of advanced glycation endproducts with their receptors/ binding proteins. J Biol Chem Vol. 269, pp. 9889-9897.

[141] Yung, L.M., Leung, F.P., Yao, X., Chen, Z.Y. & Huang, Y. (2006). Reactive oxygen species in vascular wall. Cardiovascular and Hematological Disorders Vol. 6, pp. 1-19.

[142] Zivić, S., Vlaski, J., Kocić, G., Pesić, M., Ciric, V. & Durić, Z. (2008). The importance of oxidative stress in pathogenesis of type 1 diabetes-determination of catalase activity in lymphocytes of diabetic patients. Med Pregl Vol. 61, pp. 458-463.

Chapter 9

Endoplasmic Reticulum (ER) Stress in the Pathogenesis of Type 1 Diabetes

Jixin Zhong

Additional information is available at the end of the chapter

1. Introduction

As one of the major health problems in the world, diabetes affects over 346 million people worldwide. In United States alone, according to the statistical fact sheet released 2011 by American Diabetes Association, 25.8 million children and adults accounting for 8.3% of the population are affected by diabetes. Unfortunately, the therapy of diabetes remains unsatisfied despite of extensive studies in the last decades. Diabetes can be categorized into two main types: type 1 and type 2. Type 1 diabetes mellitus, used to known as juvenile diabetes, is typically developed in children and juveniles. Despite the increasing rate of Type 2 diabetes in the United States, type 1 diabetes accounts for over 2/3 of new adolescent diabetes diagnoses. Although most commonly presented in childhood, type 1 diabetes also accounts for 5-10% cases of adult diabetes (1). Recent epidemiologic studies revealed that the incidence for type 1 diabetes in most regions of the world has increased by 2-5% (2).

Unlike type 2 diabetes, which is caused by the loss of insulin sensitivity, type 1 diabetes is caused by insulin deficiency following destruction of insulin-producing pancreatic β cells. Autoimmune-mediated β cell death has been considered as the major cause of β-cell loss in type 1 diabetes. However, the underlying mechanisms are not fully understood. Accumulating evidence suggests an involvement of endoplasmic reticulum (ER) stress in multiple biological processes during the development of type 1 diabetes. Pancreatic β cells exhibit exquisite sensitivity to ER stress due to their high development in order to secrete large amounts of insulin. There is also evidence supporting that ER stress regulates the immune cell functionality and cytokine production that is relevant to autoimmune processes in type 1 diabetes. Furthermore, β cell loss caused by autoimmune attack results in an increased ER burden on the rest pancreatic β cells and induces unfolded protein response (UPR) and ER stress, which further exacerbates β cell death. Here I will summarize the functional involvement of ER stress in the pathogenesis of type 1 diabetes and the potential underlying mechanisms.

2. Pancreatic β cell and blood glucose regulation

2.1. Blood glucose regulation by pancreas

The major cause of type 1 diabetes is loss of insulin-secreting pancreatic β cell and insulin inadequacy (3;4). For a better understanding of the pathogenesis of type 1 diabetes, the regulatory mechanisms of blood glucose by pancreaswill briefly introduced. Blood glucose level is closely regulated in order to provide a homeostatic microenvironment for tissues and organs. According to the American Diabetes Association, a normal fasting blood glucose level is between 70 to 100 mg/dL, and the recommended fasting level is to aim for 70 to 130 mg/dL and less than 180 mg/dL after meals (5). Blood glucose is monitored by the cells in the islets of Langerhans (6). Islets of Langerhans are clusters of pancreatic cells that execute the endocrine function of pancreas. They contain the following 4 types of cells, in order of abundance: β cells, α cells, δ cells, and γ cells. Pancreatic β cells and α cells make up about 70% and 17% of islet cells respectively, and both of them are responsible for the blood glucose regulation by producing insulin (β cells) and glucagon (α cells) (6). Pancreatic δ cells produce somatostatin which has a major inhibitory effect, including on pancreatic juice production. Pancreatic γ cells secrete pancreatic polypeptide that is responsible for reducing appetite.

Insulin and glucagon have opposite functions on glucose regulation. They keep blood glucose level in a normal range by coordinating with each other (Figure 1). After a meal, the digestive system breaks down the carbohydrates to small sugar molecules, mainly glucose. The glucose is then absorbed across the intestinal wall and travel to the circulating bloodstream. Pancreatic β cells sense increased blood glucose level by taking up glucose through GLUT2, a glucose transporter. The metabolism of glucose in β cells leads to the increase of ATP/ADP ratio, which causes the closing of ATP-sensitive potassium channels and further leads to the open of calcium channels on membrane. The resulting increase of intracellular calcium concentration promotes the secretion of insulin into circulation of blood. Circulating insulin then acts on cells in a variety of tissues including liver, muscle, and fat through interacting with insulin receptor on the cell membrane. Insulin signaling induces the translocation of glucose transporter GLUT4 to cell membrane of muscle cells and adipocytes, leading to the uptake of glucose into cells as an energy source. In addition, insulin signaling also stimulates the conversion of glucose into glycogen, a process called glycogenesis, in liver. Therefore, insulin lowers blood glucose level by promoting glycogenesis and glucose uptake by peripheral tissues (7). In contrast, a drop in blood glucose caused by starving or other situations like extreme exercise suppresses the secretion of insulin by β cells and stimulates α cells of pancreas to release glucagon. Glucagon acts on liver and promotes glucose production by the breakdown of glycogen to glucose (called glycogenolysis), resulting in the increase of blood glucose.

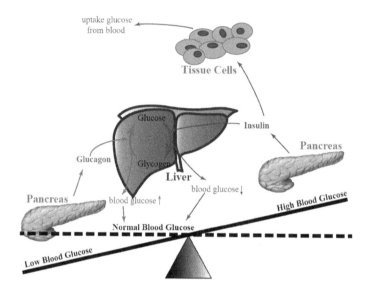

Figure 1 Homeostatic regulation of blood glucose by pancreas

Figure 1. Homeostatic regulation of blood glucose by pancreas. Pancreas is the major organ responsible for maintaining the blood glucose homeostasis. Increase of blood glucose level can be sensed by GLUT2 on β cells, a glucose transporter. The metabolism of glucose in β cells promotes the secretion of insulin into circulation of blood. Circulating insulin then increases the glucose uptake by a variety of tissues including liver, muscle, and fat. In liver, insulin signaling also stimulates the conversion of glucose into glycogen, a process called glycogenesis. Both glycogenesis and glucose uptake by peripheral tissues can lead to a decrease of glucose level in blood stream. In contrast, a drop of blood glucose level suppresses the secretion of insulin by β cells and stimulates α cells to release glucagon. Glucagon acts on liver and promotes glucose production by the breakdown of glycogen to glucose, a process called glycogenolysis, and results in the increase of blood glucose.

2.2. Pancreatic β cells and insulin biosynthesis

Either insulin deficiency or insulin inefficiency can cause diabetes. As the only cell type producing insulin, β cell plays a critical role in the development of diabetes. In type 1 diabetes, autoimmune-mediated destruction of β cell leads to insufficient insulin production and inability of cells to take up glucose. In contrast, type 2 diabetes is caused by loss of insulin sensitivity. In response to insulin resistance, the body secretes more insulin to overcome the impaired insulin action. However, pancreatic β cells fail to secrete sufficient insulin to overcome insulin resistance in some individuals, resulting in type 2 diabetes (8;9). Therefore, dysfunction of β cell exists in both types of diabetes.

Pancreatic β cell is specialized for production of insulin to control blood glucose level. In response to hyperglycemia, insulin is secreted from a readily available pool in β cells. In the meantime, the secretion of insulin activates the biosynthesis of insulin (10). Insulin is first

synthesized as preproinsulin with a signal peptide in the ribosomes of the rough endoplasmic reticulum. Preproinsulin is translocated into ER lumen by interaction of signal peptide
with signal recognition particle on the ER membrane. Preproinsulin is converted to proinsulin by removing the signal peptide forming three disulfide bonds in the ER. Proinsulin is
then translocated into Golgi apparatus and packaged into secretory granules that are close
to the cell membrane. In the secretory granules, proinsulin is cleaved into equal amounts of
insulin and C-peptide (Figure 2). Insulin is accumulated and stored in the secretory granules. When the β cell is appropriately stimulated, insulin is secreted from the cell by exocytosis (11). As the major site for protein synthesis, ER plays an important role in insulin
biosynthesis. To fulfill the requirement for secreting large amount of insulin, the pancreatic
β cells are equipped with highly developed ER, leading to the vulnerability of β cell to ER
stress (12). In type 1 diabetes, the loss of β cell increases the burden of insulin secretion on
the residual β cells. On the on hand, this compensated action is beneficial for the control of
blood glucose. On the other hand, it also increases the ER burden of residual β cells, which
further exacerbates β cell death.

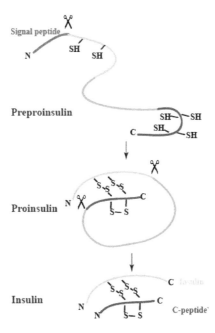

Figure 2. Biosynthesis of insulin in β cell. In the ribosomes of rough endoplasmic reticulum, insulin is first synthesized as a precursor, preproinsulin. Preproinsulin has a signal peptide that directs it to translocate into ER lumen by
interacting with signal recognition particle on the ER membrane. In ER lumen, preproinsulin is converted to proinsulin
by removing the signal peptide and forming three disulfide bonds. Proinsulin is then translocated into Golgi apparatus
and packaged into secretory granules where it is cleaved into equal amounts of insulin and C-peptide. After synthesis,
insulin is stored in the secretory granules and secreted from the cell until the β cell is appropriately stimulated.

3. Biological characterization of endoplasmic reticulum (ER) and ER stress

3.1. Endoplasmic reticulum

Endoplasmic Reticulum (ER) is an organelle of eukaryotic cells that is responsible for the facilitation of protein folding and assembly (13-15), manufacture of the membranes(16), biosynthesis of lipid and sterol, storage of intracellular Ca^{2+}, and transport of synthesized proteins in cisternae.It is a membranous network of tubules, vesicles, and cisternae that are interconnected by the cytoskeleton.The ER is well developed in endocrine cells such as β cell in which large amounts of secretory proteins are synthesized.

ER is categorized into two types: rough endoplasmic reticulum (RER) and smooth endoplasmic reticulum (SER). As featured by its name, RER looks bumpy and rough under a microscope due to the ribosomes on the outer surfaces of the cisternae. RER is in charge for protein synthesis. The newly synthesized proteins are folded into 3-dimensional structure in RER and sent to Golgi complex or membrane via small vesicles. In contrast, SER appears to have a smooth surface under the microscope as it does not have ribosomes on its cisternae. SER is responsible for the synthesis of lipids and steroids, regulation of calcium concentration, attachment of receptors on cell membrane proteins, and detoxification of drugs. It is found commonly in places such as in the liver and muscle. It is important for the liver to detoxify poisonous substances. Sarcoplasmic reticulum is a special type of SER. It is found in smooth and striated muscle, and is important for the regulation of calcium levels. It sequesters a large store of calcium and releases them when the muscle cell is stimulated.

3.2. Unfolded protein response and ER stress

ER stress is defined as the cellular responses to the disturbances of normal function of ER. The most common cause of ER stress is protein mis-folding. ER is the place where newly produced proteins fold into 3-dimensional conformation which is essential for their biological function. The sensitive folding environment could be disturbed by a variety of pathological insults like environmental toxins, viral infection, and inflammation. In addition to pathological insults, it can also be induce by many physiological processes such as overloaded protein biosynthesis on ER, For example, in case of type 1 diabetes, increased insulin synthesis in residual β cell exceeds the folding capacity of ER, resulting in the accumulation of unfolded insulin. The accumulation of unfolded or mis-folded proteins in the ER leads a protective pathway to restore ER function, termed as unfolded protein response (UPR).

Protein folding requires a serial of ER-resident protein folding machinery. A special type of proteins called chaperones is used as a quality control mechanism in the ER. As the major mechanisms to promote protein folding, chaperones assist protein folding by interacting with the newly synthesized proteins.In addition,chaperones also help to break down unfolded or incorrectly folded proteins in the ER via a process called ER associated degradation.The monitoring mechanism ensures the correct protein folding in the ER. The unfolded proteins usually have a higher number of hydrophobic surface patches than that of proteins with native conformation (17). Thus, unfolded proteins are prone to aggregate with each other in a crowed environment and directed to degradative pathway (18). Molecular chaperones in the ER preferentially interact with hydrophobic surface patches on unfolded proteins and create a private folding environment by preventing unfolded proteins from interaction and aggregation with other unfolded proteins. In addition, the concentration of Ca^{2+} in ER also impairs protein folding by inhibiting the activity of ER-resident chaperones and foldases (19-22). ER is the major site for Ca^{2+} storage in mammalian cells. The concentration of Ca^{2+} in ER is thousands times higher than that in the cytosol (23). Most chaperones and foldases in ER are vigorous Ca^{2+} binding proteins. Their activity, therefore, is affected by the concentration of Ca^{2+} in ER.

Exhaustion of the protein folding machineries or insufficient energy supply increases the accumulation of unfolded or mis-folded proteins in ER, which is responsible for the activation of UPR. UPR is a protective mechanism by which it monitors and maintains the homeostasis of ER. Various physiological and pathological insults such as increased protein synthesis, failure of posttranslational modifications, nutrient/glucose starvation, hypoxia, and alterations in calcium homeostasis, can result in the accumulation of unfolded or mis-folded proteins in ER which further causes ER stress (24).For example, altered expression of antithrombin III (25;26) or blood coagulation factor VIII (27;28), may result in the exhaustion of protein folding machinery and thus induces UPR. Some physiological processes such as the differentiation of B lymphocytes into plasma cells along with the development of highly specialized secretory capacity can also cause unfolded protein accumulation and activate UPR (29-31). In response to those physiological and pathological insults, cells initiate UPR process to get rid of the unfolded or mis-folded proteins. For instance, UPR can increase the folding capacity by up-regulating ER chaperones and foldases, as well as attenuate the biosynthetic burden through down-regulating the expression of secreted proteins (32-34). In addition, UPR also eliminates unfolded or mis-folded proteins by activating ER associated degradation process (35-37). However, once the stress is beyond the compensatory capacity of UPR, the cells would undergo apoptosis. As such, UPR and ER stress are reported to be implicated in a variety of pathological processes, including diabetes, neurodegenerative diseases, pathogenic infections, atherosclerosis, and ischemia (24;38).

In addition to protein folding, a variety of post-translational modifications including N-linked glycosylation, disulfide bond formation, lipidation, hydroxylation, and oligomerization, occur in ER. Disruption of those post-translational modifications can also result in the accumulation of incorrectly folded proteins and thereby induce UPR or ER stress. For example, glucose deprivation impairs the process for N-linked protein glycosylation and thus leads to ER stress (39).

3.3. ER stress pathways

As a protective mechanism during ER stress, UPR initiates a variety of process to ensure the homeostasis of ER. UPR can be mediated by three major pathways, which are initiated by the three transmembrane signaling proteins located on the ER membrane. Those transmembrane proteins function as a bridge linking cytosol and ER with their C-terminal in the cytosol and N-terminal in the ER lumen. The N-terminal is usually engaged by an ER resident chaperone BiP (Grp78) to avoid aggregation. When unfolded proteins accumulate in ER, chaperons are occupied by unfolded proteins and release those transmembrane signaling proteins. There are three axes of signals that are initiated by the pancreatic endoplasmic reticulum kinase (PERK), the inositol-requiring enzyme 1 (IRE1), and the activating transcription factor 6 (ATF6) respectively. The release of these proteins from BiP triggers UPR and ER stress (Figure 3).

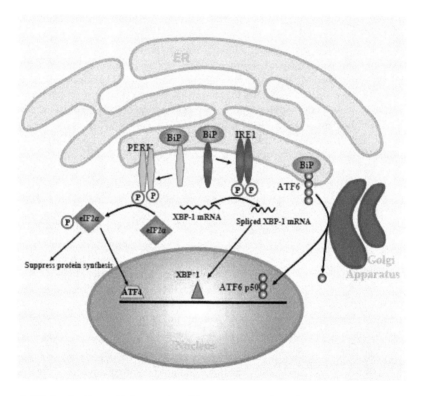

Figure 3. UPR signal pathways. Under normal condition, PERK, IRE1, and ATF6 binding to the ER chaperone BiP to remain inactive state. Upon the accumulation of unfolded proteins, BiP preferentially binds to the unfolded proteins, leading to the release of PERK, IRE1, and ATF6. PERK becomes oligomerized and activated once released from BiP, and subsequently phosphorylates eIF2α. The phosphorylation of eIF2α results in the suppression of the overall transcription of mRNAs and selectively enhanced transcription of genes implicated in UPR such as the ATF4 mRNA. Similar to PERK, IRE1 is dimerized and activated after released from BiP. Activated IRE1 induces XBP-1 by enhancing the splicing of its mRNA. XBP-1 enhances UPR by regulating the transcription of its target genes. The detachment of ATF6 from BiP results in the translocation of ATF6 to the Golgi apparatus and cleavage of ATF6. Cleaved ATF6 then translocates into the nucleus and initiates the transcription of target genes.

PERK/eIF2α/ATF4 axis: PERK is a type I transmembrane Ser/Thr protein kinase uniquely present in ER. In response to ER stress, the binding of unfolded proteins to BiP leads to the release of PERK from BiP. Once released from BiP, PERK becomes oligomerized and auto-phosphorylated. As a result, PERK inactivates eukaryotic initiation factor 2α (eIF2α) by the phosphorylation of Ser51 to inhibit mRNA translation and protein load on ER (34;40). In ad-dition, phosphorylated eIF2α also promotes the expression of stress-induced genes includ-ing the transcription factors ATF4 and CCAAT/enhancer binding protein (C/EBP) homologous protein (CHOP) (41). Deficiency of PERK results in an abnormally elevated protein synthesis in response to the accumulation of unfolded proteins in ER.

IRE1/XBP-1 axis: IRE1 is another axis of signal involved in UPR. There are 2 isoforms of IRE1: IRE1α and IRE1β. IRE1α is expressed in most cells and tissues, while IRE1β is restrict-ed in intestinal epithelial cells (42;43). Once disassociated with BiP, IRE1 becomes activated. Activated IRE1 possesses endoribonuclease activity and cleaves 26 nucleotides from the mRNA encoding X-box binding protein-1 (XBP-1), resulting in the increased production of XBP-1 (44). XBP-1 is a transcriptional factor belonging to basic leucine zipper transcription factorfamily. It heterodimerizes with NF-Y and enhances gene transcription by binding to the ER stress enhancer and unfolded protein response element in the promoters of targeted genes involved in ER expansion, protein maturation, folding and export from the ER, and degradation of mis-folded proteins (44-49). In addition, IRE1α also mediates the degradation of ER-targeted mRNAs, thus decreasing the ER burden (50).

ATF6 axis: The third axis of ER stress signal is mediated by ATF6. Unlike PERK and IRE1 which oligomerize upon UPR, ATF6 translocates into the Golgi apparatus after released from BiP. The transmembrane domain is then cleaved in the Golgi apparatus (51). The 50-kDa cleaved ATF6 is relocated into the nucleus where it binds to the ER stress response ele-ment CCAAT(N)9CCACG to regulate the expression of targeted genes. For example, once released from the ER membrane, ATF6 enhances the transcription of XBP-1 mRNA which is further regulated by IRE1 (44). In addition, ATF6 also increases the expression of the two major chaperon systems in the ER: calnexin/calreticulin and BiP/GRP94 (44;52;53).

4. The implication of ER stress in autoimmune responses

4.1. ER stress and innate immune response

The importance of innate immunity was highlighted in the pathophysiology of type 1 diabe-tes (54-57). Type 1 diabetes was initially considered a T-cell-mediated autoimmune disease (58), in which T-cell was believed as the major immune cell causing β cell destruction while the involvement of innate immune response has been ignored for a long time. However, re-cent studies suggest a critical role of innate immune responses in the development of type 1 diabetes (54;55). As the first line of defense mechanism, innate immunity is implicated in the initiation as well as the progression of autoimmune responses against pancreatic β cell.

Innate immune response is regulated by elements of the UPR pathway (59). For example, Cyclic-AMP-responsive-element-binding protein H(CREBH), an ER stress-associated tran-scription factor, regulates the expression of serum amyloid P-component and C-reactive

protein, the two critical factors implicated in innate immune responses. Like ATF6, CREBH is an ER-membrane-bound protein. In response to ER stress, CREBH release an N-terminal fragment and transit to nucleus to regulate the expression of target genes. Innate immune response, in turn, regulates the expression of CREBH through inflammatory cytokines such as IL-1β and IL-6 (60). The development of dendritic cells, the major innate immune cells, is also regulated by ER stress response (61). High levels of mRNA splicing for XBP-1 are found in dendritic cell, and mice deficient in XBP-1 show defective differentiation of dendritic cell. Both conventional (CD11b⁺ CD11c+
) and plasmacytoid dendritic cells (B220⁺ CD11c+
) are decreased by >50%. Dendritic cells deficient for XBP-1 are vulnerable to ER stress-in-duced apoptosis (61). Moreover, the secretion of inflammatory cytokine IL-23 by dendritic cell also involves ER stress response. CHOP, a UPR mediator, can directly bind to the *IL-23* gene and regulate its transcription. ER stress combined with Toll-like receptor (TLR) ago-nists was found to markedly increase the mRNA of IL-23 p19 subunit and the secretion of IL-23, while knockdown of CHOP suppressed the induction of IL-23 by ER stress and TLR signaling (62).

The association of ER stress with innate immune response is confirmed in many disease models. Richardson and coworkers reported that innate immune response induced by *P. aeruginosa* infection causes ER stress in *C. elegans*, and loss-of-function mutations of XBP-1 lead to larval lethality (63). In consistent with that, polymorphisms of *XBP-1* gene were found to be associated with Crohn's disease and ulcerative colitis in humans (64), the two autoimmune diseases share similar properties with type 1 diabetes. Lack of XBP-1 in intesti-nal epithelial cells may induce Paneth cell dysfunction which further results in impaired mucosal defense to *Listeria monocytogenes* and increased sensitivity to colitis (64).

In addition to IRE1/XBP-1 axis, PERK/eIF2α/ATF4 axis of UPR is also associated with innate response. TLR signaling, the most important innate signaling pathway, can induce selective suppression of the PERK/eIF2α/ATF-4/CHOP axis of UPR pathway (65). The activation of TLR decreases eIF2α-induced ATF4 translation. For instance, pretreatment of LPS, an ago-nist for TLR4, attenuated ATF4/CHOP signaling and prevented systemic ER stress-induced apoptosis in macrophages, renal tubule cells, and hepatocytes (65). In contrast, loss of Toll-IL-1R-containing adaptor inducing IFN-β (TRIF), an important adapter for TLR signaling, abrogated the protective effect of LPS on renal dysfunction and hepatosteatosis induced by ER stress, suggesting that TLR signaling suppresses ATF4/CHOP via a TRIF-dependent pathway (65).

4.2. ER stress and adaptive immune response

The presence of β cell specific autoantibodies is a marker for autoimmune diabetes (66). IRE1/XBP1 axis is required for the differentiation of antibody-producing B lymphocytes. IRE1 is necessary for the Ig gene rearrangement, production of B cell receptors, and lympho-poiesis. The expression multiple UPR components including BiP, GRP94, and XBP-1 is upregulated during the differentiation of B cells (67). Mice with a deficiency of IRE1 in hematopoietic cells have a defective differentiation of pro-B cells towards pre-B cells (68). XBP-1, an IRE1 downstream molecule, is also involved in the differentiation of B cell and antibody production by mature B cells. It was found that the engagement of B-cell receptor induces ubiquitin-mediated degradation of BCL-6, a repressor for B-lymphocyte-induced maturation protein 1 (69), while B-lymphocyte-induced maturation protein 1 negatively reg-ulates the expression of B-cell-lineage-specific activator protein (70), a repressor for XBP-1 (71). In line with these results, B lymphocytes deficient in B-lymphocyte-induced maturation protein 1 failed to express XBP-1 in response to LPS stimulation (72). The expression of XBP-1 is rapidly up-regulated when B cells differentiate into plasma cells. Furthermore, XBP-1is able to initiate plasma cell differentiation when introduced into B-lineage cells. XBP-1-deficient lymphoid chimeras have a defective B-cell-dependent immune response due to the absence of immunoglobulin and plasma cells (30). In addition to IRE1/XBP-1 axis, ATF6 axis may also implicated in the differentiation of B cells, as increased ATF6 cleavage is found in differentiating B cells (67). However, PERK axis does not seem to be involved in the B-cell differentiation and maturation (68;73).

Activation of T lymphocyte, another important adaptive immune cell, seems also involves UPR. TCR engagement, the first T cell activation signal, induces the expression of ER chap-erons including BiP and GRP94. Inhibition of protein kinase C, a serine/threonine protein kinase downstream of TCR signaling, suppresses the activation of ER stress response in-duced by T cell activation (74). IRE1/XBP-1 axis regulates the differentiation of effector CD8[+] T cell. IRE1/XBP-1 pathway is activated in effector CD8[+] T cell during acute infection. IL-2 promotes XBP-1 mRNA transcription, while TCR ligation induces the splicing of XBP-1 mRNA. The differentiation of CD8[+] T cell is reduced by suppression of XBP-1 (75). Other than IRE1/XBP-1, CHOP is also involved in the functionality of T cells. A recent report sug-gests GTPase of the immunity-associated protein 5 (Gimap5) mutation in BioBreeding dia-betes-prone rat, a model for type 1 diabetes, leads to ER stress and thus induces spontaneous apoptosis of T cells. Inhibition of CHOP protects Gimap5[-/-] T cells from ER stress-induced apoptosis (76).

4.3. ER stress regulates cytokine production

Cytokine production is an important inflammatory process in response to insults of pathogens, mutated self-antigens or tissue damage. ER stress is interconnected with the induction of inflammatory cytokines through multiple mechanisms including reactive oxygen species (ROS), NFκB and JNK (Figure 4). ROS are defined as highly reactive small molecules with unpaired electrons. They are important mediators of inflammatory response., Oxidative stress, caused by the accumulation of ROS, was confirmed to be as-sociated with ER stress (77). For example, the disulphide bond formation during the process of protein folding requires oxidizing condition (78). Therefore, increased protein folding load may lead to oxidative stress. The PERK axis of UPR is able to activate anti-oxidant pathway by promoting ATF4 and nuclear factor-erythroid-derived 2-related factor 2 (NRF2) (79;80). Therefore, deficiency of PERK markedly increases ROS accumulation in response to toxic chemicals (79;81). The IRE1 axis of UPR can activate NFκB, a key regulator in inflammation, by recruiting IκB kinase (82). As a result, loss of IRE1 reduces the activation of NFκB activation and production of TNF-α (82). In addition, the IRE1 axis can also activate JNK, and subsequently induce the expression of inflammatory genes by activating activator protein 1 (AP1) (83). ATF6, the third axis of UPR signaling, can also activate NFκB pathway and induce inflammatory response. Therefore, suppression of ATF6 reduces NFκB activation caused by BiP degradation (84).

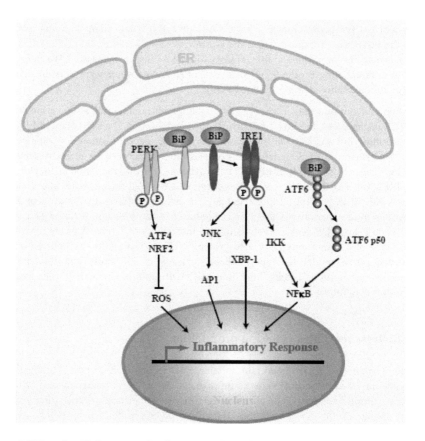

Figure 4. UPR-mediated inflammatory signaling. UPR regulates inflammation through a variety of mechanisms involving ROS, JNK, and NFκB. PERK promotes ATF4 and NRF2, which then suppress ROS production by activating antioxidant pathway. Upon activation, IRE1/TRAF2 complex recruits IKK (IκB Kinase), leading to the phosphorylation of IκBα and subsequent activation of NFκB. IRE1/TRAF2 can also activate JNK, followed by the activation of AP1. XBP-1 induced by IRE1 can also induce the expression of various genes implicated inflammation. Furthermore, cleaved ATF6 can promote inflammation via activating NFκB.

ER stress regulates the expression of cytokines, while cytokines in turn may also induce ER stress via pathways including inducible nitric oxide synthase (iNOS) and JNK. JNK pathway is activated by IL-1β. Suppression of JNK by its inhibitor SP600125 can protectβ cells from IL-1β-induced apoptosis (85). Inflammatory cytokines induce iNOS expression in β cells and produce copious amount of nitric oxygen (86).Nitric oxygen is an important mediator of β-cell death in type 1 diabetes. Excessive nitric oxygencan induce DNA damage, which leads to β cell apoptosis through p53 pathway or necrosis through poly (ADP-ribose) polymerase pathway (87). In addition, nitric oxygencan also deplete ER Ca^{2+} stores by activating Ca^{2+} channels or inhibiting Ca^{2+} pumps (88-90). Depletion of Ca^{2+} then leads to the activation of CHOP and induces ER stress and apoptosis of β cells (91;92).

4.4. ER stress in the autoimmune process of type 1 diabetes

Given the involvement of ER stress in both innate and adaptive immune systems, pathways of ER stress play a role in the autoimmune process of type 1 diabetes. For example, mice deficient in PERK, a molecule responsible for regulating UPR, are extremely susceptible to diabetes. Although the exocrine and endocrine pancreas developed normally, the *null* mice display a progressive loss of β mass and insulin insufficiency postnatally (93) (93). A severe defect of β cell proliferation and differentiation was also found in *PERK null* mice, resulting in low pancreatic β mass and proinsulin trafficking defects (94). Consistent with those observations in mice, some infant-onset diabetic cases in humans are confirmed to be associated with the mutations in PERK. For example, loss of *EIF2AK3* (the gene encodes PERK) develops Wolcott-Rallison syndrome, an autosomal recessive disorder featured by early infancy insulin-dependency and multiple systemic manifestations including growth retardation, hepatic/renal dysfunction, mental retardation, and cardiovascular abnormalities (86;95). Similarly, disruption of UPR by mutating eIF2α, the downstream molecule of PERK signaling, enhances the sensitivity to ER stress-induced apoptosis and results in defective gluconeogenesis. Mice carrying a homozygous Ser51Ala mutation for eIF2α show multiple defects in pancreatic β cells including the smaller core of insulin-secreting β cells and attenuated insulin secretion (41). Altogether, defects in PERK/eIF2α signaling render β cells highly vulnerable to ER stress in both humans and mice (87;96). In addition to PERK/eIF2α signaling, the other two pathways of ER stress, IRE1 and ATF6, are also implicated in the functionality of β cells. The activation of IRE1 signaling is involved in the insulin biosynthesis induced by hyperglycemia. Transient exposure to high glucose enhances IRE1α phosphorylation without activation of XBP-1 and BiP dissociation. IRE1α activation induced by transient exposure to high glucose induces insulin biosynthesis by up-regulating WFS1, a component involved in UPR and maintaining ER homeostasis (10;97). However, chronic exposure of β cells to high glucose may cause activation of IRE1 but with a different downstream signaling, leading to the suppression of insulin biosynthesis (10). The activation of ATF6 induced by ER stress also suppressed the expression of insulin by up-regulating orphan nuclear receptor small heterodimer partner (98).

5. The role of ER stress in β cell destruction

5.1. The involvement of ER stress in β cell destruction

Increasing evidence suggests an important role of ER stress in autoimmune-mediated β cell destruction (99;100). It was noted that β cell loss is the direct causing factor for insufficient insulin secretion in type 1 diabetes patients. Pancreatic β cells have a very well-developed ER to fulfill their biological function for secreting insulin and other glycoproteins, causing the high sensitivity of β cells to ER stress and the subsequent UPR. Severe or long-term ER stress would direct β cells undergoing apoptosis (99). As described earlier, all the three pathways of ER stress are important in the execution of β cell function and involved in the autoimmune responses during the process of type 1 diabetes.

Pro-inflammatory cytokines are believed as the major mediators contributing to ER stress in β cell mediated by autoimmune response. Autoreactive immune cells infiltrated in pancreas produce pro-inflammatory cytokines, the primary causing factor for β cell death in type 1 diabetes(101). Autoreactive macrophages and T-lymphocytes present in the pancreatic islets in the early stage of type 1 diabetes and secrete massive pro-inflammatory cytokines including IL-1β, IFN-γ and TNF-α. Pro-inflammatory cytokines have been confirmed as strong inducers of ER stress in pancreatic β cells. Insult of β cells with IL-1β and IFN-γ was reported to induce the expression of death protein 5, a protein involved in the cytokine-induced ER stress and β cell death (102). Suppression of death protein 5 by siRNA provides protection for β cells against pro-inflammatory cytokine-induced ER stress (102). In addition, stimulation of β cells with IL-1β and IFN-γ can decrease the expression of sarcoendoplasmic reticulum pump Ca^{2+} ATPase 2b, leading to subsequent depletion of Ca^{2+} in the ER (103). It has been well demonstrated that altered ER Ca^{2+} concentration induces the accumulation of unfolded proteins in ER associated with the induction of UPR and ER stress in β cells (104). Reactive oxygen species such as nitric oxygen produced during inflammation are believed to play a critical role in ER stress-induced β cell death. Excessive nitric oxygen production during insulitis induces β cell apoptosis in a CHOP-dependent manner (91).

In addition to cytokine-induced ER stress, defective protein processing and trafficking are also a direct cause of ER stress in β cell. For instance, mis-folding of insulin in β cells directly induces chronic ER stress as evidenced by the observations in Akita mice. The mutation of *Ins2* gene in Akita mouse disrupts a disulfide bond betweenα and β chain of proinsulin, leading to the mis-folding of the mutated insulin. This mutation therefore induces chronic ER stress in β cells and finally causes diabetes in Akita mouse (105). The inefficiency of protein trafficking from ER to Golgi apparatus also causes ER stress in β cells (106).

Hyperglycemia occurs only when β cells fail to compensate the increased demand for insulin. Therefore, β cells are usually "exhausted" in diabetic patients (87). The increased insulin demandrequires the remaining functional β cellsto increase insulin synthesis to compensate the decrease of β mass. The altered insulin synthesis causes ER stress in the β cells of patients with type 1 diabetes. In later case, this compensation is beneficial for control of blood glucose homeostasisin a short term.However, the long term alterations of insulin synthesis in the β cells also induce ER stress which in turn exacerbates β cell dysfunction and pro-motes disease progression. Collectively, there is convincing evidence that ER stress plays an essential role in β cell destruction during the course of type 1 diabetes.

5.2. Mechanisms underlying ER stress-induced β cell death

The primary purpose of ER stress response is to compensate the damage caused by the dis-turbances of normal ER function. However, persistence of ER dysfunction would eventually render cells undergoing apoptosis. The mechanisms underlying ER stress induced cell death are not fully elucidated, due to the fact that multiple potential participants involved but lit-tle clarity on the dominant death effectors in a particular cellular context. Generally, the process of cell death by ER stress can be illustrated in three phases: adaptation, alarm, and apoptosis (39).

The adaptation response phase is to protect cells from damage induced by the disturban-ces of ER function and restore the homeostasis of ER. As described earlier, UPR signaling involves three axes of responses: IRE1, PERK, and ATF6. These axes interact between each other and form a feedback regulatory mechanism to control the activity of UPR. The accumulation of unfolded proteins in ER results in the engagement of ER resident chaper-on BiP, and as a consequence, IRE1, PERK, and ATF6 are released from BiP. Therefore, over-expression of BiP can prevent cell death induced by oxidative stress, Ca^{2+} disturban-ces, and hypoxia (107). Upon ER stress, the transcription of BiP is enhanced by ATF6p50, the cleaved form of ATF6 (108). PERK is oligomerized and phosphorylated upon the re-lease from BiP. Activated PERK inactivates eIF2α to reduce mRNA translation and pro-tein load on ER. Therefore, PERK deficiency results in an abnormally elevated protein synthesis in response to ER stress, and renders cells highly sensitive to ER stress-induced apoptosis (109). Consistently, as a downstream molecule of PERK, eIF2α is required for cell survival upon the insult of ER stress. A mutation at the phosphorylation site of eIF2α (Ser51Ala) abolishes the translational suppression in response to ER stress (41). When re-leased from BiP, IRE1 becomes dimerized and activated. Activated IRE1 then induces XBP-1 by promoting the splicing of its mRNA (44). XBP-1 is responsible for the transcrip-tion of many adaptation genes implicated in UPR. Unlike PERK and IRE1, ATF6 translo-cates into the Golgi apparatus once released from BiP. The transmembrane domain of ATF6 is cleaved in the Golgi apparatus and is then relocated into the nucleus, by which it regulates gene expression (51).

During the alarm phase, many signal pathways are activated to alert the system. For in-stance, the cytoplasmic part of IRE1 can bind to TNF receptor-associated factor 2 (TRAF2), a key adaptor mediating TNF-induced innate immune response. TRAF2 then activates NFκB pathway via activating IKK and activates the signaling for c-Jun N-terminal kinas-es (JNK) by apoptosis signal-regulating kinase 1 (Ask1). It is reported that dominant neg-ative TRAF2 suppresses the activation of JNK in response to ER stress (110). In addition, TRAF2 is also a critical component for E3 ubiquitin-protein ligase complex (111). E3 ubiq-uitin-protein ligase complex binds to Ubc13 and mediates the noncanonical ubiquitina-tion of substrates, which is suggested to be required for the activation of JNK (112).

Furthermore, IRE1 can also activate JNK signaling by interacting with c-Jun N-terminal inhibitory kinase (JIK) (113).

Although the purpose of UPR is to maintain the homeostasis of ER, apoptosis could occur when the insult of ER stress exceeds the cellular regulatory capacity. Apoptosis is initiated by the activation of several proteases including caspase-12, caspase-4, caspase-2, and caspase-9. Studies in rodents suggest that caspase-12 is activated by IRE1 and is involved in ER stress-induced apoptosis. Mice deficient for caspase-12 are resistant to ER stress-induced apoptosis, but remain susceptible to apoptosis induced by other stimuli (114). Caspase-12 can also be activated by TRAF2, a downstream molecule of IRE1 (113). In response to ER stress, caspase-7 is translocated from the cytosol to the ER surface, and then activates pro-caspase-12 (115). Human caspase-4, the closest paralog of rodent caspase-12, can only be activated by ER stress-inducing reagents not by the other apoptotic reagents. Knockdown of caspase-4 by siRNA reduces ER stress-induced apoptosis in neuroblastoma cells, suggesting the involvement of human caspase-4 in ER stress-induced cell death (116). Similarly, caspase-2 and caspase-9 are also activated in the early phase of ER stress. Inhibition of their activation either by inhibitors or siRNA reduces ER stress-induced apoptosis (117). Other than caspase proteins, Ask1 kinase and CHOP are also critical mediators for ER stress-induced cell death. IRE1/TRAF2 complex recruits Ask1 and activates subsequent JNK signaling. The activation of JNK then induces apoptosis by inhibiting anti-apoptotic protein BCL-2 (118) and inducing pro-apoptotic protein Bim (119;120). Deficiency of Ask1 suppresses ER stress-induced JNK activation and protects cells against ER stress-induced apoptosis (121). CHOP, a transcription factor belonging to basic leucine zipper transcription factor family, can be activated by many inducers of UPR including ATF4, ATF6, and XBP-1. Upon activation, CHOP induces cells undergoing apoptosis through suppressing anti-apoptotic protein BCL-2 (122-124).

6. Conclusions and future directions

Although exogenous insulin therapy partly compensates the function of β cells, it cannot regulate blood glucose as accurately as the action of endogenous insulin. As a result, long-term improperly control of blood glucose homeostasis predisposes patients with type 1 diabetes to the development of diverse complications such as diabetic retinopathy (125-127), nephropathy (128;129), neuropathy (130-132), foot ulcers (133-135), and cardiovascular diseases (136-138). Due to the long-term health consequences of diabetes, impact of insulin dependence on life quality, and increasing appearance in both young and old populations, understanding the pathophysiology of diabetes and finding a better way to treat diabetes has become a high priority. Although the underlying mechanisms leading to type 1 diabetes have yet to be fully addressed, accumulating evidence suggests that ER stress plays a critical role in autoimmune-mediated β cell destruction during the course of type 1 diabetes. ER stress in β cells can be triggered by either autoimmune responses against β-cell self-antigens or the increase of compensated insulin synthesis. During the course of type 1 diabetes, autoreactive immune cells secrete copious amount of inflammatory cytokines, leading to excessive production of nitric oxygenand β cell destruction in an ER stress-dependent pathway. ER stress also regulates the functionality of immune cells with implications in autoimmune progression. The inadequate insulin secretion in patients with type 1 diabetes renders the residual β cells for compensated insulin secretion to maintain blood glucose homeostasis. This increase in insulin biosynthesis could overwhelm the folding capacity of ER, and exacerbate β cell dysfunction by inducing ER stress in β cells.

Although ER stress is a critical factor involved in the pathogenesis of type 1 diabetes, it should be kept in mind that the mechanisms underlying autoimmune-mediated β cell destruction in type 1 diabetes are complex, and ER stress is unlikely the exclusive mechanism implicated in disease process. Despite recent significant progress in this area, there are still many questions yet to be addressed. Are there additional factors inducing ER stress in β cells during type 1 diabetes development? Can ER stress be served as a biomarker for β cell destruction and autoimmune progression in the clinic setting? Does blockade of ER stress in immune cells attenuate autoimmune progression and protect β cells? Future studies aimed to dissect these questions would provide a deep insight for type 1 diabetes pathogenesis and would have great potential for developing novel therapeutic strategies against this devastating disorder.

Acknowledgements

This work is supported by a grant from the National Natural Science Foundation of China (81101553/H1604) to JZ. The author declares no competing financial interest.

Abbreviations

AP1, activator protein 1; Ask1, apoptosis signal-regulating kinase 1; ATF6, Activating Transcription Factor 6; C/EBP, CCAAT/enhancer binding protein; CHOP, C/EBP homologous protein; CREBH, Cyclic-AMP-responsive-element-binding protein H; eIF2α, eukaryotic initiation factor 2α; ER, Endoplasmic Reticulum; ER stress, Endoplasmic Reticulum stress; iNOS, inducible nitric oxide synthase; IRE1, inositol-requiring enzyme 1; IRS-1, insulin receptor substrate-1; JIK, c-Jun N-terminal inhibitory kinase; JNK, c-Jun N-terminal kinases; NRF2, nuclear factor-erythroid-derived 2-related factor 2; PERK, pancreatic endoplasmic reticulum kinase; RER, rough endoplasmic reticulum; ROS, reactive oxygen species; SER, smooth endoplasmic reticulum; TLR, Toll-like receptor; TRAF2, TNF receptor-associated factor 2; TRIF, Toll-IL-1R-containing adaptor inducing IFN-β; UPR, unfolded protein response; XBP-1, X box protein-1.

Author details

Jixin Zhong[1,2]

Address all correspondence to: zhongjixin620@163.com

1 Department of Medicine, Affiliated Hospital of Guangdong Medical College, Zhanjiang, Guangdong, China

2 Davis Heart & Lung Research Institute, The Ohio State University College of Medicine, Columbus, Ohio, USA

References

[1] Espino-Paisan L, Urcelay E, Concha EGdl, Santiago JL: Early and Late Onset Type 1 Diabetes: One and the Same or Two Distinct Genetic Entities? In Type 1 Diabetes Complications. Wagner D, Ed. InTech, 2011,

[2] Maahs,DM, West,NA, Lawrence,JM, Mayer-Davis,EJ: Epidemiology of type 1 diabetes. Endocrinol Metab Clin North Am 39:481-497, 2010

[3] Lehuen,A, Diana,J, Zaccone,P, Cooke,A: Immune cell crosstalk in type 1 diabetes. Nat Rev Immunol 10:501-513, 2010

[4] Zhong J, Xu J, Yang P, Liang Y, Wang C-Y: Innate immunity in the recognition of beta-cell antigens in type 1 diabetes. In Type 1 Diabetes - Pathogenesis, Genetics and Immunotherapy. Wagner D, Ed. InTech, 2011,

[5] American Diabetes Association: Standards of medical care in diabetes--2006. Diabetes Care 29 Suppl 1:S4-42, 2006

[6] Tortora GJ, Derrickson BH: Principles of Anatomy and Physiology. John Wiley & Sons Inc., 2008,

[7] Layden,VT, Durai,V, Lowe,WL: G-Protein-Coupled Receptors, Pancreatic Islets, and Diabetes. Nature Education 3:13, 2010

[8] Gerich,JE: The genetic basis of type 2 diabetes mellitus: impaired insulin secretion versus impaired insulin sensitivity. Endocr Rev 19:491-503, 1998

[9] Lillioja,S, Mott,DM, Spraul,M, Ferraro,R, Foley,JE, Ravussin,E, Knowler,WC, Bennett,PH, Bogardus,C: Insulin resistance and insulin secretory dysfunction as precursors of non-insulin-dependent diabetes mellitus. Prospective studies of Pima Indians. N Engl J Med 329:1988-1992, 1993

[10] Lipson,KL, Fonseca,SG, Ishigaki,S, Nguyen,LX, Foss,E, Bortell,R, Rossini,AA, Urano,F: Regulation of insulin biosynthesis in pancreatic beta cells by an endoplasmic reticulum-resident protein kinase IRE1. Cell Metab 4:245-254, 2006

[11] Rhodes CJ: Processing of the insulin molecule. in: D. LeRoith, S.I. Taylor, J.M. Olefsky (Eds.), Diabetes Mellitus, Lippincott Williams & Wilkins. In Diabetes Mellitus: A Fundamental and Clinical Text. 3rd ed. LeRoith D, Taylor SI, Olefsky JM, Eds. Lippincott Williams & Wilkins, 2003,

[12] D'Hertog,W, Maris,M, Ferreira,GB, Verdrengh,E, Lage,K, Hansen,DA, Cardozo,AK, Workman,CT, Moreau,Y, Eizirik,DL, Waelkens,E, Overbergh,L, Mathieu,C: Novel insights into the global proteome responses of insulin-producing INS-1E cells to different degrees of endoplasmic reticulum stress. J Proteome Res 9:5142-5152, 2010

[13] Hubbard,SC, Ivatt,RJ: Synthesis and processing of asparagine-linked oligosaccharides. Annu Rev Biochem 50:555-583, 1981

[14] Kornfeld,R, Kornfeld,S: Assembly of asparagine-linked oligosaccharides. Annu Rev Biochem 54:631-664, 1985

[15] Fewell,SW, Travers,KJ, Weissman,JS, Brodsky,JL: The action of molecular chaperones in the early secretory pathway. Annu Rev Genet 35:149-191, 2001

[16] Paltauf F, Kohlwein S.D., Henry S.A.: Regulation and compartmentalization of lipid synthesis in yeast. In The Molecular and Cellular Biology of the Yeast Saccharomyces. Jones E.W., Broach J.R., Eds. NY, Cold Spring Harbor Laboratory Press, 1992, p. 415-500

[17] Stevens,FJ, Argon,Y: Protein folding in the ER. Semin Cell Dev Biol 10:443-454, 1999

[18] Schroder,M: Endoplasmic reticulum stress responses. Cell Mol Life Sci 65:862-894, 2008

[19] Suzuki,CK, Bonifacino,JS, Lin,AY, Davis,MM, Klausner,RD: Regulating the retention of T-cell receptor alpha chain variants within the endoplasmic reticulum: Ca(2+)-dependent association with BiP. J Cell Biol 114:189-205, 1991

[20] Li,LJ, Li,X, Ferrario,A, Rucker,N, Liu,ES, Wong,S, Gomer,CJ, Lee,AS: Establishment of a Chinese hamster ovary cell line that expresses grp78 antisense transcripts and suppresses A23187 induction of both GRP78 and GRP94. J Cell Physiol 153:575-582, 1992

[21] Corbett,EF, Oikawa,K, Francois,P, Tessier,DC, Kay,C, Bergeron,JJ, Thomas,DY, Krause,KH, Michalak,M: Ca2+ regulation of interactions between endoplasmic reticulum chaperones. J Biol Chem 274:6203-6211, 1999

[22] Zhang,JX, Braakman,I, Matlack,KE, Helenius,A: Quality control in the secretory pathway: the role of calreticulin, calnexin and BiP in the retention of glycoproteins with C-terminal truncations. Mol Biol Cell 8:1943-1954, 1997

[23] Orrenius,S, Zhivotovsky,B, Nicotera,P: Regulation of cell death: the calcium-apopto-
      sis link. Nat Rev Mol Cell Biol 4:552-565, 2003

[24] Lee,AS: The glucose-regulated proteins: stress induction and clinical applications.
      Trends Biochem Sci 26:504-510, 2001

[25] Schroder,M, Friedl,P: Overexpression of recombinant human antithrombin III in Chi-
      nese hamster ovary cells results in malformation and decreased secretion of recombi-
      nant protein. Biotechnol Bioeng 53:547-559, 1997

[26] Schroder,M, Schafer,R, Friedl,P: Induction of protein aggregation in an early secreto-
      ry compartment by elevation of expression level. Biotechnol Bioeng 78:131-140, 2002

[27] Dorner,AJ, Wasley,LC, Kaufman,RJ: Increased synthesis of secreted proteins induces
      expression of glucose-regulated proteins in butyrate-treated Chinese hamster ovary
      cells. J Biol Chem 264:20602-20607, 1989

[28] Kaufman,RJ, Wasley,LC, Dorner,AJ: Synthesis, processing, and secretion of recombi-
      nant human factor VIII expressed in mammalian cells. J Biol Chem 263:6352-6362,
      1988

[29] Schroder,M, Kaufman,RJ: ER stress and the unfolded protein response. Mutat Res
      569:29-63, 2005

[30] Reimold,AM, Iwakoshi,NN, Manis,J, Vallabhajosyula,P, Szomolanyi-Tsuda,E, Grav-
      allese,EM, Friend,D, Grusby,MJ, Alt,F, Glimcher,LH: Plasma cell differentiation re-
      quires the transcription factor XBP-1. Nature 412:300-307, 2001

[31] Iwakoshi,NN, Lee,AH, Vallabhajosyula,P, Otipoby,KL, Rajewsky,K, Glimcher,LH:
      Plasma cell differentiation and the unfolded protein response intersect at the tran-
      scription factor XBP-1. Nat Immunol 4:321-329, 2003

[32] Martinez,IM, Chrispeels,MJ: Genomic analysis of the unfolded protein response in
      Arabidopsis shows its connection to important cellular processes. Plant Cell
      15:561-576, 2003

[33] Pakula,TM, Laxell,M, Huuskonen,A, Uusitalo,J, Saloheimo,M, Penttila,M: The effects
      of drugs inhibiting protein secretion in the filamentous fungus Trichoderma reesei.
      Evidence for down-regulation of genes that encode secreted proteins in the stressed
      cells. J Biol Chem 278:45011-45020, 2003

[34] Harding,HP, Zhang,Y, Ron,D: Protein translation and folding are coupled by an en-
      doplasmic-reticulum-resident kinase. Nature 397:271-274, 1999

[35] Casagrande,R, Stern,P, Diehn,M, Shamu,C, Osario,M, Zuniga,M, Brown,PO,
      Ploegh,H: Degradation of proteins from the ER of S. cerevisiae requires an intact un-
      folded protein response pathway. Mol Cell 5:729-735, 2000

[36] Friedlander,R, Jarosch,E, Urban,J, Volkwein,C, Sommer,T: A regulatory link between
      ER-associated protein degradation and the unfolded-protein response. Nat Cell Biol
      2:379-384, 2000

[37] Travers,KJ, Patil,CK, Wodicka,L, Lockhart,DJ, Weissman,JS, Walter,P: Functional and genomic analyses reveal an essential coordination between the unfolded protein response and ER-associated degradation. Cell 101:249-258, 2000

[38] Kaufman,RJ: Orchestrating the unfolded protein response in health and disease. J Clin Invest 110:1389-1398, 2002

[39] Xu,C, Bailly-Maitre,B, Reed,JC: Endoplasmic reticulum stress: cell life and death decisions. J Clin Invest 115:2656-2664, 2005

[40] Kaufman,RJ, Scheuner,D, Schroder,M, Shen,X, Lee,K, Liu,CY, Arnold,SM: The unfolded protein response in nutrient sensing and differentiation. Nat Rev Mol Cell Biol 3:411-421, 2002

[41] Scheuner,D, Song,B, McEwen,E, Liu,C, Laybutt,R, Gillespie,P, Saunders,T, Bonner-Weir,S, Kaufman,RJ: Translational control is required for the unfolded protein response and in vivo glucose homeostasis. Mol Cell 7:1165-1176, 2001

[42] Tirasophon,W, Welihinda,AA, Kaufman,RJ: A stress response pathway from the endoplasmic reticulum to the nucleus requires a novel bifunctional protein kinase/endoribonuclease (Ire1p) in mammalian cells. Genes Dev 12:1812-1824, 1998

[43] Wang,XZ, Harding,HP, Zhang,Y, Jolicoeur,EM, Kuroda,M, Ron,D: Cloning of mammalian Ire1 reveals diversity in the ER stress responses. EMBO J 17:5708-5717, 1998

[44] Lee,K, Tirasophon,W, Shen,X, Michalak,M, Prywes,R, Okada,T, Yoshida,H, Mori,K, Kaufman,RJ: IRE1-mediated unconventional mRNA splicing and S2P-mediated ATF6 cleavage merge to regulate XBP1 in signaling the unfolded protein response. Genes Dev 16:452-466, 2002

[45] Yoshida,H, Matsui,T, Yamamoto,A, Okada,T, Mori,K: XBP1 mRNA is induced by ATF6 and spliced by IRE1 in response to ER stress to produce a highly active transcription factor. Cell 107:881-891, 2001

[46] Calfon,M, Zeng,H, Urano,F, Till,JH, Hubbard,SR, Harding,HP, Clark,SG, Ron,D: IRE1 couples endoplasmic reticulum load to secretory capacity by processing the XBP-1 mRNA. Nature 415:92-96, 2002

[47] Lee,AH, Iwakoshi,NN, Glimcher,LH: XBP-1 regulates a subset of endoplasmic reticulum resident chaperone genes in the unfolded protein response. Mol Cell Biol 23:7448-7459, 2003

[48] Yoshida,H, Matsui,T, Hosokawa,N, Kaufman,RJ, Nagata,K, Mori,K: A time-dependent phase shift in the mammalian unfolded protein response. Dev Cell 4:265-271, 2003

[49] Lee,AH, Chu,GC, Iwakoshi,NN, Glimcher,LH: XBP-1 is required for biogenesis of cellular secretory machinery of exocrine glands. EMBO J 24:4368-4380, 2005

[50] Hollien,J, Weissman,JS: Decay of endoplasmic reticulum-localized mRNAs during the unfolded protein response. Science 313:104-107, 2006

[51] Ye,J, Rawson,RB, Komuro,R, Chen,X, Dave,UP, Prywes,R, Brown,MS, Goldstein,JL: ER stress induces cleavage of membrane-bound ATF6 by the same proteases that process SREBPs. Mol Cell 6:1355-1364, 2000

[52] Okada,T, Yoshida,H, Akazawa,R, Negishi,M, Mori,K: Distinct roles of activating transcription factor 6 (ATF6) and double-stranded RNA-activated protein kinase-like endoplasmic reticulum kinase (PERK) in transcription during the mammalian unfolded protein response. Biochem J 366:585-594, 2002

[53] Ni,M, Lee,AS: ER chaperones in mammalian development and human diseases. FEBS Lett 581:3641-3651, 2007

[54] Han,J, Zhong,J, Wei,W, Wang,Y, Huang,Y, Yang,P, Purohit,S, Dong,Z, Wang,MH, She,JX, Gong,F, Stern,DM, Wang,CY: Extracellular high-mobility group box 1 acts as an innate immune mediator to enhance autoimmune progression and diabetes onset in NOD mice. Diabetes 57:2118-2127, 2008

[55] Zhang,S, Zhong,J, Yang,P, Gong,F, Wang,CY: HMGB1, an innate alarmin, in the pathogenesis of type 1 diabetes. Int J Clin Exp Pathol 3:24-38, 2009

[56] Zhong J, Yang P, Wang C: Environmental Triggers and Endogenous Alarmins Linking Innate Immunity to the Pathogenesis of Type 1 Diabetes. In: Type 1 Diabetes Mellitus: Etiology, Diagnosis and Treatment. Nova Science Publishers, Inc., 2011, p. 177-206

[57] Zhong J, Xu J, Yang P, Liang Y, Wang C-Y: Innate immunity in the recognition of ? cell antigens in type 1 diabetes. In Type 1 Diabetes - Pathogenesis, Genetics and Immunotherapy. Wagner D, Ed. InTech, 2011,

[58] Pietropaolo,M, Barinas-Mitchell,E, Kuller,LH: The heterogeneity of diabetes: unraveling a dispute: is systemic inflammation related to islet autoimmunity? Diabetes 56:1189-1197, 2007

[59] Zhao,L, Ackerman,SL: Endoplasmic reticulum stress in health and disease. Curr Opin Cell Biol 18:444-452, 2006

[60] Zhang,K, Shen,X, Wu,J, Sakaki,K, Saunders,T, Rutkowski,DT, Back,SH, Kaufman,RJ: Endoplasmic reticulum stress activates cleavage of CREBH to induce a systemic inflammatory response. Cell 124:587-599, 2006

[61] Iwakoshi,NN, Pypaert,M, Glimcher,LH: The transcription factor XBP-1 is essential for the development and survival of dendritic cells. J Exp Med 204:2267-2275, 2007

[62] Goodall,JC, Wu,C, Zhang,Y, McNeill,L, Ellis,L, Saudek,V, Gaston,JS: Endoplasmic reticulum stress-induced transcription factor, CHOP, is crucial for dendritic cell IL-23 expression. Proc Natl Acad Sci U S A 107:17698-17703, 2010

[63] Richardson,CE, Kooistra,T, Kim,DH: An essential role for XBP-1 in host protection against immune activation in C. elegans. Nature 463:1092-1095, 2010

[64] Kaser,A, Lee,AH, Franke,A, Glickman,JN, Zeissig,S, Tilg,H, Nieuwenhuis,EE, Higgins,DE, Schreiber,S, Glimcher,LH, Blumberg,RS: XBP1 links ER stress to intestinal inflammation and confers genetic risk for human inflammatory bowel disease. Cell 134:743-756, 2008

[65] Woo,CW, Cui,D, Arellano,J, Dorweiler,B, Harding,H, Fitzgerald,KA, Ron,D, Tabas,I: Adaptive suppression of the ATF4-CHOP branch of the unfolded protein response by toll-like receptor signalling. Nat Cell Biol 11:1473-1480, 2009

[66] Baekkeskov,S, Nielsen,JH, Marner,B, Bilde,T, Ludvigsson,J, Lernmark,A: Autoantibodies in newly diagnosed diabetic children immunoprecipitate human pancreatic islet cell proteins. Nature 298:167-169, 1982

[67] Gass,JN, Gifford,NM, Brewer,JW: Activation of an unfolded protein response during differentiation of antibody-secreting B cells. J Biol Chem 277:49047-49054, 2002

[68] Zhang,K, Wong,HN, Song,B, Miller,CN, Scheuner,D, Kaufman,RJ: The unfolded protein response sensor IRE1alpha is required at 2 distinct steps in B cell lymphopoiesis. J Clin Invest 115:268-281, 2005

[69] Niu,H, Ye,BH, la-Favera,R: Antigen receptor signaling induces MAP kinase-mediated phosphorylation and degradation of the BCL-6 transcription factor. Genes Dev 12:1953-1961, 1998

[70] Lin,KI, ngelin-Duclos,C, Kuo,TC, Calame,K: Blimp-1-dependent repression of Pax-5 is required for differentiation of B cells to immunoglobulin M-secreting plasma cells. Mol Cell Biol 22:4771-4780, 2002

[71] Reimold,AM, Ponath,PD, Li,YS, Hardy,RR, David,CS, Strominger,JL, Glimcher,LH: Transcription factor B cell lineage-specific activator protein regulates the gene for human X-box binding protein 1. J Exp Med 183:393-401, 1996

[72] Shaffer,AL, Shapiro-Shelef,M, Iwakoshi,NN, Lee,AH, Qian,SB, Zhao,H, Yu,X, Yang,L, Tan,BK, Rosenwald,A, Hurt,EM, Petroulakis,E, Sonenberg,N, Yewdell,JW, Calame,K, Glimcher,LH, Staudt,LM: XBP1, downstream of Blimp-1, expands the secretory apparatus and other organelles, and increases protein synthesis in plasma cell differentiation. Immunity 21:81-93, 2004

[73] Gass,JN, Jiang,HY, Wek,RC, Brewer,JW: The unfolded protein response of B-lymphocytes: PERK-independent development of antibody-secreting cells. Mol Immunol 45:1035-1043, 2008

[74] Pino,SC, O'Sullivan-Murphy,B, Lidstone,EA, Thornley,TB, Jurczyk,A, Urano,F, Greiner,DL, Mordes,JP, Rossini,AA, Bortell,R: Protein kinase C signaling during T cell activation induces the endoplasmic reticulum stress response. Cell Stress Chaperones 13:421-434, 2008

[75] Kamimura,D, Bevan,MJ: Endoplasmic reticulum stress regulator XBP-1 contributes to effector CD8+ T cell differentiation during acute infection. J Immunol 181:5433-5441, 2008

[76] Pino,SC, O'Sullivan-Murphy,B, Lidstone,EA, Yang,C, Lipson,KL, Jurczyk,A, diIorio,P, Brehm,MA, Mordes,JP, Greiner,DL, Rossini,AA, Bortell,R: CHOP mediates endoplasmic reticulum stress-induced apoptosis in Gimap5-deficient T cells. PLoS One 4:e5468, 2009

[77] Malhotra,JD, Kaufman,RJ: Endoplasmic reticulum stress and oxidative stress: a vicious cycle or a double-edged sword? Antioxid Redox Signal 9:2277-2293, 2007

[78] Tu,BP, Weissman,JS: Oxidative protein folding in eukaryotes: mechanisms and consequences. J Cell Biol 164:341-346, 2004

[79] Harding,HP, Zhang,Y, Zeng,H, Novoa,I, Lu,PD, Calfon,M, Sadri,N, Yun,C, Popko,B, Paules,R, Stojdl,DF, Bell,JC, Hettmann,T, Leiden,JM, Ron,D: An integrated stress response regulates amino acid metabolism and resistance to oxidative stress. Mol Cell 11:619-633, 2003

[80] Cullinan,SB, Zhang,D, Hannink,M, Arvisais,E, Kaufman,RJ, Diehl,JA: Nrf2 is a direct PERK substrate and effector of PERK-dependent cell survival. Mol Cell Biol 23:7198-7209, 2003

[81] Cullinan,SB, Diehl,JA: PERK-dependent activation of Nrf2 contributes to redox homeostasis and cell survival following endoplasmic reticulum stress. J Biol Chem 279:20108-20117, 2004

[82] Hu,P, Han,Z, Couvillon,AD, Kaufman,RJ, Exton,JH: Autocrine tumor necrosis factor alpha links endoplasmic reticulum stress to the membrane death receptor pathway through IRE1alpha-mediated NF-kappaB activation and down-regulation of TRAF2 expression. Mol Cell Biol 26:3071-3084, 2006

[83] Davis,RJ: Signal transduction by the JNK group of MAP kinases. Cell 103:239-252, 2000

[84] Yamazaki,H, Hiramatsu,N, Hayakawa,K, Tagawa,Y, Okamura,M, Ogata,R, Huang,T, Nakajima,S, Yao,J, Paton,AW, Paton,JC, Kitamura,M: Activation of the Akt-NF-kappaB pathway by subtilase cytotoxin through the ATF6 branch of the unfolded protein response. J Immunol 183:1480-1487, 2009

[85] Wang,Q, Zhang,H, Zhao,B, Fei,H: IL-1beta caused pancreatic beta-cells apoptosis is mediated in part by endoplasmic reticulum stress via the induction of endoplasmic reticulum Ca2+ release through the c-Jun N-terminal kinase pathway. Mol Cell Biochem 324:183-190, 2009

[86] Delepine,M, Nicolino,M, Barrett,T, Golamaully,M, Lathrop,GM, Julier,C: EIF2AK3, encoding translation initiation factor 2-alpha kinase 3, is mutated in patients with Wolcott-Rallison syndrome. Nat Genet 25:406-409, 2000

[87] Oyadomari,S, Mori,M: Roles of CHOP/GADD153 in endoplasmic reticulum stress. Cell Death Differ 11:381-389, 2004

[88] Messmer,UK, Brune,B: Nitric oxide-induced apoptosis: p53-dependent and p53-independent signalling pathways. Biochem J 319 (Pt 1):299-305, 1996

[89] Viner,RI, Ferrington,DA, Williams,TD, Bigelow,DJ, Schoneich,C: Protein modification during biological aging: selective tyrosine nitration of the SERCA2a isoform of the sarcoplasmic reticulum Ca2+-ATPase in skeletal muscle. Biochem J 340 (Pt 3): 657-669, 1999

[90] Xu,KY, Huso,DL, Dawson,TM, Bredt,DS, Becker,LC: Nitric oxide synthase in cardiac sarcoplasmic reticulum. Proc Natl Acad Sci U S A 96:657-662, 1999

[91] Oyadomari,S, Takeda,K, Takiguchi,M, Gotoh,T, Matsumoto,M, Wada,I, Akira,S, Araki,E, Mori,M: Nitric oxide-induced apoptosis in pancreatic beta cells is mediated by the endoplasmic reticulum stress pathway. Proc Natl Acad Sci U S A 98:10845-10850, 2001

[92] Xu,L, Eu,JP, Meissner,G, Stamler,JS: Activation of the cardiac calcium release channel (ryanodine receptor) by poly-S-nitrosylation. Science 279:234-237, 1998

[93] Harding,HP, Zeng,H, Zhang,Y, Jungries,R, Chung,P, Plesken,H, Sabatini,DD, Ron,D: Diabetes mellitus and exocrine pancreatic dysfunction in perk-/- mice reveals a role for translational control in secretory cell survival. Mol Cell 7:1153-1163, 2001

[94] Zhang,W, Feng,D, Li,Y, Iida,K, McGrath,B, Cavener,DR: PERK EIF2AK3 control of pancreatic beta cell differentiation and proliferation is required for postnatal glucose homeostasis. Cell Metab 4:491-497, 2006

[95] Araki,E, Oyadomari,S, Mori,M: Endoplasmic reticulum stress and diabetes mellitus. Intern Med 42:7-14, 2003

[96] Mathis,D, Vence,L, Benoist,C: beta-Cell death during progression to diabetes. Nature 414:792-798, 2001

[97] Fonseca,SG, Fukuma,M, Lipson,KL, Nguyen,LX, Allen,JR, Oka,Y, Urano,F: WFS1 is a novel component of the unfolded protein response and maintains homeostasis of the endoplasmic reticulum in pancreatic beta-cells. J Biol Chem 280:39609-39615, 2005

[98] Seo,HY, Kim,YD, Lee,KM, Min,AK, Kim,MK, Kim,HS, Won,KC, Park,JY, Lee,KU, Choi,HS, Park,KG, Lee,IK: Endoplasmic reticulum stress-induced activation of activating transcription factor 6 decreases insulin gene expression via up-regulation of orphan nuclear receptor small heterodimer partner. Endocrinology 149:3832-3841, 2008

[99] Eizirik,DL, Cardozo,AK, Cnop,M: The role for endoplasmic reticulum stress in diabetes mellitus. Endocr Rev 29:42-61, 2008

[100] Laybutt,DR, Preston,AM, Akerfeldt,MC, Kench,JG, Busch,AK, Biankin,AV, Biden,TJ: Endoplasmic reticulum stress contributes to beta cell apoptosis in type 2 diabetes. Diabetologia 50:752-763, 2007

[101] Eizirik,DL, Colli,ML, Ortis,F: The role of inflammation in insulitis and beta-cell loss in type 1 diabetes. Nat Rev Endocrinol 5:219-226, 2009

[102] Gurzov,EN, Ortis,F, Cunha,DA, Gosset,G, Li,M, Cardozo,AK, Eizirik,DL: Signaling by IL-1beta+IFN-gamma and ER stress converge on DP5/Hrk activation: a novel mechanism for pancreatic beta-cell apoptosis. Cell Death Differ 16:1539-1550, 2009

[103] Cardozo,AK, Ortis,F, Storling,J, Feng,YM, Rasschaert,J, Tonnesen,M, Van,EF, Mandrup-Poulsen,T, Herchuelz,A, Eizirik,DL: Cytokines downregulate the sarcoendoplasmic reticulum pump Ca2+ ATPase 2b and deplete endoplasmic reticulum Ca2+, leading to induction of endoplasmic reticulum stress in pancreatic beta-cells. Diabetes 54:452-461, 2005

[104] Rutkowski,DT, Kaufman,RJ: A trip to the ER: coping with stress. Trends Cell Biol 14:20-28, 2004

[105] Ron,D: Proteotoxicity in the endoplasmic reticulum: lessons from the Akita diabetic mouse. J Clin Invest 109:443-445, 2002

[106] Preston,AM, Gurisik,E, Bartley,C, Laybutt,DR, Biden,TJ: Reduced endoplasmic reticulum (ER)-to-Golgi protein trafficking contributes to ER stress in lipotoxic mouse beta cells by promoting protein overload. Diabetologia 52:2369-2373, 2009

[107] Liu,H, Bowes,RC, III, van de,WB, Sillence,C, Nagelkerke,JF, Stevens,JL: Endoplasmic reticulum chaperones GRP78 and calreticulin prevent oxidative stress, Ca2+ disturbances, and cell death in renal epithelial cells. J Biol Chem 272:21751-21759, 1997

[108] Haeri,M, Knox,BE: Endoplasmic Reticulum Stress and Unfolded Protein Response Pathways: Potential for Treating Age-related Retinal Degeneration. J Ophthalmic Vis Res 7:45-59, 2012

[109] Harding,HP, Zhang,Y, Bertolotti,A, Zeng,H, Ron,D: Perk is essential for translational regulation and cell survival during the unfolded protein response. Mol Cell 5:897-904, 2000

[110] Urano,F, Wang,X, Bertolotti,A, Zhang,Y, Chung,P, Harding,HP, Ron,D: Coupling of stress in the ER to activation of JNK protein kinases by transmembrane protein kinase IRE1. Science 287:664-666, 2000

[111] Zheng,C, Kabaleeswaran,V, Wang,Y, Cheng,G, Wu,H: Crystal structures of the TRAF2: cIAP2 and the TRAF1: TRAF2: cIAP2 complexes: affinity, specificity, and regulation. Mol Cell 38:101-113, 2010

[112] Habelhah,H, Takahashi,S, Cho,SG, Kadoya,T, Watanabe,T, Ronai,Z: Ubiquitination and translocation of TRAF2 is required for activation of JNK but not of p38 or NF-kappaB. EMBO J 23:322-332, 2004

[113] Yoneda,T, Imaizumi,K, Oono,K, Yui,D, Gomi,F, Katayama,T, Tohyama,M: Activation of caspase-12, an endoplastic reticulum (ER) resident caspase, through tumor ne-

crosis factor receptor-associated factor 2-dependent mechanism in response to the ER stress. J Biol Chem 276:13935-13940, 2001

[114] Nakagawa,T, Zhu,H, Morishima,N, Li,E, Xu,J, Yankner,BA, Yuan,J: Caspase-12 mediates endoplasmic-reticulum-specific apoptosis and cytotoxicity by amyloid-beta. Nature 403:98-103, 2000

[115] Rao,RV, Hermel,E, Castro-Obregon,S, del,RG, Ellerby,LM, Ellerby,HM, Bredesen,DE: Coupling endoplasmic reticulum stress to the cell death program. Mechanism of caspase activation. J Biol Chem 276:33869-33874, 2001

[116] Hitomi,J, Katayama,T, Eguchi,Y, Kudo,T, Taniguchi,M, Koyama,Y, Manabe,T, Yamagishi,S, Bando,Y, Imaizumi,K, Tsujimoto,Y, Tohyama,M: Involvement of caspase-4 in endoplasmic reticulum stress-induced apoptosis and Abeta-induced cell death. J Cell Biol 165:347-356, 2004

[117] Cheung,HH, Lynn,KN, Liston,P, Korneluk,RG: Involvement of caspase-2 and caspase-9 in endoplasmic reticulum stress-induced apoptosis: a role for the IAPs. Exp Cell Res 312:2347-2357, 2006

[118] Yamamoto,K, Ichijo,H, Korsmeyer,SJ: BCL-2 is phosphorylated and inactivated by an ASK1/Jun N-terminal protein kinase pathway normally activated at G(2)/M. Mol Cell Biol 19:8469-8478, 1999

[119] Putcha,GV, Le,S, Frank,S, Besirli,CG, Clark,K, Chu,B, Alix,S, Youle,RJ, LaMarche,A, Maroney,AC, Johnson,EM, Jr.: JNK-mediated BIM phosphorylation potentiates BAX-dependent apoptosis. Neuron 38:899-914, 2003

[120] Lei,K, Davis,RJ: JNK phosphorylation of Bim-related members of the Bcl2 family induces Bax-dependent apoptosis. Proc Natl Acad Sci U S A 100:2432-2437, 2003

[121] Nishitoh,H, Matsuzawa,A, Tobiume,K, Saegusa,K, Takeda,K, Inoue,K, Hori,S, Kakizuka,A, Ichijo,H: ASK1 is essential for endoplasmic reticulum stress-induced neuronal cell death triggered by expanded polyglutamine repeats. Genes Dev 16:1345-1355, 2002

[122] McCullough,KD, Martindale,JL, Klotz,LO, Aw,TY, Holbrook,NJ: Gadd153 sensitizes cells to endoplasmic reticulum stress by down-regulating Bcl2 and perturbing the cellular redox state. Mol Cell Biol 21:1249-1259, 2001

[123] Matsumoto,M, Minami,M, Takeda,K, Sakao,Y, Akira,S: Ectopic expression of CHOP (GADD153) induces apoptosis in M1 myeloblastic leukemia cells. FEBS Lett 395:143-147, 1996

[124] Zinszner,H, Kuroda,M, Wang,X, Batchvarova,N, Lightfoot,RT, Remotti,H, Stevens,JL, Ron,D: CHOP is implicated in programmed cell death in response to impaired function of the endoplasmic reticulum. Genes Dev 12:982-995, 1998

[125] Bandurska-Stankiewicz,E, Wiatr,D: [Programme preventing vision loss due to diabetes]. Klin Oczna 109:359-362, 2007

[126] Cheung,N, Wong,TY: Diabetic retinopathy and systemic vascular complications. Prog Retin Eye Res 27:161-176, 2008

[127] Studholme,S: Diabetic retinopathy. J Perioper Pract 18:205-210, 2008

[128] Monhart,V: [Diabetes mellitus, hypertension and kidney]. Vnitr Lek 54:499-504, 507, 2008

[129] Navarro-Gonzalez,JF, Mora-Fernandez,C: The role of inflammatory cytokines in diabetic nephropathy. J Am Soc Nephrol 19:433-442, 2008

[130] Boulton,AJ: Diabetic neuropathy: classification, measurement and treatment. Curr Opin Endocrinol Diabetes Obes 14:141-145, 2007

[131] Cornell,RS, Ducic,I: Painful diabetic neuropathy. Clin Podiatr Med Surg 25:347-360, 2008

[132] Otto-Buczkowska,E, Kazibutowska,Z, Soltyk,J, Machnica,L: [Neuropathy and type 1 diabetes mellitus]. Endokrynol Diabetol Chor Przemiany Materii Wieku Rozw 14:109-116, 2008

[133] Gardner,SE, Frantz,RA: Wound bioburden and infection-related complications in diabetic foot ulcers. Biol Res Nurs 10:44-53, 2008

[134] Malgrange,D: [Physiopathology of the diabetic foot]. Rev Med Interne 29 Suppl 2:S231-S237, 2008

[135] Ochoa,O, Torres,FM, Shireman,PK: Chemokines and diabetic wound healing. Vascular 15:350-355, 2007

[136] Anselmino,M, Gohlke,H, Mellbin,L, Ryden,L: Cardiovascular prevention in patients with diabetes and prediabetes. Herz 33:170-177, 2008

[137] Inoguchi,T, Takayanagi,R: [Role of oxidative stress in diabetic vascular complications]. Fukuoka Igaku Zasshi 99:47-55, 2008

[138] Marwick,TH: Diabetic heart disease. Postgrad Med J 84:188-192, 2008

Permissions

The contributors of this book come from diverse backgrounds, making this book a truly international effort. This book will bring forth new frontiers with its revolutionizing research information and detailed analysis of the nascent developments around the world.

We would like to thank Alan Escher and Alice Li, for lending their expertise to make the book truly unique. They have played a crucial role in the development of this book. Without their invaluable contribution this book wouldn't have been possible. They have made vital efforts to compile up to date information on the varied aspects of this subject to make this book a valuable addition to the collection of many professionals and students.

This book was conceptualized with the vision of imparting up-to-date information and advanced data in this field. To ensure the same, a matchless editorial board was set up. Every individual on the board went through rigorous rounds of assessment to prove their worth. After which they invested a large part of their time researching and compiling the most relevant data for our readers. Conferences and sessions were held from time to time between the editorial board and the contributing authors to present the data in the most comprehensible form. The editorial team has worked tirelessly to provide valuable and valid information to help people across the globe.

Every chapter published in this book has been scrutinized by our experts. Their significance has been extensively debated. The topics covered herein carry significant findings which will fuel the growth of the discipline. They may even be implemented as practical applications or may be referred to as a beginning point for another development. Chapters in this book were first published by InTech; hereby published with permission under the Creative Commons Attribution License or equivalent.

The editorial board has been involved in producing this book since its inception. They have spent rigorous hours researching and exploring the diverse topics which have resulted in the successful publishing of this book. They have passed on their knowledge of decades through this book. To expedite this challenging task, the publisher supported the team at every step. A small team of assistant editors was also appointed to further simplify the editing procedure and attain best results for the readers.

Our editorial team has been hand-picked from every corner of the world. Their multi-ethnicity adds dynamic inputs to the discussions which result in innovative outcomes. These outcomes are then further discussed with the researchers and contributors who give their valuable feedback and opinion regarding the same. The feedback is then collaborated with the researches and they are edited in a comprehensive manner to aid the understanding of the subject.

Apart from the editorial board, the designing team has also invested a significant amount of their time in understanding the subject and creating the most relevant covers. They scrutinized every image to scout for the most suitable representation of the subject and create an appropriate cover for the book.

The publishing team has been involved in this book since its early stages. They were actively engaged in every process, be it collecting the data, connecting with the contributors or procuring relevant information. The team has been an ardent support to the editorial, designing and production team. Their endless efforts to recruit the best for this project, has resulted in the accomplishment of this book. They are a veteran in the field of academics and their pool of knowledge is as vast as their experience in printing. Their expertise and guidance has proved useful at every step. Their uncompromising quality standards have made this book an exceptional effort. Their encouragement from time to time has been an inspiration for everyone.

The publisher and the editorial board hope that this book will prove to be a valuable piece of knowledge for researchers, students, practitioners and scholars across the globe.

List of Contributors

Thomas Frese and Hagen Sandholzer
Department of Primary Care, Medical School, Leipzig, Germany

Didier Hober, Famara Sané, Karena Riedweg, Ilham Moumna, Anne Goffard, Laura Choteau and Enagnon Kazali Alidjinou
Université Lille 2, CHRU, Laboratoire de Virologie/ EA3610, 59037 Lille, France

Rachel Desailloud
UPJV CHU, Service d'Endocrinologie-Diabétologie-Nutrition, 80054 Amiens, France

Hakon Hakonarson
Center for Applied Genomics, Children's Hospital of Philadelphia, Pennsylvania, USA
Department of Pediatrics, The University of Pennsylvania School of Medicine, Philadelphia, Pennsylvania, USA

Marina Bakay and Rahul Pandey
Center for Applied Genomics, Children's Hospital of Philadelphia, Pennsylvania, USA

Mohamed M. Jahromi
Pathology Department, Salmaniya Medical Complex, Ministry of Health, Manama, Kingdom of Bahrain

Soltani Nepton
Physiology Department, Faculty of Medicine, Hormozgan University of Medical Science, Iran

Morihito Takita and Nigar Seven
Baylor Research Institute, Islet Cell Laboratory, Dallas, USA

Marlon F. Levy and Bashoo Naziruddin
Baylor Simmons Transplant Institute, Dallas, USA

Philip Newsholme and Kevin Keane
School of Biomedical Sciences, Curtin University, Western Australia

Paulo I Homem de Bittencourt Jr.
Department of Physiology, Institute of Basic Health Sciences, Federal University of Rio Grande do Sul, Porto Alegre, Brazil
National Institute of Hormones and Women's Health, Brazil

Mauricio Krause
Institute of Technology Tallaght and Institute for Sport and Health, UCD Dublin, Ireland
School of Public Health and Physiotherapy, UCD Dublin, Ireland

Donovan A. McGrowder
Department of Pathology, Faculty of Medical Sciences, The University of the West Indies, Mona, Kingston, Jamaica

Lennox Anderson-Jackson
Radiology West, Montego Bay, Jamaica

Tazhmoye V. Crawford
Health Policy Department, Independent Health Policy Consultant, Christiana, Manchester, Jamaica

Jixin Zhong
Department of Medicine, Affiliated Hospital of Guangdong Medical College, Zhanjiang, Guangdong, China
Davis Heart & Lung Research Institute, The Ohio State University College of Medicine, Columbus, Ohio, USA

Printed in the USA
CPSIA information can be obtained
at www.ICGtesting.com
JSHW011813301024
72690JS00002B/64